# A HISTORY OF OCCUPATIONAL HEALTH AND SAFETY

## Wilbur S. Shepperson Series in Nevada History
### Series Editor: Michael Green (UNLV)

Nevada is known politically as a swing state and culturally as a swinging state. Politically, its electoral votes have gone to the winning presidential candidate in all but two election since 1912 (it missed in 1976 and 2016). Its geographic location in the Sun Belt; an ethnically diverse, heavily urban, and fast-growing population; and an economy based on tourism and mining make it a laboratory for understanding the growth and development of postwar America and postindustrial society. Culturally, Nevada has been associated with legal gambling, easy divorce, and social permissiveness. Yet the state also exemplifies conflicts between image and reality: It is a conservative state yet depends heavily on the federal government. Its gaming regulatory system is the envy of the world but resulted from long and difficult experience with organized crime. And its bright lights often obscure the role of organized religion in Nevada affairs. To some who have emphasized the impact of globalization and celebrated or deplored changing moral standards, Nevada reflects America and the world; to others, it affects them.

This series is named in honor of one of the state's most distinguished historians, author of numerous books on the state's immigrants and cultural development, a longtime educator, and an advocate for history and the humanities. The series welcomes manuscripts on any and all aspects of Nevada that offer insight into how the state has developed and how its development has been connected to the region, the nation, and the world.

*Charcoal and Blood: Italian Immigrants in Eureka, Nevada,*
*and the Fish Creek Massacre*
SILVIO MANNO

*A Great Basin Mosaic: The Cultures of Rural Nevada*
JAMES W. HULSE

*The Baneberry Disaster: A Generation of Atomic Fallout*
LARRY C. JOHNS AND ALAN R. JOHNS

*A History of Occupational Health and Safety: From 1905 to the Present*
MICHELLE FOLLETTE TURK

# A HISTORY OF OCCUPATIONAL HEALTH AND SAFETY

## FROM 1905 TO THE PRESENT

Michelle Follette Turk

UNIVERSITY OF NEVADA PRESS *Reno & Las Vegas*

University of Nevada Press | Reno, Nevada 89557 USA
www.unpress.nevada.edu
Copyright © 2018 by University of Nevada Press
All rights reserved
Cover photograph © Fotosearch

LIBRARY OF CONGRESS CATALOGING-IN-PUBLICATION DATA
Names: Turk, Michelle Follette, 1981– author.
Title: A history of occupational health and safety : from 1905 to the present /
    by Michelle Follette Turk.
Description: Reno : University of Nevada Press, [2017] | Series: Wilbur S. Shepperson series
    in Nevada history | Includes bibliographical references and index.
Identifiers: ISBN 978-1-943859-70-2 (cloth : alk. paper) | ISBN 978-1-943859-71-9 (e-book) |
    LCCN 2017038083 (print) | LCCN 2017038533 (e-book)
Subjects: | MESH: Occupational Health—history | Occupational Injuries—history |
    Occupational Diseases—history | History, 20th Century | History, 21st Century |
    Nevada
Classification: LCC T55 (print) | LCC T55 (e-book)| NLM WA 11 AN2 | DDC 363.11—dc23
LC record available at https://lccn.loc.gov/2017038083

FIRST PRINTING

Manufactured in the United States of America

*For Don*

# CONTENTS

*Illustrations follow page 168.*

# ACKNOWLEDGMENTS

Like any book, the inspiration for this one has a story behind it. I grew up in a medical family. One grandfather was a trauma surgeon in Las Vegas, Nevada, the other, an internist in Santa Monica, California. One grandmother and several aunts were nurses. My uncle was a cardio-thoracic and transplant surgeon. When I was thirteen my surgeon grandfather, Kirk V. Cammack Jr., flew me to Las Vegas to watch him perform a double mastectomy at University Medical Center (UMC) to help me research for a school science project on cancer. It was at that moment I decided I wanted to be a doctor.

I did become a doctor eventually, but not the medical kind. During college I became fascinated with medical history, especially regarding medicine in Las Vegas. My grandfather had moved to Nevada in 1961 and established a successful practice as the second board certified surgeon in the state. He was a colorful character, a towering 6-foot 3-inch cowboy from Rock Springs, Wyoming, with flaming red hair and a sharp wit. When I was a small child he filled my head with stories of the Wild West of medicine in Nevada, stories that sounded more like tall tales than reality. He told me about extracting a ruptured appendix on his pool table in his basement, traveling outside town for house calls to see his "desert rats," about treating cowboy patients in the back of saloons, and performing comp surgeries at Sunrise Hospital for the mob contingent and other Las Vegas icons of the 1960s. From an early age, I idolized his unique approach to medicine, and came to view Las Vegas medicine in the same light. My perspective shifted when my mother passed away from intracranial bleeding while I finished up my undergraduate degree. After receiving substandard care at a Las Vegas hospital, she died on the operating table. Her experience left me with many questions: How did Las Vegas, a growing metropolis with millions of residents, have such second-rate health care? When my grandfather moved to town, the medical community held so much promise, recruiting young, talented physicians from across the country to create innovative medical programs. Somewhere along the way, the quality of care flatlined.

As my questions grew, inspiration for this book began. I started with a paper on the medical history of Hoover Dam, but soon realized that Las Vegas medicine was fundamentally connected with the region's major industries. At the same time, I formed a better understanding of why my mother died. After slipping at work, she had torn ligaments in both knees and her orthopedic surgeon chose to reconstruct them both at the same time. When her workers' compensation coverage ended, she stopped physical therapy and had to return to work; she developed a blood clot soon after that probably traveled through her heart to her brain. Acquiring this understanding gave me closure as well as new perspective regarding the importance of health and safety in the workplace. Thus, my topic shifted to focus on occupational health. The move created an opportunity not only to evaluate the development of health and safety in the twentieth century American workplace but also to better understand the state of medicine in the Las Vegas area.

Researching, writing, and rewriting this book for nearly a decade, I am indebted to so many people that I will certainly fail to thank everyone. To those not mentioned here, I apologize and appreciate your time and contributions.

I first wish to thank my mentors. Hal Rothman had a special role in this book, helping me find my voice. He taught me how to write history, but more importantly, he always believed in me even when others did not. His strong conviction drove me to complete this book. I am grateful for the short time I had with him.

After Hal's passing, I was fortunate to gain a mentor and friend in David Wrobel. He enthusiastically supported me in my work. David is a great role model and scholar, and I hope to match his dedication to history of the American West.

Eugene Moehring also played an important role in this project, especially in the development and editing process, and prodding me to publish this book. I thank him for providing important expertise on the history of Nevada. I value the time he spent editing my work and even grew to love his red pen.

I would also like to recognize David Tanenhaus, Andy Kirk, and Robert Futrell for reading versions of this manuscript at various stages. I am grateful for the friendship of Mike Green, always answering my questions and teaching me how to navigate Nevada's archives. During the rewrites, I was fortunate to have Chris Sellers and Janet Greenlees review my manuscript and help sharpen my work. It was with their excellent guidance that I found my voice, inspiring the concept of occupational health regimes. I am deeply appreciative for the generous time that they gave.

An important component of this book was my archival research, from newspapers to state and government reports, oral histories, industry materials, and other primary sources. For nearly two years I sat in the Special Collections at University of Nevada, Las Vegas, examining their incredible collections, scanning documents and listening to interviews on cassette tapes. I used a huge percentage of the archives in this book, from employee documents in the Union Pacific Collection, Basic Magnesium Inc. Collection, and Sands and Dunes Hotel Collections, to litigation resources in the Baneberry Collection and the MGM Fire Collection, and decades of correspondence between Senator Howard S. Cannon and his constituents.

In the process, the Special Collections became my second home. A special thank you to its wonderful staff, especially Su Kim Chung, Thomas Summers, and Delores Brownlee. I would also like to recognize the Nevada State Museum in Las Vegas and the role the McNamee Collection played in this book, offering insight into employer liability cases from the railroad years to the 1970s. Crystal Van Dee and Paul Carson were exceedingly helpful, allowing me to come early and stay late in the archives.

My research on Hoover Dam was conducted primarily at the Boulder City Museum and Historical Association, a crucial resource for scholars of Hoover Dam. I would like to thank Dennis McBride, as well as Shirl Naegle and Judith Irons, for providing key documents and perspective on the dam experience. I am also indebted to the Atomic Testing Museum as well as the Nevada Test Site Oral History Project, the hard work of Mary Palevsky, Andy Kirk, Leisl Carr Childers, and others. I would like to individually thank Mary for inviting me to tour the test site twice for my research. Thank you to Randy Thompson at the National Archives at Riverside, the University of California at Berkeley's Bancroft Library, and the University of California at San Diego's Mandeville Special Collections Library for accommodating my research trips. I am also beyond grateful for financial support I received to fund this project, including the Harold L. and Judith Boyer History Student Scholarship, the Charles Redd Center Summer Award, and the President's Fellowship at the University of Nevada, Las Vegas.

Finally, I wish to recognize my parents, children, and husband for their love and encouragement. I started my research before I became a mother, and having two boys during the rewriting process had a profound effect on this book. I am thankful to Logan and Heath for inspiring me to be a better scholar and mother. Don, thank you for believing in me and helping me achieve my dreams. You are my everything. I dedicate this book to you.

# A HISTORY OF OCCUPATIONAL HEALTH AND SAFETY

# INTRODUCTION

Harold "Rusty" Billingsley started his workday like any other. October 5, 2007, was a typical fall day in Las Vegas, sunny and warm. After arriving at the CityCenter construction site, he began his job as an ironworker. CityCenter was the hottest megaresort project on the Las Vegas Strip. To replace the Boardwalk Hotel and Casino, architect César Pelli had designed an urban metropolis that spanned sixty-six acres. With a projected cost of $4 billion, plans detailed three boutique high-rise hotels, 550,000 square feet of retail shops, and 1,650 condominium units. When CityCenter opened in December 2009, it was the largest privately financed construction project in American history, costing an estimated $8.5 billion. MGM Mirage president Jim Murren called the megaresort an "exciting departure [from the past and] the next evolution of Las Vegas."[1]

CityCenter was part of a $32 billion construction boom on the Strip during the 2000s, along with the Wynn and Encore, Palazzo, Trump International, Cosmopolitan, Fontainebleau, and Echelon. Each competed to create the next greatest experience on the Strip, delivering it as quickly as possible. Since the Strip's inception, construction had always moved at a rapid pace. In 1946 contractor Del Webb faced considerable pressure from Benjamin "Bugsy" Siegel to complete the Flamingo on time. During the construction of the International and MGM Grand from 1967 to 1973, Taylor Construction Company encountered steep penalties for missing deadlines and received bonuses for finishing early. To manage the 1990s megaresort construction boom, crews built the massive structures in phases. After imploding the Sands in 1996, the Las Vegas Sands Corporation mapped out a master plan with contractor Pernini Building Company that spanned more than a decade. In 1999 the corporation unveiled the first phase, the Venetian, and in 2003, the Venezia. In 2008 the Las Vegas Sands Corporation opened the Palazzo and began constructing a condominium tower.

The 2000s megaresort construction boom followed a more aggressive timeline. MGM Mirage tasked Pernini to complete CityCenter and Cosmopolitan in three years, which meant building eight high-rise towers at the same time. Reminiscent of Hoover Dam nearly a century earlier, the nature of work reached a new level of complexity. To avoid costly penalties, Pernini instructed its crew to work rapidly under very crowded conditions. With everything happening at once, "everyone [was] fighting for real estate," one foreman complained. Confronted by a labor shortage, Pernini also hired out-of-town workers, inexperienced in the demands of dense megaresort construction. The risky conditions stressed and exhausted the workers. According to the same foreman, MGM Mirage was "just asking for someone to make an error."[2]

On October 5, 2007, the CityCenter site bustled with activity as Harold Billingsley worked on the second floor. Nicknamed Rusty for his red hair, he was a highly experienced journeyman ironworker. Billingsley began ironwork in the 1990s, supporting the construction of the towering Stratosphere. He loved adventure and the job provided plenty of thrills. Described as an adrenaline junkie by his family, Billingsley enjoyed balancing on high beams and other dangerous elements. In 2006, he joined Pernini's crew at the Cosmopolitan site and began working seventy hours a week. But the work scared him. The job involved the alignment of support columns, and even though he took safety classes, Billingsley repeatedly said that he did not feel secure. Eventually, his anxiety impelled him to request a job transfer to CityCenter. On October 5 he had worked there for less than a month. Walking along a skeletal frame of temporary metal decking, Billingsley tripped. Three safety measures, outlined by Occupational Safety and Health Administration (OSHA) guidelines, should have protected him. First, the decking should have caught him, but there was a three-by-eleven-foot hole at that exact spot. Billingsley surged forward and fell through. Second, a safety harness should have stopped his fall. It was not attached. Third, OSHA guidelines required temporary flooring or netting underneath, but neither was in place. A simple trip ended his life. Billingsley fell fifty-nine feet to his death. It was the fourth fatality at CityCenter in eight months.[3]

Death shrouded the CityCenter and Cosmopolitan projects since early 2007. In February a 7,300-pound wall collapsed and crushed two workers. In August an elevator struck and killed an operating engineer. In November a beam broke and an apprentice ironworker fell to his death with his safety harness attached to the beam. The following January, an iron post collapsed and a safety engineer plummeted five stories. The Palazzo, Trump, Fontainebleau, and Echelon experienced similar tragedies. By mid-2008 the Strip's dangerous working conditions were infamous. Enduring the most fatalities, CityCenter workers started calling the construction site City Cemetery and Cemetery Center.[4]

In eighteen months there were twelve fatalities at CityCenter, Cosmopolitan, Trump International, Palazzo, Fontainebleau, and Echelon. Every six weeks, a worker died. Employees of Pernini accumulated the majority, with a total of nine. CityCenter alone had six causalities. Not since Hoover Dam had a construction project in southern Nevada caused so many deaths. In early 2008 *Las Vegas Sun* reporter Alexandra Berzon began investigating the unusual number of fatalities. By the end of the year, she had written fifty-three stories and twenty-one editorials. Her series documented the cramped, rushed, and unsafe conditions, and revealed the cozy relationship between federal and state regulatory agencies and the contractors. In fact, OSHA weakened safety requirements, and when the Nevada Occupational Safety and Health Administration (Nevada OSHA) investigated the deaths, it withdrew or reduced violations at informal, private meetings with management without families present or union representation. The workers' other advocate, the local unions, also failed to rally support. Berzon's reporting, coupled with editorials by David Clayton and Matt Hufman, led to congressional hearings and reforms in occupational health. The workers also forced changed. Outraged by the *Las Vegas Sun* revelations, seven thousand men and women working at CityCenter and Cosmopolitan walked out in June 2008, shutting down the site. Pernini quickly negotiated a truce. By the end of the day, it had agreed to establish a rigorous, ten-hour health and safety training class and periodic safety assessments. The combination of events produced an ethos shift in Strip construction, favoring health and safety. The final casualty occurred on June 16, 2008, at the Echelon site. After that, the deaths stopped.[5]

In her series, Berzon refers to the twelve Strip construction deaths as reflecting a disturbing trend in Las Vegas. During the 1990s megaresort boom, she writes, only nine construction workers died. By the 2000s Las Vegas "pinned its addiction to growth" and a subsequent "body count emerged."[6] The death count was indeed disturbing, but the trend was a historical tradition in Nevada and the United States as a whole, joining the nation's long and unfortunate history of exposing workers and the public to hazardous work. The history of occupational health is a subject that transcends traditional historiography, blending medical, labor, political, environmental, legal, and social history into one narrative. Workplace hazards are not only an employment problem, they also have political, social, economic, and environmental implications. The genre of occupational health history developed after industrialization, with most literature focusing on the evaluation of the so-called dangerous trades. Following the direction of Italian physician Bernardino Ramazzini, often referred to as the father of occupational health after penning *Diseases of Workers* in 1713, traditional writings chronicled a linear progression of discovery and innovation in workplace safety. Most early historians worked in the field, documenting individual, pioneering practitioners that developed innovative methods to deal with industrialism. As noted by historians Christopher Sellers and Joseph Melling, this model has not held up well because the stories typically resulted in only limited victories.[7]

Despite the creation of an extensive network of regulatory agencies, laws, and safety procedures, workplaces continued to be dangerous. Occupational health history has since evolved from this model, emerging as a dynamic field documenting important history relevant to present-day problems. Most existing literature concentrates on a specific industry or health concern and is national in scope, covering relatively short periods. A vast majority also covers the origins of occupational health during the late nineteenth and early twentieth centuries, ignoring the development during the mid and late twentieth century.[8]

This book departs from the scholarship, focusing on place as a subject rather than health concern or industry. It is a localized, long-term study that examines how occupational health developed in Nevada, and more particularly in the Las Vegas area. By taking this approach, it considers the history of health and safety in twentieth-century America. An influence for this book is Linda Nash's *Inescapable Ecologies*, an innovative study that uses place to discuss the ecological history of bodies in the California Central Valley. Putting place at the center of the story allows for a broader context of how industry operates, and uncovers the importance of location in shaping health regulation and attitudes. Although the narrative retains a chronological order, it is not a linear history, but instead contemplates the complex relationship between health, people, workplaces, and place.

Until recently, the history of occupational health has been an almost neglected subject. A contribution to the growing scholarship is Christopher Sellers and Joseph Melling's *Dangerous Trades*, which provides a useful theatrical framework to conceptualize this history. Sellers and Melling propose using an "industrial hazard regime," the informal and formal arrangements by which "public bodies, private interests, and civic mobilizations handle danger and damage associated with an industry." In short, hazards rarely stay within the boundaries of work. Employees are usually the first casualty, but there is also a sociocultural side that involves the employer, medical experts, government officials, reformers, and the community. Furthermore, damages affect human beings and the environment via pollution and agricultural or ecological damage. Sellers and Melling find that the neglected parts of each regime give way to the worst hazards, forcing historical change. This framework is particularly useful because it allows for an assessment of how and why the regimes varied and evolved across time and place.[9]

Since the focus of this book is occupational health history, and not only the history in dangerous trades, I have modified this framework slightly to an occupational health regime. The adjustment still provides an understanding of the hazards, as well as the various measures undertaken to address them, but also explains how the work, and health and safety programs, fit within each regime. Borrowing parts of historian Michelle Murphy's concept of regimes of perceptibility, an occupational health regime also takes into account the interactions and beliefs of occupational health among the various actors. How did the employers, employees, medical and public health practitioners, the community, and the local, state, and federal governments interact and respond to the hazards? I am particularly interested in how the medical sphere—company physicians, community doctors, nurses, hospitals, and public health professionals—conceptualized and framed their respective medical realms, the evolving field of occupational health, and the impact of hazardous work. Since a core feature of occupational health is medicine, it seemed fitting to apply an extra-medical approach. I found that it revealed a rich history of Nevada industry, community, and health networks, and law and state building throughout the century.

The benefit of a long-term study is that it allows historians to evaluate how occupational health differed from one period to the next. Each occupational health regime in Nevada operated in three general periods. The initial era occurred from the beginning of industrialization to 1945, and is the subject of the first three chapters of the book, covering the railroad industry, the construction of Hoover Dam, and the manufacture of magnesium during World War II. During the nineteenth century, the Industrial Revolution encouraged a dramatic transition from agriculture to new manufacturing processes, profoundly changing the nature of work. The technology used advanced machinery, significantly increasing production. It was efficient, but it was dangerous work, with labor paying the highest price. Even though the first congressional reports on workplace hazards began in the late 1830s, health and safety standards and employer liability still did not exist. Departing from English common law, American courts developed the doctrine of assumed risk, which understood that workers in a free market consented to all potential hazards before accepting employment. Workplace accidents were therefore a part of the process and not the employers' fault. With the assumed risk doctrine, employers were not morally required to protect workers. More importantly, employers were also protected by legal precedent.[10]

In 1842 *Farwell v. Boston & Worcester Railroad Corp.* held that employees could not recover damages because compensation for injuries created a moral hazard in the workplace, rewarding employee carelessness instead of preventing it. Subsequent cases broadened this defense. In 1905 *Lochner v. New York* held that the right to free contract was implicit in the due process clause of the Fourteenth Amendment. In this landmark decision, the Supreme Court determined that law could not protect workers, calling injury compensation an "unreasonable, unnecessary, and arbitrary interference with the right and liberty of the individual to contract."[11]

Although Farwell and Lochner barred employer liability, several factors influenced a shift toward health and safety in the early twentieth century. The first was simple economics. Business was not profitable if employee injuries or deaths stopped work. The railroad, iron, lumber, and steel industries quickly discovered this, and invested in new technology to improve productivity doubling as safety measures. Some big firms developed basic safety programs, and offered informal health-care plans with company physicians on the payroll. Besides offering medical care, the doctors screened employees to determine appropriate jobs for body types, and excluded applicants with physical impairments. The physicals documented preexisting ailments and the state of an employee's overall health, which proved useful in compensation hearings.[12]

The new initiatives worked; healthier workforces improved production and reduced workplace accidents. Besides economics, maternal protectionism also became an important consideration. Historian Allison Helper characterized the early industrial health movement as taking an environmentalist world view to protect women and the human race. Sickness in the workplace came to be viewed as an environmental condition, or something contracted at work, and could potentially hurt a woman's reproductive system. Since workplace hazards were a threat to procreation, they needed to be removed either by correcting the condition or by barring women from the work.[13]

Industrial health and hygiene emerged as an informal movement during progressivism, first propagating the idea that the federal and state governments were obligated to provide information about workplace hazards and chemicals.[14] On March 25, 1911, the Triangle Shirtwaist Company fire in New York City killed 146 garment workers, most of them young, recent Jewish and Italian immigrant women. With the doors locked and no fire escapes, a common practice to prevent theft and unapproved breaks, the imprisoned employees suffocated and burned to death, or fell and jumped from the building. The tragedy infuriated the public and spurred the growth of the influential International Ladies Garment Workers' Union (ILGWU), but it did not encourage real safety reform.[15] A year later, the Esch Act passed, the first occupational health legislation in the United States, placing a high prohibitive tax on white phosphorus matches. It was a marked success, significantly reducing cases of phosphonecrosis, a necrosis of the jaw bone common among match workers. Dr. Alice Hamilton was the first American physician to devote her career to the cause during the Progressive Era, focusing on the effects of industrial metals on the human body. Her innovative methodology relied on inspections, and surveys of employees and local physicians in mines, lead and mercury works, and munitions factories, meticulously researching, publishing, and politicizing unsafe conditions through the objectivity of science.[16]

The work of Alice Hamilton, John R. Commons, Florence Kelley, and others inspired state and federal progressive reforms, including the creation of the Public Health Service (PHS) and Department of Labor (DOL), and the establishment of an assortment of health laws and workmen's compensation in forty-six states by 1921. Workmen's compensation in particular appealed to employers and employees alike. Instead of suing for damages, the law automatically compensated workers at a fixed rate, making costs more predictable and decreasing the risk of labor conflict. Eventually, all jurisdictions adopted the gender-neutral term "workers' compensation," but the term "workmen's" reflected its true nature in the early 1900s; it compensated only dependent widows, not widowers.[17] Until the 1930s workmen's compensation was an employee's primary means to seek damages for workplace injuries or deaths. It first appeared in 1908 in the Federal

Employers' Liability Act (FELA), providing benefits to workers engaged in interstate commerce; in 1910 New York passed the first state compensation statute. Still, most statutes had flaws, overlooking farm and domestic workers, and small companies, and workplace diseases like silicosis. Labor unions were particularly active in the amendment process; the Wisconsin State Federation of Labor (WSFL) helped the state of Wisconsin implement the most progressive laws in the nation. Recognizing the financial opportunity, private insurance companies entered the market as well, briskly selling compensation policies before and after World War I. Legal precedent also made it easier to prove employers' liability and distribute workmen's compensation payments—a dramatic shift from nineteenth-century practices. By 1932 most states had authorized the progressive Wisconsin system, with only Arkansas, Florida, Mississippi, and South Carolina lacking workmen's compensation laws.[18]

During World War I the industrial health movement stalled due to production needs. During the war injuries and fatalities were astonishingly high, with an estimated thirty thousand deaths in 1917 alone. The federal government recognized the problem, founding the Working Condition Service to help states inspect factories and limit risks, but it made little difference. During the conservative interwar years, rates remained unchanged, but a new kind of activism developed in the American university system. As historian Christopher Sellers has shown, schools such as Harvard, Yale, Johns Hopkins, Columbia, and the University of Pennsylvania opened industrial hygiene laboratories to study workplace hazards. The laboratories offered expertise to companies as neutral and apolitical mediators in industrial disease disagreements. Departing from progressive methods of inspections, surveys, physical examinations, and legislation, the researchers shifted industrial health from the field to the laboratory, and from humans to animals. The move depoliticized workplace safety, giving shape to modern regulatory practices. Founded in 1918, the industrial hygiene division at Harvard was one of the most important sites of research. The fatigue laboratory contributed greatly to health and safety at Hoover Dam, conducting on-site studies concerning the high number of workers dying from heat exhaustion.[19]

In 1929 the United States plummeted into economic depression, and stopped virtually all industrial production and construction. The shift prompted widespread unemployment, but the employed were only slightly better off. Most work opportunities required temporary, unskilled labor with low wages and little career advancement. To retain jobs, employees regularly ignored safety standards, subjecting themselves and coworkers to dangerous working conditions. The harmful effects of industrial diseases—carbon monoxide, silica, lead poisoning, and others—were well documented but consistently overlooked. A report at the 1936 United Auto Workers' convention indicated that in the seven years since 1929, 13,000 cases of lead poisoning had occurred in auto factories, and management made no attempt to ventilate or remove toxins from the work site. Manufacturing, mining, and construction workers experienced similar conditions.[20]

The most extreme case of employer negligence occurred near Gauley Bridge, West Virginia at the Hawk's Nest Tunnel. In 1930 the Rinehart and Dennis Company instructed workers to dry drill a diversion tunnel embedded with silica as part of a hydroelectric project. Federal and state mining laws prohibited dry drilling, but the project was not considered mining and therefore was not subject to its safety standards. The silica exposure killed as many as fifteen hundred workers, the highest loss of human life in American workplace history.[21]

After 1932 the Roosevelt administration urged industry to move toward safer working conditions. Improvements in technology and public policy helped, with most large firms institutionalizing health and safety programs, and employing engineers to improve efficiency.[22] Workers also benefited from New Deal legislation, but the federal role mainly provided service and information to state agencies. In the 1940s mobilization for World War II impeded real change. Employment opportunities certainly reduced the unemployment rate, but they also increased workplace injuries. After the attack on Pearl Harbor in late 1941, companies recruited inexperienced workers to fill the massive production needs. Given little instruction in safety, they lacked familiarity with working in heavy industry, and were a danger to themselves and coworkers. The conditions worsened as mobilization intensified and factories extended the workweek and instituted speedups to increase production. The high rate of accidents and injury-related absenteeism eventually slowed production, and health and safety had become a higher priority by the end of the war.[23]

The second era in occupational health history went from the end of World War II to the 1970s, and is the subject of the fourth chapter of the book covering nuclear testing. During this period, industrial health transformed into occupational health, a term that better described health and safety in all workplaces, and became linked to the intersections between the workplace, the community, and the environment. After the war, the federal government lost interest in industrial health, for the most part because of the perception that it challenged an employer's right to control work procedures. The private sector consequently exercised complete control over its workplaces during the 1950s. As shown by historians Gerald Markowitz and David Rosner, this occurred simultaneously with the rise of scientific authority. Following the war, laboratories emerged as the only avenue to diagnose workplace diseases, and not the independent diagnoses of primary physicians, and shifted from prominent universities to bureaucracies like the Food and Drug Administration (FDA) and private corporate research facilities. Under the latter model, companies tested their chemicals on site, guaranteeing greater control over the research outcomes.[24]

By the late 1950s Americans became increasingly skeptical with industry's ability to protect human health and the environment. Radioactive fallout raised an initial alarm, highlighting the dangers of nuclear testing, and later, chemical pollution surrounding industrial plants, and toxic pesticides and household products. It became clear that federal–state partnership could no longer deal with America's dangerous trades. Although additional federal laws were passed, most only covered specific industries. Historians commonly date the appearance of environmental public awareness with the publishing of Rachel Carson's *Silent Spring* in 1962, a book that connected industry to human health and the environment. Carson revealed that the hazards rarely stayed within the confines of the workplace; chemicals flowed to the earth, and traveled from rivers to fish to bloodstreams to breastmilk, slowly poisoning us and our children. Suddenly, dangerous trades were no longer only a worker's problem. They affected us all. The cultural revelation prompted a symbolic switch in name, from industrial health to occupational health, allowing for health and safety in all workplaces, and protecting the community and environment from harm.[25]

A combination of environmental activism and the Vietnam War brought occupational health into the national discussion. By the 1960s, 14,000 employees died a year and 2.2 million were unable to work due to injuries or illnesses sustained on the job. Industry-specific statutes were still being passed but did little good. In 1965 the National Foundation of the Arts and Humanities Act established labor standards for professional performers, personnel, laborers, and mechanics, declaring that the program would not fund unsanitary or dangerous projects that threatened employee health and safety. A year later, Congress passed the Metal and Nonmetallic Mine Safety Act, setting up procedures for developing health and safety standards in metal and metallic mines, yearly inspections, and education and training programs. Much like during World War II, the Vietnam War forced the issue, putting significant pressure on industrial production. A sharp increase in accidents and deaths drove labor unions to stage strikes across the nation. Activists demanded information about workplace hazards, safety and health statutes, and what injuries and illnesses were covered by the law. Their pursuit revealed significant gaps in coverage. For example, the 1936 Walsh–Healey Public Contracts Act authorized inspections of companies under federal contract, but in practice it covered few workers and was difficult to enforce. Moreover, private interests established most safety standards under the auspices of voluntary safety commissions. The era culminated in the passage of the Occupational Safety and Health Act (OSHA) and the National Institute for Occupational Safety and Health (NIOSH) in 1970, the first time the federal government established regulatory and research agencies completely devoted to workplace health and safety. The Act also guaranteed access to information about substances they worked with and the possibility of harmful results, and confirmed that employers and the government were responsible for the well-being of American workers.[26]

The third era in occupational health history began in an environmentally conscious, post-OSHA America, and is the subject of the fifth chapter covering the service industry. After the 1970s occupational accidents were no longer considered a part of the job; the installation of health and safety standards could remove risk. Laissez-faire became fully rejected as well, replaced by the assumption that employers and the government were obligated to protect workers. Employees also earned the right to know about occupational hazards and diseases, and could improve their own conditions.[27]

During the 1970s the American workplace had evolved as well, marked by a dramatic decline in industrial work due to automation and imports. Multinational corporations also responded to environmentalism and OSHA by moving hazardous manufacturing overseas. The shift terminated thousands of American jobs, mostly in the steel and automotive industries. But as the economy deindustrialized, employment in services, research and information technology, health care, and finance grew. In comparison to radiological, chemical, mechanical, and construction hazards, postindustrial workplaces appeared dramatically safer. The indoor buildings had carpeted floors, air conditioning and heating, and seemed clean and well maintained. But as historian Michelle Murphy has shown, the pleasant features "only captured the bodily experience." Postindustrial workplaces still functioned like a factory, extracting productivity in a materially arranged setting.[28]

In the process, employees faced similar hazards to industrial workers, but the risks were harder to define and interpret. For example, energy conservation during the 1970s reduced the infiltration of outside air, adding to an accumulation of indoor air contaminants in office buildings. Many employees developed health problems associated with their time spent at work, but did not have specific diseases or chemical exposures to measure. As noted by Murphy, environmental politics shifted indoors when building-related illnesses entered the conversation, creating new problems in health and safety.[29]

A second, important component of the third era extends the parameters of this book. When multinational corporations moved their businesses to developing nations, many opened factories employing harmful processes strictly prohibited at home, a reprehensible practice that endangered foreign workers. By the 1990s manufacturing also became defined by American companies subcontracting out the most dangerous jobs. If a foreign worker died, only the subcontracting firm was held accountable. Christopher Sellers and Joseph Melling argue that an era developed out of the efforts to contend with these double standards abroad.[30]

Using this periodization, I have put Nevada at the center to provide a broader context in which industry operates, examining the importance of place in influencing health and safety regulation and attitudes. A core thread is also the development of notions of responsibility, the assumption that employers and the government were obligated to protect workers.[31]

Each chapter explores the work, conditions, and hazards at an industrial or postindustrial site, along with the health and safety procedures implemented. No other locale in the United States contains such a wide assortment of workplaces—the railroad, dam construction, chemical manufacturing, nuclear testing, and service—which offers unique opportunities to evaluate the development of health and safety in twentieth-century America. My goal is to provide a deeper understanding of the development of occupational health, and to evaluate workplace disasters and responses to inform future crises. I recognize that using place has its drawbacks, because harm to workers occurred during the construction of all railroads, dams, and construction sites, and the nuclear and service industries. Nevada is not unique in that respect. Focusing on a single location might also miss important developments occurring elsewhere in the United States. That being said, this book represents a history of occupational health. Place allows the opportunity to explain one state's relationship with occupational health, and how its attitudes in relation to health and safety evolved over time.

Nevada is fascinating for historical study. It is truly a state of contradictions. The state slogan is "Battle Born," but soldiers never fought on its soil. It is politically conservative, yet allows legalized gambling and prostitution. Eighty-seven percent of the state is federal land that houses water, defense, and industrial projects, yet residents pride themselves on state sovereignty and individualism. It is the seventh largest state in geographical size, but has a population of only several million, ranking thirty-fifth in population nationally.[32] These contradictions alone have made it difficult for occupational health to succeed.

Nevada began protecting its residents' health in 1893, establishing the State Board of Health in response to a cholera outbreak in the eastern United States. The first statute to protect workers passed in 1909, establishing the State Inspector of Mines. At the time, Nevada ranked sixth in production of gold, silver, copper, and lead, with dividends amounting to more than the mines in Montana, Arizona, Idaho, and Alaska combined. Three years prior to that statute, the state's output was smaller than any one of those states. Although the boom increased production and profits, it also brought attention to mining's dangerous working conditions. In a special legislative session in 1909, Lieutenant and Acting Governor Denver S. Dickerson tasked the inspector to compel the mining industry to provide "the fullest protection possible of the health" of all miners.[33] Not surprisingly, inspections did not receive a warm welcome. Managers complained that regulations placed unrealistic burdens on them, but the complaints eventually subsided when they discovered the new standards saved lives and boosted production levels.[34]

In line with the progressive reform, Nevada established its first compensation statute in 1913. Beginning in 1911, Governor Tasker Oddie addressed the legislature with the idea, stressing that labor unrest was due to "the universal defeat of justice in the matter of compensating the victims of accidents and fatalities" and that Nevada needed to establish a "rational system of atonement."[35] Legislators subsequently passed the Nevada Industrial Insurance Act of 1913, authorizing a state-run regulatory agency that maintained and dispersed insurance funds. Named the Nevada Industrial Commission (NIC), it eventually provided medical and hospital treatment to employers without healthcare plans as well. The following year, legislators established a labor commissioner to facilitate "just contractual relations" to prevent the "defrauding of workmen," monitor working conditions, and enforce eight-hour workday regulations and the recently passed statewide ban on child labor.[36]

In all appearances, the state positioned itself to be a major advocate for working people during the twentieth century. In a few isolated cases, this was true. The Inspector of Mines was an important ally to Hoover Dam workers, vigorously protesting against the use of gasoline-fueled trucks underground during the construction of the project's diversion tunnels. But for the most part, Nevada consistently failed to protect its workers throughout the century and continuously suffered large-scale workplace disasters. Why did this happen? Answering this question inspired the exploration of this book.

There are no easy answers. What the book reveals is that occupational health history is not a story of progress defined by an ahistorical constant: a health and safety movement trying to protect workers versus an unapologetic private sector. The benefit of a long-term, localized study is that it shows that a single, constant movement did not exist. The occupational health regimes were diverse in Nevada, varying from one period to the next, and the differences are an important part of understanding this history.

## NOTES

1. Several articles cover the inception of CityCenter. See Liz Benson, "MGM Plans Massive Strip Project," *Las Vegas Sun,* Nov. 10, 2004 (incl. "exciting departure"); "MGM Mirage Picks Pernini to Build CityCenter," *Las Vegas Sun,* May 13, 2005; "Boardwalk Closing to Clear Way for CityCenter," *Las Vegas Sun,* Sept. 16, 2005; T. R. Witcher, "How One Giant Casino Could Turn Around Las Vegas," *Time* (Sept. 29, 2009).

2. See Alexandra Berzon, "Pace Is the New Peril," *Las Vegas Sun,* Mar. 30, 2008 (incl. "everyone [was] fighting" and "just asking"). This article is part of a Pulitzer-winning series written by Berzon that reveals the lax safety standards at CityCenter and other properties on the Las Vegas Strip.

3. Berzon covers the death of Harold Billingsley in her *Las Vegas Sun* series. In her series see "Pace Is the New Peril"; "OSHA Goes Easy," Mar. 31, 2008; "Not in This City," Apr. 1, 2008. See also Brian Haynes, "Iron Worker Falls to Death on Strip," *Las Vegas Review-Journal* (hereafter *Review-Journal*), Oct. 6, 2007; Arnold Knightly, "Workers Walk Off Job," *Review-Journal,* June 3, 2008.

4. Additional articles on the Strip construction deaths include David Kihara, "Two Workers Killed at Project CityCenter," *Review-Journal,* Feb. 7, 2007; "Construction Worker Plunges to Death," *Review-Journal,* Nov. 28, 2007; Francis McCabe, "Worker Killed on Strip Project," *Review-Journal,* Aug. 10, 2007; Tony Illia, "Rise in Construction Deaths Alarm Many, But Work Goes On," *Review-Journal,* Aug. 26, 2007; Arnold Knightly and Howard Stut, "Worker Dies on Strip," *Review-Journal,* June 17, 2008.

5. Berzon, "Pace Is the New Peril"; Berzon, "Construction Worker Dies at Echelon," *Las Vegas Sun,* June 16, 2008; Mary Watters, "Lessons Learned from Las Vegas," *Occupational Health and Safety,* June 3, 2009; Robert Gavin, "9 Deaths at Pernini Stir Questions," *Boston Globe,* Sept. 10, 2008; "*Las Vegas Sun* Wins Pulitzer Prize," *Las Vegas*

*Sun,* Apr. 20, 2009; Marshall Allen, "Sun Wins the Pulitzer Prize: Worker Safety Coverage Honored for Public Service," *Las Vegas Sun,* Apr. 21, 2009; Tina Susman, "5 Pulitzers for *NY Times*: Vegas Paper's Reporting on Worker Deaths Also Honored," *Chicago Tribune,* Apr. 21, 2009.

6. Berzon, "Pace Is the New Peril" (incl. "pinned its" and "body count," n.p.).

7. See Christopher Sellers and Joseph Melling, eds., *Dangerous Trade: Histories of Industrial Hazard Across a Globalizing World* (Philadelphia: Temple University Press, 2012), 3.

8. For scholarship on the history of occupational health in the United States, see Ronald Bayer, ed., *The Health and Safety of Workers: Case Studies in the Politics of Professional Responsibility* (New York: Oxford University Press, 1988); Daniel Berman, "Why Work Kills: A Brief History of Occupational Safety and Health in the United States," *International Journal of Health Services* 7 (1977): 63–87; Claudia Clark, *Radium Girls: Women and Industrial Health Reform, 1910–35* (Chapel Hill: University of North Carolina Press, 1997); Jacqueline Corn, *Protecting the Health of Workers: The American Conference of Governmental Industrial Hygienists* (Cincinnati, OH: American Conference of Governmental Industrial Hygienists, 1989); Corn, *Response to Occupational Health Hazards* (New York: Van Nostrand Reinhold, 1992); Steve Fox, *Toxic Work: Women Workers at GTE Lenkurt* (Philadelphia: Temple University Press, 1991); Allison Helper, *Women in Labor: Mothers, Medicine, and Occupational Health in the United States, 1890–1980* (Columbus: Ohio State University Press, 2000); Bennett Judkins, *We Offer Ourselves as Evidence: Toward Workers' Control of Occupational Health* (New York: Greenwood, 1986); Gerald Markowitz and David Rosner, *Deadly Dust: Silicosis and the Politics of Occupational Disease in Twentieth-Century America* (Princeton, NJ: Princeton University Press, 2003); Markowitz and Rosner, *Deceit and Denial: The Deadly Politics of Industrial Pollution* (Berkeley: University of California Press, 2006); Markowitz and Rosner, eds., *Dying for Work: Workers' Safety and Health in Twentieth-Century America* (Bloomington: Indiana University Press, 1987); Markowitz and Rosner, *Lead Wars: The Politics of Science and the Fate of America's Children* (Berkeley: University of California Press, 2014); Markowitz and Rosner, "The Early Movement for Occupational Safety and Health, 1900–1917," in *Sickness and Health in America,* ed. Judith Walzer and Ronald Numbers (Madison: University of Wisconsin Press, 1997); Markowitz and Rosner, "The Limits of Thresholds: Silica and the Politics of Science, 1935–1990," *American Journal of Public Health* 85, no. 2 (1995): 253–62; Dorothy Nelkin and Michael Brown, *Workers at Risk: Voices for the Workplace* (Chicago: University of Chicago Press, 1984); Christopher C. Sellers, "Factory as Environment: Industrial Hygiene, Professional Collaboration and the Modern Sciences of Pollution," *Environmental History Review* 18, no. 1 (1994): 55–83; Sellers, *Hazards of the Job: From Industrial Disease to Environmental Health Science* (Chapel Hill: University of North Carolina Press, 1997); Helen E. Sheehan and Richard P. Wedeen, *Toxic Circles: Environmental Hazards from the Workplace to the Community* (New Brunswick, NJ: Rutgers University Press, 1993); Barbara Ellen Smith, *Digging Our Own Graves: Coal Miners and the Struggle over Black Lung Disease* (Philadelphia: Temple University Press, 2004); Paul Weindling, ed., *The Social History of Occupational Health* (London: Croom Helm, 1985).

9. Sellers and Melling, *Dangerous Trade,* 3–6, 197–201 (incl. "industrial hazard regime" and "public bodies," 4).

10. For more on American accident law during the nineteenth and early twentieth centuries, see John Fabian Witt, *The Accidental Republic: Crippled Workmen, Destitute Widows, and the Remaking of American Law* (Cambridge, MA: Harvard University Press,

2004); William Novak, *The Peoples' Welfare: Law and Regulation in Nineteenth-Century America* (Chapel Hill: University of North Carolina Press, 1996).

11. Farwell v. Boston & Worcester R.R. Corp, 45 Mass. 49 (Mass. 1842); Lochner v. New York, 198 U.S. 45 (1905) (incl. "unreasonable").

12. Physical examinations also became an important component in the life insurance industry. See Audrey Davis, "Life Insurance and the Physical Examination: A Chapter in the Rise of Medical Technology," *Bulletin of the History of Medicine* 55 (1981): 392–406; Angela Nugent, "Fit for Work: The Introduction of Physical Examinations in Industry," *Bulletin of the History of Medicine* 57 (1983): 578–95.

13. Allison Helper argues that the relationship between motherhood and the workplace, and the utilization of gender differences in occupational health, had a lasting effect on working women, hindering their ability for employment advancement throughout the twentieth century. See Helper, *Women in Labor*.

14. Progressivism addressed economic and social reform during the late nineteenth and early twentieth centuries, with reformers responding to industrialization and its social by-products. See Richard Hofstadter, *The Age of Reform: From Bryan to FDR* (New York: Knopf, 1955); Gabriel Kolko, *The Triumph of Conservatism* (New York: Free Press of Glencoe, 1963); Samuel Hays, *The Response to Industrialism, 1885–1914* (Chicago: University of Chicago Press, 1957); Robert Wiebe, *The Search for Order* (New York: Hill & Wang, 1967); Daniel T. Rodgers, "The Search of Progressivism," *Reviews in American History* 10, no. 4, *The Promise of American History: Progress and Prospects* (Dec. 1982), 113–32.

15. See Richard A. Greenwald, *The Triangle Fire, Protocols of Peace, and Industrial Democracy in Progressive Era New York* (Philadelphia: Temple University Press, 2005).

16. See Alice Hamilton, *Exploring the Dangerous Trades: The Autobiography of Alice Hamilton* (Boston: Northeastern University Press, 1985 [1943]).

17. Early forms of workmen's compensation did not apply to working women. As such, husbands of deceased working women could not bring claims for compensation. See Witt, *Accidental Republic*, 133–34; Wengler v. Druggists' Mutual Insurance Co., 446 U.S. 142 (1980).

18. See FELA, 34 Stat. 232 (1906); FELA, 35 Stat. 65 (1908); 1910 New York Laws Ch. 674 § 219a; Andrew E. Kersten, *Labor's Home Front: The American Federation of Labor During World War II* (New York and London: New York University Press, 2006), 171–72. For further discussion of employers' liability and the origins of workmen's compensation, see also Witt, *Accidental Republic*; and Price Fishback and Shawn Kantor, *A Prelude to the Welfare State: The Origins of Workers Compensation* (Chicago: University of Chicago Press, 2000).

19. For more on industrial hygiene moving from the field to university laboratories during the 1920s, see Sellers, *Hazards of the Job*; and Michelle Murphy, *Sick Building Syndrome and the Problem of Uncertainty* (Durham, NC, and London: Duke University Press, 2006).

20. Richard C. Barth, Patricia D. George, and Ronald H. Hill, *Environmental Health and Safety for Hazardous Waste Sites* (Fairfax, VA: American Industrial Hygiene Association, 2002), 3.

21. See Markowitz and Rosner, *Deadly Dust*, 96; and Martin Cherniack, *The Hawk's Nest Incident: America's Worst Industrial Disaster* (New Haven, CT: Yale University Press, 1986).

22. The Civil Works Administration promoted safety engineers and occupational health programs consisting of safety requirements, first-aid training, and education. At the same time, the Public Works Administration (PWA), Works Progress Administration (WPA), and the National Recovery Administration (NRA) created safety organizations, mandating all work to follow specific safety codes. In 1934 the DOL established a committee to develop health and safety standards for the NRA, including machinery protection, physical examinations, and injury reporting. While most programs were discontinued or brief, they helped spread the safety movement to the private sector. See Mark Aldrich, *Safety-First: Technology, Labor and Business in the Building of Work Safety, 1870-1939* (Baltimore: Johns Hopkins University Press, 1997), 156-57.

23. Aldrich, *Safety-First*, 166, 271-72.

24. See Markowitz and Rosner, *Deadly Dust*, 179, 188-90; Murphy, *Sick Building Syndrome*, 90; David Hounshell and John Kenley Smith, *Science and Corporate Strategy: Du Pont R&D, 1902-1980* (Cambridge, UK: Cambridge University Press, 1988) also provides a case study documenting the history of corporate research labs.

25. Rachel Carson, *Silent Spring* (New York: Houghton Mifflin Company, 2002 [1962]); Linda Nash, *Inescapable Ecologies: A History of Environment, Disease, and Knowledge* (Berkeley: University of California Press, 2006), 157-58.

26. Markowitz and Rosner, *Deceit and Denial*, 156-57, 159, 164.

27. Corn, *Response*, 1-2.

28. Murphy, *Sick Building Syndrome*, 57-59 (incl. "only captured," 57).

29. Occupational Safety and Health Administration, *OSHA Technical Manual (OTM)*, OSHA Instruction TED 01-00-015, Section III: Chapter 2, "Indoor Air Quality Investigation," www.osha.gov/dts/osta/otm/otm_iii/otm_iii_2.html.

30. Sellers and Melling also use periodization to conceptualize industrial hazard history on the global scale. See *Dangerous Trade*, 202-4.

31. For scholarship that developed the thread of notions of responsibility in occupational health history, see Clark, *Radium Girls*; Corn, *Protecting*; Corn, *Response*; Markowitz and Rosner, "Early Movement."

32. Michael Bowers, *The Nevada State Constitution: A Reference Guide* (Westport, CT: Greenwood Press, 1993). In 2015 the U.S. Census Bureau estimated that the population of Nevada was 2,890,845.

33. "Governor's Message to the Legislature," *Appendix to the Journals of the Nevada State Senate and Assembly* (hereafter *Appendix*), 24th Sess., Vol. 1 (Carson City, NV: State Printing Office [hereafter SPO], 1909) (incl. "the fullest," 19).

34. "Report of the State Board of Health," *Appendix*, 17th Sess., Vol. 1 (Carson City, NV: SPO, 1895), 3-4; "Report of Inspector of Mines," *Appendix*, 25th Sess., Vol. 2 (Carson City, NV: SPO, 1911), 5-7.

35. "Governor's Message to the Legislature," *Appendix*, 25th Sess., Vol. 1 (incl. "the universal defeat" and "rational system," 29).

36. "Report of the Nevada Industrial Commission: Reviewing the Administration of the Nevada Industrial Act for the Period of Three Years—July 1, 1913, to June 30, 1916" (Carson City, NV: SPO, 1917), 5; "Report of Commissioner of Labor," and "Governor's Message to the Legislature," *Appendix*, 28th Sess., Vol. 1 (Carson City, NV: SPO, 1917), 5-9, 26 (incl. "just contractual relations" and "defrauding of workmen," 26).

# 1

# THE RAILROAD

THE STORY OF WORK in Las Vegas begins in 1905 with the railroad. The industry embarked on a challenging task, constructing a railway between Salt Lake City and Los Angeles. The two cities were separated by sparsely populated desert, with high temperatures, limited water, and no infrastructure, so the carrier determined that it needed to establish a railway station and yard at the halfway point. Las Vegas was founded during the first period of occupational health history, a time when concerns for employee health and safety were beginning to emerge. Industrial capitalism brought conflict and volatility to the United States, prompting workplace violence, economic depression, corruption, increased social stratification, and insecurity, and eroded the nation's democratic institutions. There was no workplace more unsafe than those in America, and the railroad industry was one of the most dangerous.[1]

Borrowing technological knowledge from Europe, Americans rapidly developed the railroad during the nineteenth century. The first continental carrier, Baltimore & Ohio Railroad (B&O), was completed in 1828, and by 1873 American companies operated the largest railroad network in the world, with more than seventy thousand miles of track. The railroad industry borrowed from European technology to shape all aspects of railroad transportation, including safety. Those companies' choices, along with limited federal regulation, created a unique American institution that was considerably more dangerous than European counterparts. In 1901 the fatality rate per thousand American railroad workers was more than double the rate per English workers. Indeed, railroading was a dangerous trade because it was a developing industry; Europeans endured numerous accidents during the development process as well. As shown by historian Mark Aldrich, the main difference between the European and American railroad culture is that American carriers traded expensive capital and labor for accidents, running more freight than passenger cars and coupling with links and pins instead of the expensive European method, by hook and chain.[2]

Railroad management officials believed they were not responsible for health and safety because accidents were the workers' fault. Edward Dickinson, general manager of the Union Pacific Railroad (UPRR), commented, "Fully 90% of railway derailments and wrecks are caused by careless, or rather willful, disobedience of well-defined rules and regulations on the part of some employee."[3] At least initially, labor shared this viewpoint, consenting that all hazards were negotiable only before starting the job. After workers were on the job, hazards were part of their contract.

*Farwell v. Boston & Worcester R.R. Corp.* made it impossible for employees to recover damages from their employer even if a coworker contributed to an injury.[4] *Farwell* influenced courts in Massachusetts and across the nation to develop a series of doctrines that made it nearly impossible for workers to seek the law for insurance against the risks of work. Often, courts found that coworkers were not liable if an injured worker was guilty of contributory negligence. Employers also were required only to exercise care. While obligated to warn employees of dangerous conditions, they were not required by law to remedy those conditions. According to historian John Fabian Witt, the combination of these nineteenth-century policies created an "'unholy trinity' of rules that made it difficult for injured employees to recover damages from their employers."[5]

By the last decades of the nineteenth century, after outrunning the capacity to handle its tracks, the railroad entered a new phase. With management directing capital toward new construction rather than existing lines, radical cutbacks forced supervisors to run their workers and equipment until they fell apart.[6] The policies eventually prompted regulators, managers, and workers to campaign for better equipment and tighter regulation. In 1873 Eli H. Janney patented the automatic knuckle coupler, which replaced the link and pin method, and in 1887 George Westinghouse modified the train brake to work on long freights. The technological advances not only improved productivity but also fostered safer working conditions. Historians regard both developments as the most significant safety inventions in American railroads from the end of the Civil War to 1900.[7] Congress established the Interstate Commerce Commission (ICC), which published railroad fatality statistics. The figures revealed the extraordinary risk of trainmen on the job.[8] A subsequent campaign for safety culminated in the Federal Safety Appliance Act of 1893, the first federal law that sought to improve worker safety. The act required all railroad companies to install air brakes and automatic couplers on all trains. It took nearly a decade for the new equipment to reach most carriers, but this equipment has been credited with the decline of trainmen accidents in the early twentieth century.[9]

It was during this period of occupational health history that the railroad arrived in southern Nevada. Even though it had an abundant water supply and fertile ground for crops, settlers found it hard to achieve long-term settlement in the region. In 1855 Brigham Young instructed Mormon missionaries to establish a homestead in Las Vegas, but the mission disbanded in 1858. In the late nineteenth century, Nevada emerged from a twenty-year economic depression after the discovery of various mineral lodes in central and eastern parts of the state. Still, state politics continued to favor the northern mining industry.[10]

The location of southern Nevada nevertheless elevated the region to prominence. There was no link between Salt Lake City and Los Angeles, and U.S. Senator William A. Clark of Montana wanted to enter the railroad business. Clark was a corrupt mining and banking entrepreneur from Montana, described by author Mark Twain: "[He is as] rotten a human being as can be found anywhere under the flag…[and is] a shame to the American nation."[11]

The UPRR's Southern Pacific Railroad also recognized the benefits of building a rail between Salt Lake City and Los Angeles. The UPRR was founded under wartime pressure in 1862 to link the Pacific Ocean. By the 1890s it had declared bankruptcy and a group of financiers bought the company. Headed by Edward Harriman, the financiers forced major improvements, a vision that ultimately created the modern American railroad system. The UPRR had proposed building a southwestern route, but the company abandoned the plan during the bankruptcy process. Consequently, Clark won title to the land. In 1900 Clark chartered the San Pedro, Los Angeles, & Salt Lake Railroad Company (later shortened to the Los Angeles and Salt Lake Railroad, or LA&SL), organizing a construction company to build the line. Harriman, however, still intended to build the track. In March 1901 Harriman and Clark filed their claim in court, and began simultaneously constructing lines in the Clover Creek Canyon, a narrow ravine near Caliente, Nevada.[12]

Conflict between the two lines soon became unavoidable. The UPRR heavily recruited its rival's crews, offering a significant pay raise, and swept their opponents off the grade. In response, the LA&SL erected barbed wire and barricades. The mood was restless, with both sides anxious to avoid violence—but a clash was inevitable. Some newspapers reported an all-out war, but with the exception of a few bloody noses and harassment allegations, work continued without significant interruption. Eventually, the courts interceded, shutting down track production on both sides until the companies reached a compromise. In 1902 Clark agreed to operate the railroad in exchange for furnishing the UPRR with a 50 percent stake in the company. In early 1905 workers completed the railway in Jean, Nevada, and special trains began running. Passenger service began on May 1, 1905.[13]

Finishing the track marked a significant milestone for southern Nevada. The line inspired the creation of a town somewhere between Salt Lake and Los Angeles: In 1902 Clark bought Helen Stewart's two-thousand-acre ranch in the Las Vegas Valley with the intention of establishing a company town. After completing the track, he organized an auction for commercial and residential lots, forming a subsidiary, the Las Vegas Land & Water Company (LVL&W), to handle all land transactions. Las Vegas became a major transshipment site virtually overnight, storing and loading supplies from California and Utah onto wagons traveling northwest to construction camps. The town also benefited from Clark's decision to establish another railroad, the Las Vegas and Tonopah Railroad, in 1907.[14]

The first occupational health regime to coalesce in Las Vegas dealt with the dangers associated with working in and living near the railroad industry. The turn of the century marked a time of transition for railroad health and safety. The industry as a whole boomed, forcing carriers to upgrade existing lines to accommodate a rise in passenger and freight traffic. Yet the expansion increased the frequency of accidents. Even though carriers invested in high-tech brakes, couplers, signals, and other safety measures, worker and passenger fatalities rose 30 and 60 percent, respectively. During the first years of the LA&SL's operation, the ICC reported more than 5,000 workers killed and 75,286 workers injured in railroad accidents nationwide, an increase of 755 killed and 8,577 injured from previous years. Congress responded to the spike in injuries and deaths by passing the Accident Reports Act, which required carriers to report to the ICC all accidents involving injury or losses of more than $150. To reduce negative publicity, carriers studied how to improve technology, and invested in better track, communication devices, and control features. They also created comprehensive safety programs and public positions on safety, hiring the American Railway Association (ARA) to speak on its behalf. The combination of higher accident costs to employers due to new compensation laws and stricter employer liability, and the establishment of safety programs eventually improved conditions. Worker fatalities steadily declined after 1910.[15]

Still, accidents were frequent across the state of Nevada, most likely because it hosted a number of dangerous industries in remote locations. Most industries also lacked comprehensive health and safety programs until the 1920s. In 1944 Reno physician Dr. M. Rollin Walker recalled the struggle of regulating health and safety in the Nevada workplace: "The question arising concerning industrial injuries and occupational diseases is a very live one today. In 1911 such questions and discussions were just in their adolescent stage. Injuries were fairly simple, but questions concerning disorders supposed to be due to the occupation had received so little attention that only a few physicians and surgeons were conversant.... Even in so sparsely settled a State as Nevada it is apparent that the old order must give way to a broader concept, a more centralized control and administration in industry, education, and public health."[16]

From 1913 to 1916 there were 4,145 accidents in all industry classes. Mining involved the most risk, with 4.84 out of 1,000 workers experiencing a fatal accident each year, and 205 out of 1,000 suffering some form of injury. In contrast, only 1.49 out of 1,000 railroad workers experienced a fatal accident, and 84.82 out of 1,000 suffered some form of injury.[17]

The LA&SL was a dangerous operation, but the workers willingly gambled with their lives. The risks of working versus the risks of not working was a common predicament among employees at the turn of the century.[18] Workers knew the job could cause injury or death, but they also knew that not receiving a paycheck presented greater consequences, such as the inability to provide food and shelter to their families. The employee demographic was typical of western towns depending on industries other than mining. Most of the population descended from at least one parent who had immigrated from the United Kingdom or elsewhere in Europe, and who had themselves immigrated from another state. The hiring process was prejudiced, with the most difficult and most dangerous labor allocated to minorities. In the quest for cheap labor, the railroad employed Japanese laborers, forcing them to sleep outside the city limits in construction cars or the repair shops, and shuffling Mexican and Native American laborers to camps outside of town. There were very few blacks, with only sixteen reported in the 1910 census of Las Vegas, and most worked in Block 16 and 17, the northern section of the townsite along Stewart Street that legally served liquor without licensing restrictions. Conflict among the diverse railroad crew was common. In early 1905, the *Las Vegas Age* reported on fights involving Caucasian workers and the "swarthy sons of Japan," and instances between Italians and Greeks working for the railroad south of town, writing, "Judge Brennan was engaged in a legal sponsor for the Greeks and Dan V. Noland appeared for the banana sellers." In this incident, he fined the parties involved $10. In 1912 a Mexican laborer was murdered by a coworker, cut "from ear to ear with a sharp instrument," dragged by the arms twenty feet, and his body placed between the railroad tracks. A switch engine later ran him over.[19]

Laborer conflict was a universal problem in railroading, but the work itself presented even more of a hazard. In 1908 alone, 281,641 employees in the United States were injured at work and more than twelve thousand killed.[20] The biggest risks at the LA&SL were human error and equipment failures. Miscalculations operating machinery on the train and in the yards, fatigue, limited work experience, and inadequate hazard awareness caused most accidents. Derailments, caused by weaknesses in road equipment, erratic desert storms, axle failures, inability to enforce speed, and track debris were particularly menacing. Derailments plagued the railroad industry throughout the nineteenth century, but steadily declined due to technological advancements. However, the economic upswing of 1897 reversed the trend, increasing passenger and freight traffic. In 1902 there were 1,609 derailments nationwide. In 1920 the total was 11,172. But although derailments increased, improvements in technology helped casualties decline. The railroad industry also increasingly moved toward scientific technology to improve reliability, and rises in traffic and costs encouraged investments to improve track and roadbed.[21]

Desert storms caused the majority of derailments on the LA&SL. Large clouds dumped rain on the track, splintering the roadbed and prompting washouts. As a result of these washouts, trains plunged off bridges, a recurrent and costly problem.[22] From January 1 to June 15, 1910, a succession of storms suspended traffic due to washouts. The line became impassable for hundreds of miles, requiring the carrier to continuously rebuild the track throughout the year. In 1907 trainman Lou Martin described a dramatic derailment twenty-five miles outside Caliente. After heavy rainfall had washed away the roadbed, he saw three cars "topple into the river." Martin unsuccessfully tried to save two carloads of horses before the water submerged them. He and his crew eventually gave up and walked back to Caliente, passing around a quart of alcohol. Martin recalled that it was "all they could do to get that liquor away from me." Several months later, workers found portions of the train as far away as Moapa Valley. They did not find the engine until a year later, completely covered in deep mud.[23]

Faulty track, wheels, and electrical wires also caused a considerable amount of derailments. The railroad cited bad steel and construction defects for these accidents, while manufacturers countered that the train weights, speed, and improper maintenance were to blame. While en route, a defective electrical wiring burst into flames on a sleeping Pullman car in 1926. The train stopped immediately and evacuated the passengers, and firefighters subdued the blaze except for a small, smoldering section on the roof. Assuming the risk had passed, several passengers boarded the train to collect their belongings and were subsequently smothered by carbon monoxide poisoning that had been produced by toxins in the curtains and cushions. All of them died. In a trial to determine if there had been negligence, a jury found the LA&SL innocent of all criminal activity but determined that it had not followed proper safety precautions. The jury mandated outfitting all trains with large fire extinguishers, thus establishing that the existing protocol of small hand pumps was not adequate enough to safeguard lives.[24]

As with most workplaces, human error caused the most accidents prompted by fatigue, limited work experience, and inadequate hazard awareness. Trainmen often reported crush injuries when they carelessly switched operating doors and hatches, and loaded cars. Miscommunication was also a common problem, especially when workers had limited lines of sight. Oncoming trains frequently struck trackwalkers, employees working in pairs that were responsible for tightening bolts and clearing off track debris. Train operators did not see them until it was too late for them to stop. In 1918 a train hit trackwalker A. R. Nelson outside Las Vegas. Company physician Dr. John Fuller was on call and attempted to save his life, but the man was "delivered to [him] in an injured condition." Although there was no damage to his torso, he eventually succumbed to skull fractures, experiencing "two open wounds on the head from which brain matter was protruding" and "bleeding from both wounds and from the nose."[25]

Traditional construction-type accidents also afflicted workers on the roadbed and railway yards. Hoisting cranes frequently toppled over while repairing flat cars and washouts, and engine oil tanks exploded, fatally burning workers. On one occasion a foreman caught his shirt sleeve in a concrete mixer and was pulled in. The mixer whirling him around broke almost every bone in his body, and he died several hours later. Workplace violence attributed to deaths as well: During track construction, a worker found postmortem remains of a man in his bunk. At first it appeared the man had died of natural causes, but a Los Angeles coroner later determined it had been murder. Someone allegedly had committed the crime after the UPRR paid off the man to quit Clark's crew.[26]

Train collisions were one of the most visible threats of the job. After the railroad industry began limiting the use of single tracks and enhanced signaled crossings, head-on collisions were less frequent, but reduced visibility due to weather and poor communication still proved fatal. In 1907 a crew worked all night to fix a washout in Caliente. Rushing to finish the job, they forgot to move several cars loaded with timber on the main line and failed to communicate that the washout had not been fixed. Without warning, a passenger train crashed into the loaded freight cars. Workers jumped off the train and track to save themselves. The incident killed four people and "horribly mangled others," according to the Las Vegas Age, injuring fifty. Company physicians Hal Hewetson and Roy Martin quickly arrived at the scene, treating fractures and performing amputations. Las Vegas residents were furious about the accident, with the Las Vegas Age demanding a "thorough investigation [be made] in interest of humanity" for the railroad's negligence.[27]

Of course, passengers were not always passive victims. Even though the LVL&W attempted to control the type of businesses established in Las Vegas, Fremont Street quickly emerged as the town's central business district and premier attraction for vice. Passengers with layovers could legally drink alcohol, gamble, or pay for sex with a prostitute—activities prohibited in most towns. Afterwards, many returned to the train station in a delirious state. They frequently fell off the unfenced platform or tried to board moving trains. In 1917 a passenger tried to board a moving freight and the train decapitated him. Citing that "booze-related deaths" were "very common" in Las Vegas, the Las Vegas Age reported that the passenger had been drinking heavily in the local saloons for "several days."[28]

The trains also regularly hit trespassers. During the early twentieth century vagabonds or hobos became a nuisance for the railroad industry. Many trespassers fell and experienced fatal injures while attempting to board a moving train or were crushed by heavy freight cargo. As the casualties rose, carriers began a campaign that publicized the dangers of trespasser evil. Its motives were a mix of humanitarianism, economics, and politics. Trespassing was especially problematic in southern Nevada because it housed a transcontinental highway, with migrant workers hitching rides to California. In 1914 alone the LA&SL reported killing sixteen trespassers and injuring thirty. The carrier blamed trespassers for the widespread belief that American railways were dangerous, calling them a "menace to the lives of train-men." This was partially true. Indeed, most trespasser deaths were completely preventable, and were not caused by railroad negligence. Unfortunately, there was very little the railroad could do. It was diffi-cult to discourage trespassing in a legal manner, because federal laws on the matter did not exist and magistrates tended not to prosecute offenders.[29]

Las Vegas residents were also subject to railroad-related casualties, mostly due to unfenced lines and unguarded crossings. Traditionally, crossings were problematic only in urban settings involving horses, wagons, and pedestrians. But after the arrival of the automobile, rural areas became much more dangerous. The loud noise of early automo-biles certainly impaired hearing, but most drivers also operated the vehicles at high speeds. Both factors increased the danger, especially in instances of obstructed visibility. In 1910 annual fatalities at crossings to nontrespassers rose nationally. In response, the railroad industry installed bells at heavily traveled crossings to warn motorists, and placed "Stop, Look, Listen" announcements in local newspapers.

As a rural town, Las Vegas was especially susceptible to such ac-cidents. In 1938 a train struck a light Ford truck on Charleston Boule-vard, killing the driver and seriously injuring his small daughter. The accident occurred due to inadequate railroad crossing protection: An arm on the railroad crossing sign had broken off, and residents had complained about it for years. The accident revealed that the LA&SL had an obligation to protect the community. The family of the victims ultimately sued the carrier for damages, forcing it to update all cross-ing signs and safety measures throughout the town.[30]

As a transcontinental and transient workplace and community, public health concerns also threatened southern Nevada. The State Board of Health found it difficult to regulate industrial hygiene in Ne-vada industries as a whole because most were temporary enterprises.

In 1911 the Board of Health started publishing vital statistics to learn more about its disease epidemics. Clark County began reporting its findings in 1913, with Dr. Roy Martin serving as the chairman of Clark County's State Board of Health. The statistics ultimately revealed that Clark County was not the most dangerous county in the state; Washoe County had that distinction, leading in accidental deaths and suicides.[31]

At first the LA&SL and its company town enjoyed relatively fair public health, but the conditions deteriorated by the 1930s due to environmental weathering, age, economic depression, and an influx of population during the construction of Hoover Dam. The yards were cramped, and the terminal was overcrowded and subject to air and water contamination. Communicable diseases were a threat to the population, especially influenza, pneumonia, and tuberculosis. Las Vegas experienced its first public health endemic in 1918–19, with the so-called Spanish flu.[32]

Since the 1600s a major human influenza outbreak has occurred approximately three times a century. There are four types of known influenza viruses: A, B, C, and D, named for the order in which they were discovered. Influenza A infects both animals and humans, while influenza B is a human virus. Both types cause seasonable epidemics in humans nearly every winter in the United States. Influenza C is a mild respiratory illness in both humans and swine, and influenza D has only been detected in swine, cattle, sheep, and goats. All major flu pandemics in humans have been caused by influenza A, a virus with potentially 144 different subtypes. The three combinations that have produced the most outbreaks are H1N1, H2N2, and H3N2.[33] Some of these strains resemble an ordinary flu, but others mutate. This happened in 1918, one of the deadliest disease events in human history. In one year, more humans died globally from an H1N1 virus that originated from avian influenza A than had died during all of World War I.[34]

The first outbreak in the United States occurred at Camp Funston, a U.S. Army training camp located on Fort Riley in Kansas, on March 4, 1918. Within several days, hundreds were ill, with cases reported in every state. While the first wave of the virus was highly contagious, it was not lethal. During the next year, it mutated and spread rapidly, infecting an estimated 500 million people worldwide, 25 to 30 percent of the population. Death estimates range from 20 million to 100 million, with 675,000 Americans among the dead. Like most western states, the second wave hit Nevada hard. The first cases reached Reno and Las Vegas in the fall of 1918 and soon the State Board of Health reported that there was "scarcely a village or hamlet that did not pay toll to it in human life." In total, it sickened nearly 5,000 and killed 734 Nevada residents. Fatalities were few in uncomplicated cases, but patients who developed pneumonia had a high death rate. The high mortality of healthy people was unique to the 1918 pandemic, as there was no vaccine to protect against the disease and no antibiotics, a discovery by Alexander Fleming a decade later, to treat secondary bacterial infections.[35]

To fight the disease, the State Board of Health quarantined patients, and instructed everyone to wear masks, use disinfectants, and limit public gatherings. The precautions were not particularly successful. In the end, most Nevadan doctors cited that widespread anxiety worsened the problem, reducing their patients' natural resistance. The State Board of Health even reported that "fear should have been entered into the death certificates." Dr. Rupert Blue, surgeon general of the Public Health Service, shared the sentiment, commenting that the virus killed only five thousand Americans and the others succumbed to "fear and worry."[36]

As a transient railroad town, the pandemic swept across Las Vegas. Dr. Hal Hewetson had been drafted to military service during the war, serving in the Medical Department. When he returned home in October 1918, he arrived to a shocking sight. The disease had already sickened 150 residents, with five new cases reported daily, mostly accompanied by pneumonia. As the sick toll rose, local doctors were understaffed and overwhelmed, and there was not enough burial space or coffins to accommodate the dead. In December 1918 ten new cases were reported daily and fifty people had died.[37]

The LA&SL enforced control measures to fight the disease, including isolation, new personal hygiene requirements, the use of disinfectants, and forbidding public gatherings. The railroad also issued a hygiene list to employees:

1. Ventilators in office should be kept freely open, and if there is heat in the building the temperature of the quarters would not be permitted to go over 68 degrees.
2. At noon all windows of offices should be opened and the rooms cleared of all clerical help possible during lunch time.
3. Avoid crowds and congregating in groups.
4. Elevators should not be crowded.
5. Everyone coughing and sneezing should do so in handkerchiefs.
6. Use individual drinking cups.
7. Keep hands clean by frequently washing, as they are conveyers of disease germs.
8. Do not visit anyone suffering from "Influenza," "Pneumonia," and "Epidemic Colds."
9. Remember that the germs of "Flu" and "Pneumonia" are found in the discharges from the mouth and nose of not only those so infected, often in persons who seem to be healthy.
10. Avoid getting feet and clothing wet.
11. Protect others by observing these health rules just as you would have others protect you.[38]

The public health measures did not isolate the virus, but by the end of 1919 it naturally became less lethal and gradually disappeared from Las Vegas.[39]

Apart from the flu pandemic, the Las Vegas community enjoyed mostly good health. Respiratory diseases, such as pneumonia and tuberculosis, were the biggest menace, contributing to 20 percent of all deaths in Nevada. But there were no large-scale epidemics, thanks to newly established national and statewide public health precautions, and advances in immunizations. The Public Health Service instructed communities and industries to protect their water supply from sewage and industrial waste to prevent cholera and typhoid fever, and monitored neighborhoods for disease-carrying mosquitoes and flies. Additionally, the State Board of Health distributed smallpox, diphtheria, and other vaccines to Clark County. Consequently, death rates in diphtheria declined significantly; Clark County reported only two fatal cases in 1927. But while the vaccinations were beneficial to their health, many residents declined them, citing that poor protection of vaccination sores and impurities could cause injury or death. Many people were also wary of modern advances in medicine.[40]

Las Vegas's first industrial health system emerged during a time in American history when employers began to combine their interests with workers to respond to the risk of working. As Christopher Sellers, Joseph Melling, and other historians have shown, injury at work became a more visible concern at the turn of the century due to the growth of statistical analysis and scientific knowledge concerning workplace hazards, productivity, and profits.[41] Employers, physicians and public health advocates, and progressive reformers worked alongside insurance companies, eager to limit costs, founding an industrial hygiene movement that raised the specter of job safety and urban epidemics. As the most visible and dangerous American work site, railroad industry regulation was at the forefront. In 1907 unions, including the Brotherhood of Locomotive Engineers and Trainmen, lobbied for improved safety regulation of locomotives and freight cars, helping institute federal and state legislation that required three brakemen per freight train. Although intended as safety standards, the laws also averted layoffs since technological advances like air brakes eliminated the need for labor. Laws that regulated train lengths had similar intentions. In 1910 the railroad formed the Bureau of Railway Economics to limit these efforts, publishing pamphlets to present their cause. Although twenty states passed crew laws and one passed a law with regard to train length, the industry held off similar legislation at the federal level. In general, most progressive railroad safety legislation was moderately advantageous to workers at best.[42]

While national developments improved health and safety, the first occupational health regime emerged in Las Vegas, beginning with the institution of an industrial health program at the LA&SL. In 1913 the railroad founded a Safety-First campaign designed to end small accidents. First introduced at the Chicago and North Western Railroad in 1910, Safety-First was the creative effort of claim agent Ralph Richards. Since most workers died as a result of minor accidents, he proposed a commonsense program that advocated limiting carelessness to reduce casualties. Richards created the motto, "It is better to cause a delay than an accident." The slogan was genius, implying that safety was the most important part of the job.[43]

By all appearances, employers' top priority was their employees' health. Of course, this was not always the case. At first, the Safety-First program was difficult to implement, because many managers continued to focus on production numbers. But when the technical press began publicizing it, Safety-First appeared in most railroad health and safety programs. Ultimately, the broadening of industrial health was tied to economics. Safety-First corresponded with the FELA, making workplace injuries very expensive. FELA administered the conditions where an injured worker of any interstate railroad could receive compensation against his employer. It also made several key changes to the law, abolishing the rule established by *Farwell v. Boston & Worchester Railroad Corp.* (1842) that employers were not liable for a coworker's contributory negligence. Moreover, workers could now receive damages even if an injury resulted from personal negligence. Decades prior, the railroad industry took chances with long working hours and cheap equipment. Facing mounting financial obligations, it had to encourage safety after the 1910s.[44]

Workplace safety at the LA&SL reflected national trends. From 1905 to 1913 the workers on the railroads around the country experienced high accident rates and loosely followed safety procedures. But rising media scrutiny, traffic density, and collisions encouraged the railroad to install modern safety equipment. It invested in automatic signals and major extensions in block signaling, improving the ability to communicate and control trainmen. In 1916 the LA&SL spent more than $400,000 on a block-signal system. The improvements were very effective: Collisions decreased significantly, and by 1922 the railroad had blocked nearly 45 percent of the main track and installed 21 percent with automatic signals. To augment the new equipment, the LA&SL also announced the inauguration of its Safety-First campaign. General manager H. G. Nutt wrote a bulletin for employees: "We are each of us, in truth, our brother's keeper, and once convinced of the seriousness of the situation and the large field for intelligent effort, we believe that all will lend to the movement that mutual helpfulness and cordial cooperation which is so essential to the success of any undertaking."

He described the Safety-First campaign as removing "the causes of fatalities and accidents."[45] Nutt appointed a committee on safety and efficiency, which conducted studies on the cause and prevention of accidents, and provided important recommendations. In 1914 the LA&SL was submitting annual reports to the Federal Safety and Efficiency Bureau, revealing that employees were able to benefit from 50 percent of the recommendations. Although sixteen trespassers had died in 1914, there had been no passenger fatalities and only three worker deaths. More importantly, only thirty workers had incurred injuries on the job, a one-third reduction from the previous year. Although the Safety-First campaign could not remedy the problem with trespassers, the railroad had achieved real results within a year.[46]

After the UPRR acquired the railroad, it expanded the Safety-First campaign to comply with the newly instated ICC regulations. The campaign greatly enhanced conditions on the railroad. The company formed a safety department, headquartered in Los Angeles, that hosted monthly meetings. In 1924 alone it held 99 meetings, made 2,149 safety recommendations, and published 1,579 safety bulletins for workers. The UPRR also created signal tests to demonstrate efficiency, observing signals by trains and engine crews, telegraphers, and dispatchers. To improve medical care, it also built an emergency hospital in Los Angeles. Although it was used only for short-term trauma, the hospital temporarily housed employees with serious injuries and illnesses en route to a main hospital. Finally, the UPRR improved overall maintenance of the equipment and track, rehabilitating the main line and branches. It replaced bridges, installed firefighting equipment, rehabilitated decayed buildings, oiled tracks to settle the dust, and built safety railings. In southern Nevada, the company replaced zinc-treated redwood ties with creosoted ties, reducing general maintenance cost and bettering the track conditions; it also continuously improved its equipment, purchasing heavier steel and applying higher standards for material. It organized inspections, using research from Omaha on detecting broken metals, and investigated failures due to material or human error. Overall, the UPRR's acquisition of the LA&SL greatly improved worker health and safety. By modernizing and adhering to stricter safety procedures, the company reduced engine

failures, railway breakage, and personal injuries, improving conditions for both workers and the public.[47]

The UPRR promoted workplace safety within this occupational
health regime in several ways. First, it drew on the analogy that health
and safety resembled a baseball game: Players needed to follow the
rules of the game, and hiring a new employee was comparable to
choosing a player for the team. Someone with inferior sportsmanship
would not be appointed to the first baseman position, and a player
violating the rules of a game would be ejected. This was also the case
in hiring a skilled trainman or terminating an employee for inferior
work.[48]

Second, the UPRR involved employees in various contests that
promoted workplace safety. It submitted its units—the UPRR, Oregon
Short Line, Oregon–Washington Railroad and Navigation Company,
and the LA&SL—in the nationwide contests for the E. H. Harriman
Memorial Medal and National Safety Council Award. Throughout the
1920s the UPRR consistently won the E. H. Harriman Memorial Medal
for Class A American Steam Railroads, and the National Safety Council
recognized the LA&SL with an individual award. From 1923 to 1927 the
LA&SL also established a Group D safety record: only 3.49 accidents
per million man-hours worked, which was one of the lowest ever at-
tained in the classification.[49]

To create healthy competition, the UPRR also established a systemwide program to promote safety. Founded in 1921, the Safety Banner
Contest awarded the railroad line with the lowest number of injuries
to employees, passengers, and contractors, and the lowest amount of
time lost as the result of an accident. The contest was very popular
among workers and did a "great deal of good in stimulating interest
in the safety movement," according to the railroad's general solicitor,
A. S. Halsted. The program, however, was also slightly counterproduc-
tive. Since ICC classifications reported only injuries requiring more
than three days of lost work, competitive workers often returned to
the jobs before fully healing. Halsted called it a "serious problem" and
stressed that "fraud should not be condoned." During its first year
participating, the LA&SL won second place, with 4,998 injuries, nar-
rowly losing to the main UPRR line. In 1936 workers had also begun

participating in a systemwide Safety Emblem Contest with awards for individuals with no operating accidents for that year.[50]

Overall, the various safety contests worked well to promote health and safety in the railroad industry. The ARA calculated that in 1923 there were 1,866 fatalities and 148,146 injuries nationally among railroad workers. In 1929 the numbers had dropped to 606 fatalities and 28,706 injuries. But by the 1930s, the National Safety Council declared the safety movement had "passed the 'rah rah' stage" and needed redirection. Since most workers did not want to get hurt, it suggested that programs actually teach safety procedures rather than focusing on enthusiasm for accident prevention. The UPRR countered that its program was not based on enthusiasm: the program actively promoted worker safety. Indeed, the company was right. After decades of slaughter, the American railroad industry as a whole had become one of the safest industries in the nation.[51]

Besides instituting safety programs, the railroad established a community designed to reinforce productivity and create a sense of community. When founding Las Vegas, Clark promised to encourage and foster its development. In doing so, he created a unique company town. Most company towns controlled every aspect of their employees' lives, furnishing rented housing, establishing curfews and strict rules, and issuing scrip, as in the copper and coal-mining towns of White Pine County, Nevada or West Virginia and Pennsylvania. While Las Vegas did not use scrip, the railroad was behind every other feature as the town's major employer and builder. The LA&SL's vision was like a master-planned community, offering a railroad station and repair shops, ice houses, a meeting hall, a public school, an opera house, social and fraternal organizations, and churches. Under its subsidiary the LVL&W, the company carved the Las Vegas townsite of the 1,800-acre Stewart Ranch, organizing it into forty five-by-six blocks with 1,200 lots separated by twenty-foot alleys.[52]

Each block was specified by a number with specific rules for development written into the land deeds. On only two blocks, 16 and 17, were shops allowed to sell alcohol; most deeds had a temperance clause that prohibited the sale of liquor. After the two-day action for commercial and residential lots, Clark predicted, "In a year from now we shall have churches and schools, and the tents of settlement will have given way to substantial buildings for business purposes and places of permanent abode."[53]

With a population of only a thousand until a decade later, Las Vegas materialized as a typical small town that reinforced the occupational health regime. Local businessmen invested in development projects, banding together to create a safe, healthy, and profitable community. In June 1905 a gasoline stove fire at the Chop House Bill's restaurant spread to three adjacent buildings, inspiring local business owners to hold a fundraiser to found a volunteer fire brigade. A sanitary committee promoted public health, successfully lobbying the railroad to back a bond issue that built mains and ten septic tanks to help eliminate cesspools and toilet holes. In 1906 local businessmen also opened an electric company, the Consolidated Power and Telephone Company, ending the dangerous practice of lighting the town with gas lamps. The LVL&W also took development initiative, paving Fremont Street and oiling secondary streets to reduce dust, and building a network of redwood pipes to supply the steam engines with water. The water lines also protected the town from fire, with several hydrants installed throughout the town. Still, poor water pressure was a persistent problem. When several fires erupted in 1919, the pressure was "of little, if any value in controlling the fires," according to Walter Bracken, head agent of the LVL&W. In 1924 the LVL&W provided additional material and labor to install nineteen additional fire hydrants to expand fire protection in the town. The railroad also helped found a centralized government in southern Nevada, influencing the creation of Clark County in 1909, with Las Vegas as the county seat.[54]

A key aspect of the company town was to provide comfortable, clean employee housing, but there was a catch. In 1912 the railroad had determined that homeowners created better workers than free housing recipients, so it designed a system where employees could apply for mortgages based on their salaries. According to general manager H. G. Nutt, the strategy was designed to attract "a more desirable class of men" to their workforce.[55] In an area known as Railroad Row, the company reserved blocks along South Second, South Third, and South Fourth Streets. Bracken called it the "most attractive [place to live] in

Las Vegas." The railroad planned on erecting 120 cottages from 1909 to 1912, but ended up building only sixty-four. In each case, the LVL&W initially rented out the house, after which the employee applied for a loan to purchase. The system afforded the company "a very handsome profit," according to Bracken. More-privileged employees could plan their own residences. In 1914 Dr. Hal Hewetson bought several lots in Block 29. After drawing up a blueprint, the LVL&W Company provided materials and labor to build the structure for $2,600. At completion, Hewetson entered a contract of lease for sixty months with privilege to purchase at the end of that period.[56]

Clark's company town went according to plan except for one major problem: the railroad could not limit liquor sales to only Blocks 16 and 17 due to a provision allowing any business with a hotel room to sell alcohol. Consequently, hotels and liquor stores along Fremont Street and elsewhere took advantage of the opportunity. The business district became a destination that countered the railroad's goals of promoting worker health and, above all, productivity. After work, employees flocked to the Fremont saloons to gamble, often staying there all night. Exhausted and fatigued, they performed poorly on the job the next day, and workplace intoxication became a regular problem. Bracken called the gambling craze "or curse" more dangerous than the "social evil or run shops" to the railroad, citing that output suffered because of "loss of sleep resulting from [the workers'] rest period being spent at the gaming table."[57]

The Queen of Block 16 was the Arizona Club, an elite saloon and gambling hall. Neighboring businesses were not as respectable. While most concentrated on liquor and gambling, the Star Saloon, Double O, and Arcade included back rooms for prostitutes. Eventually, most Fremont Street establishments offered prostitution, with the area emerging as one of the most infamous red-light destinations in the West. Sam Gay, a bouncer at the Arizona Club, and later, a deputy for Lincoln County, recalled Fremont Street's early years: "From 1905–1910, Las Vegas was a rough and tumble western town. Five men dead for breakfast one Sunday morning and ten men wounded."[58]

After Clark sold his interest to the UPRR in May 1920, the transfer of power put the town into a predicament.[59] The new leadership, located in Omaha and New York, was less paternalistic and more concerned with profits. The UPRR immediately fired sixty repair shop employees, and by the summer of 1922, a strike was inevitable. Local workers supported a nationwide strike, effectively stopping most train lines. Violence flared in Las Vegas when strikebreakers arrived to town. Pickets gathered to "intimidate" and "put fear" in strikebreakers, according to one witness. The railroad tried to fix the situation, filing a restraining order against picketing interference, and separating strikebreakers from strikers in the rooming houses. The federal court also served a temporary injunction. Regardless, strikers continued to harass strikebreakers. Nightly shootings occurred and a trainmaster was assaulted, tarred, and feathered. The assailants were identified, but they fled town before being formally charged. The wife of a strikebreaker was also assaulted by four women. The women beat her with their "hands, sticks, bottles, or whatever was available" as their husbands cheered them on.[60]

With the trains stopped, the local economy took a significant blow. The UPRR punished the town after the strike, moving its repair yards to Caliente and costing Las Vegas more than three hundred jobs. The town soon recovered, though, with the economy remaining fairly strong throughout the 1920s. The strike proved that the UPRR needed to establish authority in Las Vegas, but Fremont Street inhibited its ability to do so. In the 1920s the eight-hour workday was practically universal in the railroad industry, increasing the amount of workers' leisure time. The UPRR quickly noticed the danger of leisure in Las Vegas. With Prohibition, the law abolished casino gambling, but speakeasies masqueraded as clubs. To counter the problem, the UPRR decided to develop a "broader and more wholesome relationship," determining that Fremont Street fostered poor work ethic and "dissatisfaction and unrest of the masses." It founded social welfare clubs that instilled "a sincere appreciation of the employees' obligation" to perform "faithful and loyal service to their daily work." The clubs offered sporting teams and entertainment features that encouraged healthy social relationships to rival the "demoralizing influence" of Fremont. Still, it did little good, and most workers continued enjoying the Las Vegas night life.[61]

While the industrial health program and community were important contributions to the occupational health regime, the central
component was the establishment of medical resources under the direction of the two physicians, Hal Hewetson and Roy Martin. Arriving
in October 1904, Hewetson opened Las Vegas's first hospital, at first
only a tent near Fremont Street. He was an accomplished physician:
he graduated from the University of Pennsylvania's medical school
with honors, and organized a chair of pathology and bacteriology at
the University of Omaha. However, during his tenure teaching he contracted tuberculosis and moved to the West to treat the disease. The
desert climate healed him, and in 1901 he assumed a full-time position with the UPRR, joining the LA&SL in 1903. Hewetson stayed in Las
Vegas until his death in 1930.[62]

Unlike Hewetson, the railroad did not recruit Roy Martin. Martin was a thirty-two-year-old entrepreneur who enjoyed a moderate
streak of luck selling real estate in Oklahoma. Real estate, however,
was a summer job. Martin was a physician, earning his medical degree
in 1903 from the University Medical College in Kansas City, Missouri.
Intrigued by the American West and its financial potential, he heard
about the Goldfield boom and decided to try his luck at mining, settling on the Bullfrog Mining District in Rhyolite, Nevada. Martin had
a short layover in Las Vegas and locals informed him that Bullfrog was
a has-been district. But the news did not discourage Martin. He met
a disillusioned physician who offered to sell him a medical practice
for $10, the cost of a railroad ticket to Los Angeles. Since Martin did
not have the money, he challenged the fastest sprinter in town to a
foot race. He won the race, bought the practice, and remained in Las
Vegas for thirty-eight years. Martin became the chief surgeon for the
Las Vegas and Tonopah Railroad to augment his income as a local physician, holding the position until the railroad closed in 1919.[63]

The two physicians were important assets to a region without a
medical infrastructure. In fact, the state lagged as a whole. In Governor John Sparks's annual address to the legislature of 1907, he stressed
the importance of the railroad industry to Nevada. But he also knew
it involved risk, remarking that it took "nerve [and a] great deal of
money [to construct a railroad] under prevailing conditions" in the

state. Nevada stretched for "hundreds of miles or more before an object of uncertainty can be reached at the other end." The greatest concern of the LA&SL was the lack of medical facilities in southern Nevada, a common theme among carriers in the American West. There were simply no clinics or hospitals to care for workers and passengers. As a result, the remote setting inspired the creation of a uniquely western form of employee-funded hospital care.[64]

Since its founding, the railroad industry was obligated to provide medical care to employees due to the hazardous nature of the work.[65] At first they offered casual programs, hiring a doctor or contracting with local physicians. But there were no formal contracts. By the late nineteenth century, liability concerns and labor conflict encouraged most companies to establish formal medical systems. As shown by historian Mark Aldrich, three distinct forms of medical organizations emerged in the 1880s reflecting the various geographic and economic conditions of each line. The first form was found in the East and Midwest. Most railroad companies made contractual arrangements with local physicians, but did not build company-run hospitals or require employees to contribute to health plans. The system also covered only work-related injuries, not illnesses. The second form, first instituted by the B&O and usually found in large carriers, was a mutual-benefit society. Following strike agitation in 1877 and an employee petition demanding benefits, the B&O Relief Association began offering optional health care and workmen's compensation to current employees, and mandatory participation to new ones. The program contracted out with existing hospitals to provide free medical care. All members were entitled to care for injuries and illnesses from several hundred doctors practicing on the B&O route, as well as relief payment for injuries. The program greatly reduced lawsuits because employees that sued the company fortified benefits. During World War I similar mutual-benefit societies covered nearly 30 percent of all railroad workers.[66]

The third form was found in the West. Due to low population density, western railroad carriers faced an almost complete lack of medical resources. They consequently developed employee-funded health organizations that provided medical services and built company-run hospitals. The carriers had two motives. While humanitarianism motivated this workplace advancement, the carriers also wanted to maintain a healthy labor force to protect their assets and increase profit potential. The Central Pacific Railroad was the first railroad to create a medical organization, patterning its health plan and hospital after the U.S. Marine Hospital Service. In the late 1860s it employed a salaried chief surgeon and division/district surgeons, and contracted with local talent for major emergencies. The company also established a temporary hospital in Sacramento and, by 1870, had built a permanent structure with 125-bed capacity. For health-care benefits, the Central Pacific charged employees $0.50 per month. The plan provided free medical care for ailments apart from preexisting conditions or venereal diseases. All workers were required to participate except for Chinese workers, who were explicitly excluded. Eventually, improvements in American hospital care prompted most large western railroads to emulate this model. In 1879 the Missouri Pacific and Texas Pacific Railroad set up identical services, and in 1882 the Northern Pacific Railroad established a hospital association and built facilities in Brainerd, Minnesota and Missoula, Montana. In 1883 the Denver and Rio Grande Railroad joined forces with the Colorado Fuel & Iron Company to build a hospital in Salida, Colorado. The next carriers to follow suit were the Santa Fe, Wabash, Milwaukee, Great Northern, and UPRR. During World War I hospital plans provided medical care to nearly 2 million railroad employees and employed 10 percent of American physicians on a full- or part-time basis.[67]

The desert landscape of Las Vegas posed similar problems for Senator Clark, with the added bonus of high heat and limited water. The town's location forced the establishment of a medical infrastructure in his company town, a move that was entirely voluntary; the NIC did not require industries to furnish medical care and hospitals until 1917. The founding of the railroad in Las Vegas also antedated the advent of workmen's compensation for interstate railroad employees. Clark's mining company helped fund a miner's hospital in Butte, Montana, without a legal mandate. Even before the town site auction, the LA&SL had established rudimentary first aid services. Hewetson arrived in 1904, setting up a medical tent with four cots in the railroad yard. When the railroad completed a permanent structure in 1905, it officially established a medical department for "the care of sick and injured employees, but without gain or profit." For employment consideration, workers contributed each month to a health fund to receive medical benefits. In 1925 the payroll deduction was $0.75 per month. In the mid-1940s it was $3 per month. The workers also signed a release that discharged the company "of all liability of every character on account of any act or omission [connected to any] hospital, physician, surgeon, nurse, or any employee connected." The monthly contributions often did not meet expenses, and management provided additional funds to ensure continued function.[68]

Practicing medicine in early Las Vegas was "pretty primitive" according to Dr. John Fuller, a surgeon practicing in town from 1910 to 1917. Hewetson and Martin rarely performed surgeries because they had limited medical supplies and the desert heat made it difficult to properly monitor a patient's body temperature. The standard procedure was to stabilize and send patients to Los Angeles. During dire emergencies, the physicians carried out surgeries at 4:00 A.M. in operating rooms located in the back of the hospital, under shady trees, and with the windows open. Hewetson usually treated only railroad workers and whites, while Martin's practice was less discriminatory, making house calls in Las Vegas and driving to Mesquite, Moapa, Overton, and Death Valley. He also cared for minorities, traveling on horseback to visit the Paiute Indian Reservation, and visiting Mexican railroaders and U.S. Gypsum workers in Arden. The trips could be "wild," according to his daughter Mazie Martin Jones, because most of the injuries he treated were gunshot and knife wounds.[69]

For the first few years, the railroad workers maintained remarkably good health. There were no epidemics of smallpox, diphtheria, typhoid, or scarlet fever. Hewetson remained the only LA&SL physician until Fuller arrived. On the night of Fuller's arrival, the little town amazed him. He described a vibrant full moon and a desert that seemed to "pulsate with violet light glowing against the surrounding mountains." From Fremont Street, Fuller could see Block 16, the red-light district, which he referred to as "the girls down the line." "If a townsman was down on his luck," he recalled, "[the prostitutes] were always ready to pass the hat to help them out." On one occasion, Fuller picked up a woman hitchhiker out of "desert courtesy," even though he "knew what she was." When the doctor reached the outskirts of town, the woman "insisted on getting out…because it would hurt [his] reputation to be seen in her company."[70]

In 1910 Fuller recalled that there were no trained nurses, only untrained male attendants, and the medical facilities. The hospital did not have x-ray, laboratory, or decent surgery facilities. Hewetson eventually rented a building to use as a hospital for $40 per month to hospitalize patients. Still, he sent the most severe cases to Los Angeles or Salt Lake City. The doctors would accompany patients in the hope of keeping them alive until they reached the city. In one case, a worker's eye had been knocked out of the socket, and Hewetson continued to treat him throughout his transfer to Los Angeles. Los Angeles surgeons removed the worker's eye, relieving a constant hemorrhage. Since the worker made no claim for workmen's compensation, the LA&SL allowed him to draw his salary as usual, and met all railroad and hospital expenses.[71]

Since southern Nevada had limited medical resources, the LA&SL had a predicament with regard to providing health care. At the time, the norm among employers was to treat employees only, and not their families. But since Las Vegas was in such a remote location, the carrier made an exception, allowing families access to the doctors and hospital that they paid for out of pocket. Fuller rode his bicycle around town to make house calls and deliver babies. Roy Martin also opened the town's first private hospital, the Las Vegas Hospital, to better accommodate family members. The *Las Vegas Age* described the hospital as modest, but said it "met the requirements of the community, the railroad, and surrounding mining camps." In 1920 the Las Vegas Hospital upgraded its technology, installing an x-ray machine similar to the equipment of any metropolitan hospital. Doctors practicing in both hospitals regularly worked together, traveling to the various railroad sites to treat workers for heat exhaustion or other injuries.[72] Once, Fuller went to Moapa to treat railroad workers "overcome with heat." He found one man dead and another barely breathing, although "rigor mortis had already set in." The doctor was not surprised both had died, given the scorching desert heat.[73]

As an enhancement to this medical care, several world-class physicians also moved to Las Vegas to get a divorce. Nevada's famously liberal divorce laws required only a six months' residency. Beginning in 1906, several well-publicized cases in Reno revealed the state's lenience on the issue. The law permitted divorces on vague grounds such as mental cruelty. Entrepreneurs quickly capitalized on the industry, opening dude ranches or hotels designated for at least one of the parties in a marriage to establish residency and obtain a hassle-free divorce. The marriage industry flourished as well because Nevada did not require a waiting period or medical examinations. While Reno remained the divorce and marriage center, Las Vegas also capitalized on the industry. In 1918 Dr. Silas Lewis, a prominent New York surgeon, arrived in Las Vegas. Described as a "middle aged, distinguished looking man wearing a Van Dyke beard" by the *Las Vegas Age,* he brought along his two children and a young nurse, and became associated with the Las Vegas Hospital. Local residents were flattered that a prominent physician chose to practice in Las Vegas, especially since World War I had created a scarcity of doctors and nurses. Lewis was ultimately instrumental in helping the town fight the Spanish flu. Nonetheless, he remained in Las Vegas for only six months; the doctor obtained a divorce from his wife, scandalously married his young nurse, and left town to establish a practice in Beverly Hills.[74]

During the 1920s, rumors of a proposed dam project nearby enticed physicians to move to Las Vegas, further expanding the medical infrastructure. Martin hired Dr. Forest Mildren, and bought the Palace Hotel to convert the building into a new hospital. The new Las Vegas Hospital opened in 1920, complete with eight rooms and operating facilities. Hewetson also convinced the LA&SL to build a new hospital for workers. The doctor recognized that Las Vegas needed to modernize and reflect medical standards in Los Angeles. He proposed that for an extra $21 per week, an updated facility could provide modern first aid and surgical care to employees. In the end, it would be a minimal cost to the company to improve their care. The railroad complied and remodeled a former rooming house. The new Hewetson Hospital had fourteen beds, a nursery, and a separate wing for indigents, and Hewetson lived on the ground floor of the building. Both the Las Vegas

Hospital and Hewetson Hospital adequately served the Las Vegas community until Hoover Dam construction began in 1931, demanding larger facilities.[75]

A final, important aspect of the occupational health regime that formed around the LA&SL was a legal contingent. At the turn of the century, personal injury suits were gaining momentum, a marked difference from the previous century. Moreover, personal injury suits rarely occurred in remote industrial areas because most attorneys typically lived in urban settings. After the Civil War, however, the number of lawyers skyrocketed, especially among first- and second-generation immigrants. The legal profession expanded nearly 150 percent from 1870 to 1900. From 1890 to 1900, the number of native-born lawyers with immigrant parents also grew 80 percent. The lawyers created a new group of professionals associated with the working class. As their numbers grew, competition inspired a new type of business. The lawyers lacked traditional connections, so they solicited injured workers to file personal injury claims. Several such lawyers created a system of runners who provided case leads, paying off both workers and policemen. Others committed fraud, fabricating claims and accepting questionable settlements under the table. Corporate defenders also developed comparable unethical strategies, exploiting overlapping jurisdiction rules of the federal and state courts. Some railroad companies paid employees not to testify on a coworker's behalf, and insurance agents approached injured workers to sign off on settlements. Defense attorneys also struck corrupt bargains with the plaintiffs' counsel. By the twentieth century, personal injury litigation had developed a nasty reputation. Elon R. Brown, a New York politician and lawyer, observed in 1908 that personal injury litigation was "marked by a lower tone of professional ethics of the Bar," and contributed to the opinion that litigation, lawyers, and judges were "speculative" and "haphazard." Likewise, an LA&SL official referred to lawyers as "sharks" that got hold of workers.[76]

In response to rising personal injuries costs, the LA&SL established a legal department in 1913, headed by attorney Frank R. McNamee. The son of Irish immigrants, McNamee moved from the mining boomtown Eureka, Nevada, in 1883 and was admitted to the Nevada Bar in 1895. He served as district attorney for Lincoln County from 1896 to 1903, practicing in both Delmar and Caliente. His son, Leo, passed the Nevada Bar and was elected district attorney of Lincoln County in 1910, opening a law office in Pioche. When Las Vegas was named the Clark County seat over Searchlight in 1909, father and son founded McNamee & McNamee, opening offices in Los Angeles in 1912 and Las Vegas in 1913. In 1915 the railroad appointed Frank as general attorney because of his experience with Nevada law, and Leo as assistant general attorney. The McNamees became a staple of the Las Vegas legal community, retained by the LA&SL and later, Six Companies, Inc., the builders of Hoover Dam. After the UPRR assumed control of the railroad, the two worked alongside the company's legal team until 1946. McNamee & McNamee remained open in Las Vegas until 1978 and spanned four generations.[77]

The LA&SL's legal department typically fought claims rather than settle, basing its cases on the general principles of American employers' liability law. In 1910 journalist John Gitterman wrote about the dangers of working in the railroad industry, revealing that fatalities were a part of daily operations and the American court system mishandled accident litigation. Most importantly, he exposed the law of American employers' liability. If a person objected to working in hazardous conditions, he or she had the privilege of quitting. A worker was "not a slave" and could not "be compelled under his broiler, or have his head scraped off while attempting to couple cars."[78]

American employers' liability was therefore based on the assumption of risk, as the Latin phrase "volenti non fit injuria," puts it: "There is no injury to one who consents." An 1895 tort law handbook explained, "No action can be maintained for damages resulting from conduct suffered by consent."[79] The McNamees based their cases on this doctrine. In 1917 a sixteen-year-old worker injured his eye while grinding an emery wheel, and doctors were forced to remove it. Frank McNamee determined that the case would be based on two important details. One, whether the minor was warned of the danger, and two, if the railroad had offered him safety goggles. McNamee believed that the assumption of risk was "dependent upon the servant's knowledge," but could be negated since the worker was a minor and did not fully comprehend the dangers of employment. In the end, the court determined that the employee had assumed all risks at employment and could not recover damages. He concluded the verdict was just because the "disobedience of rules or orders [do not] merit negligence" on the employers' fault.[80]

Personal injury suits rarely provided compensation, but workers had other options. Prior to 1913, the LA&SL offered life and disability insurance through the National Causality Company. After the creation of the NIC in 1913, the company accepted the Nevada Industrial Insurance Act and allowed employees to purchase additional coverage with Pacific Mutual Life Insurance Company.[81]

If an employer rejected the NIC provisions, the courts automatically assumed that all workplace injuries were caused by employer negligence. Leo McNamee consequently advised that it was "almost compulsory" for Nevada industries to accept the provisions.[82] However, when the UPRR assumed control, it rejected the NIC since it was a larger, nationally run carrier. In 1917 the company established its own plan, covering life, permanent disability, accident, and health insurance, offering it to employees at a "very low cost [and] without medical examination," providing workers were under sixty years of age and had not lost any time due to illness. The UPRR payroll deducted the cost, $0.60 per month. Employees could purchase additional policies from several private insurance carriers.[83]

The final option for LA&SL workers was the FELA, which awarded damages to injured employees engaged in interstate commerce. FELA had several drawbacks, though. Workers could collect compensation only if their injuries occurred while they engaged in commerce between states, not commerce within one state. It therefore raised legal questions regarding the boundaries of interstate and intrastate commerce. From 1908 to 1934, the Supreme Court decided forty-five cases on whether an injury occurred within interstate or intrastate lines. The decisions created contradictory legal precedents. Pumping water on an interstate train was determined to be interstate commerce, but loading coal on the same train was considered to be intrastate commerce. A nighttime watchman of an interstate train was engaged in interstate commerce. If he received an injury while pursuing stolen goods from the train, it was intrastate commerce. FELA ultimately created a lot of confusion. Distinguishing between interstate and intrastate commerce for statutory or constitutional purposes was pointless, and many attorneys determined it an unworkable concept.[84]

The LA&SL had set protocol after each workplace-related accident. The Legal Department immediately prepared to contest any form of compensation. Employees filed with the NIC if the injury occurred intrastate or with FELA if interstate. To be safe, most employees filed under both. After each filing, Frank and Leo McNamee determined "whether or not the employer and employee were engaged in interstate commerce at the time of the injury." Because the UPRR had rejected the NIC, FELA was a much cheaper option. After one repairman slipped on loose gravel at a railroad quarry, the District Court held the rock was intended to repair roadbeds in Nevada. Therefore, he had engaged in intrastate commerce. This was not good for the UPRR; the state automatically assumed that employers were negligent, citing "the burden of proof…upon the employer to rebut the resumption of negligence."[85] The McNamees did not have a case. Their only option was to argue that the injury occurred interstate and the repairman assumed the risk of the job. The UPRR's chief attorney, Fred E. Pettit Jr., advised them to settle because a judgment could be far more expensive. This pattern was typical in workmen's compensation cases in Nevada. According to Frank McNamee, employers were "deprived of all ordinary defenses on account of not accepting the Compensation Act" under state law. Unless the company exercised "great and extraordinary care" to prevent an injury, it was guilty of even slight negligence.[86]

In the late 1920s the American railroad industry had made significant strides to protect its workforce, but the industrial health movement was at a crossroads. Federal agencies such as the Public Health Service enjoyed broad power to oversee workplaces during World War I, but its powers shifted to state and local agencies during the conservative 1920s. The enforcement of workmen's compensation laws also proved difficult. The federal government supported business development during the 1920s thanks to the friendly relationship between the various Republican administrations and big business. Employers held off reformers by lobbying sympathetic lawmakers, actively contesting suits in court, and hiring physicians to question whether workers' diseases could be traced to the workplace rather than to the neighborhood and home. In most cases, judges ruled in favor of management, a trend that discouraged personal injury litigation. Still, legal pressures forced many big employers to invest in safety and fund academic research at industrial hygiene departments at Harvard, Yale, Johns Hopkins, Columbia, and the University of Pennsylvania. The laboratories provided expertise to companies as neutral and apolitical mediators in legal disagreements, depoliticizing workplace safety and giving shape to modern regulatory practices.[87]

In the late 1920s the occupational health regime had waned as the Las Vegas medical infrastructure struggled to provide for the growing community. Hewetson retired, and the railroad contracted health care out to Dr. Ferdinand Ferguson and Dr. R. D. Balcom, transferring over the Hewetson Hospital.[88]

Ferguson and Balcom also provided insurance to families, organizing the Guaranteed Medical Service, Inc., a plan that offered medical, surgical, and dental care at a yearly cost. Even so, the situation continued to worsen for local medicine. After experiencing financial woes, Martin closed the Las Vegas Hospital. The closing could not have come at a worse time. The announcement that a dam would be built thirty miles away prompted a sudden immigration, spiking the population tenfold. After years of relative success, the existing occupational health regime could not accommodate the new residents. Moreover, under the new leadership of the UPRR, the LA&SL had gradually relinquished its paternalistic responsibility to Las Vegas. To manage its public health, the town turned to the understaffed and underfinanced county health department. In 1930 Dr. J. C. Landenberger, chief surgeon of the UPRR, visited Las Vegas, calling it "probably the most unsanitary in the country" and if not the worst, "a decidedly close race for honors." The *Evening Review-Journal* agreed, reporting that health violations existing downtown "would not be permitted in no other city in the United States" and declaring Las Vegas was "courting disaster to the health of the community."[89]

The situation prompted action from two factions of the Las Vegas community. In 1931 Martin, Ferguson, and Balcom formed the Las Vegas

Hospital Association. The doctors pulled together their resources and constructed a two-story hospital with thirty-five beds, a laboratory, maternity ward, x-ray machine, five treatment rooms, and an operating room with a tilting table and lighting system. Dr. John R. McDaniel and Dr. Clare W. Woodbury later joined the Las Vegas Hospital Association and Dr. Forest Mildren, feeling mistreated by his associates, severed professional ties and opened the Mildren Clinic.[90]

In the same year a local chapter of the American Legion, a congressionally chartered veteran organization, launched a campaign to fund a hospital for the treatment of Nevada's veterans. Only nine states did not have a Veterans Bureau Hospital in 1931. All but four had federally funded medical institutions, such as naval hospitals or services provided by the Public Health Service. Three of the remaining four—South Carolina, Vermont, and Delaware—contracted with private hospitals to care for disabled veterans. Nevada had the dubious distinction of being the only state in the nation with no medical resources for veterans.

On January 23, 1931, the American Legion presented its case to the Subcommittee on World War Veterans in Washington, DC, stressing the need for hospital services based on an impending reclamation project in the region. In 1928 Congress passed the Swing–Johnson Bill, authorizing the construction of a dam at Black Canyon. In early 1931 southern Nevada's veteran population ranged between 5,400 and 7,000 men, and the legion anticipated that the Boulder Dam situation would increase this number.[91] Their concern had merit, as Swing–Johnson authorized the U.S. Employment Service to give employment preference to veterans who served in World War I, the Spanish-American War, and the Philippine-American War. Since Las Vegas did not have the medical resources to accommodate them all, the construction of a Veterans Bureau Hospital seemed like the logical solution.[92]

The campaign worked, and Congress allocated $625,000 to the state of Nevada for a veterans' hospital. Location requirements included at least thirty acres for a building site, and close proximity to city water, sewerage, power, and electricity. Reno, Ely, and Las Vegas each built its case for the hospital. The Las Vegas Chamber of Commerce appointed a committee to help the American Legion, and solicited the UPRR for help, requesting a land donation that would be "repaid from a financial as well as moral standpoint." The UPRR accepted, authorizing the LVL&W to donate or require a minimal charge for more than twenty acres north of the railroad yard.[93]

The American Legion prepared its case contingent on Las Vegas being the most practical location in Nevada. It had an existing railroad line and water supply, and would have access to cheap power after Hoover Dam was completed. From a need standpoint, the region also had no veteran facilities, and at least fifteen hundred veterans lived in southern Nevada, western Arizona, and western Utah. During the construction of the dam, the committee forecasted a sharp increase in this number, with a veteran workforce of 50 percent or higher.[94]

Most importantly, the railroad's medical infrastructure had outgrown its capacity to serve the health needs of the community. The American Legion described Las Vegas medicine as "extremely inadequate" and "entirely wanting." While the personalized care of Hal Hewetson and Roy Martin had been highly regarded, the hospitals never fully modernized, and were "completely reliant on southern California," and also were "crowded beyond capacity." The group cited a case in which it took forty-five days for a local veteran to get a hospital bed. Since Southern California's veterans' hospital was full, he settled on traveling to Wyoming. This was a common scenario. The American Legion called the inadequate hospital situation in the American Southwest "notorious."[95]

One of the most interesting aspects of the case is that the American Legion included letters of support from local physicians, revealing how medical professionals during the early 1930s perceived the desert and its effect on human health. After practicing in Las Vegas for nearly three decades, Roy Martin wrote, "I am somewhat of an authority on conditions that affect the health of the people residing here. To say 'the climate is healthy' is entirely inadequate. It is much more than that." Ferdinand Ferguson noted that Clark County's death rate was "one-half" the national average, that infections were "very rare" and mortality "practically negligible," and that his patients enjoyed outdoor life "at all times of the year." R. D. Balcom listed the climate as "conducive to the cure of tuberculosis," and Forest Mildren attested it was better suited for a tuberculosis sanitarian than Arizona and New Mexico. John McDaniel considered the locale great for nephritis, asthmatics, and sinus conditions. There was also an absence of fog, smoke and dust in the air, and a high percentage of sunshine, which accelerated patient recovery time. These observations were in stark contrast to how people would come to view the environment only a few years later, considering the Las Vegas area during dam construction more like a hostile wasteland that killed rather than healed. Perhaps because he was new to town, interim railroad doctor Dr. H. C. Vander Meulen departed from the climate argument, writing that southern Nevada needed a hospital because of the dam. He predicted that Las Vegas would become a "resort and tourist center [and experience] industrial growth," and forecasted the hazards confronting workers at the dam: "Already we are handicapped in caring for disabled veterans and this is going to increase."[96]

Las Vegas lost the bid to Reno, and the city did not receive a veterans' health-care system until 1972, and a hospital until 2012. The episode contributed to a North–South split in the Nevadan medical community, a common theme throughout the twentieth century.[97]

While it is impossible to determine if a veterans' hospital would have saved lives at Hoover Dam, one thing was clear: the existing occupational health regime in Las Vegas could not support the health and safety of dam workers. Under these conditions, the Boulder Canyon Project began.

## NOTES

1. Aldrich, *Safety-First*, xx.

2. See Aldrich, *Death Rode the Rails: American Railroad Accidents and Safety, 1828–1965* (Baltimore: Johns Hopkins University Press, 2006), 10, 15; Great Britain Board of Trade, *General Report on Accidents* (London, various years) in Aldrich, *Death Rode the Rails*; Aldrich, "The Peril of the Broken Rail: The Carriers, the Steel Companies, and Rail Technology, 1900–1945," *Technology and Culture* 40, no. 2 (1999): 263–91. For a history of the B&O, see James Dilts, *The Great Road: The Building of Baltimore and Ohio, the Nation's First Railroad, 1828–1853* (Stanford, CA: Stanford University Press, 1993). See also Thomas Hughes, "Evolution of Large Technological Systems," in *The Social Construction of Technological Systems*, eds. Wiebe Bijker, Thomas P. Hughes, and Trevor Pinch (Cambridge, MA: MIT Press, 1987), 51–83; Robert Shaw, *Down Brakes: A History of Railroad Accidents, Safety Precautions, and Operating Practices in the United States of America* (London: Macmillan, 1961); Steven Usselman, "Air Brakes for Freight Trains: Technological Innovation in the American Railroad Industry, 1869–1900," *Business History Review* 58

(1984): 30–50; John White, *The American Railroad Freight Car* (Baltimore: Johns Hopkins University Press, 1993) for a history of health and safety in the railroad industry.

3. Maury Klein, *Union Pacific: Birth of a Railroad, 1862–1893* (New York: Double-day & Company, 1987) (incl. "Fully 90%," 503).

4. Railroad engineer Nicholas Farwell's right hand was crushed on the job due to a switchman's carelessness. The court held that a worker could not recover compensation from his employer for injuries caused by a coworker. Essentially, the injured worker was in as good of a position as his employer to monitor the work of his peer. The ruling held that allowing Farwell to recover damages would create a moral hazard in the workplace. See Farwell v. Boston & Worcester R.R. Corp.; Christopher L. Tomlins, "A Mysterious Power: Industrial Accidents and the Legal Construction of Employment Relations in Massachusetts, 1800–1850," *Law and History Review* 6, no. 2 (Fall 1988).

5. Aldrich, *Safety-First*, 31; Witt, "The Federal Employers' Liability Act," in *Major Acts of Congress*, ed. Brian K. Landsberg (New York: Macmillan, 2003) (incl. "'unholy trinity,'" n.p.).

6. Maury Klein, *Union Pacific: The Rebirth, 1894–1969* (New York: Doubleday 1989), 503.

7. For a history of George Westinghouse's inventions regarding air and water brakes, see Quentin R. Skrabec Jr., *George Westinghouse: Gentle Genius* (New York: Algora, 2006). See also John H. White Jr., "America's Most Noteworthy Railroaders," *Railroad History* 154 (Spring 1986): 9–15, for an overview of notable technological inventions.

8. Prior to the establishment of the ICC, state governments were not completely inactive. In the 1850s the New York State Railroad Commission began publishing casualty lists. For information about the founding of the ICC, see Interstate Commerce Act, 24 Stat. 379 (1887). See also Aldrich, *Safety-First*, 9; and Richard D. Stone, *The Interstate Commerce Commission and the Railroad Industry* (New York: Praeger, 1991).

9. Federal Safety Appliance Act, 27 Stat. 531 (1893); Aldrich, *Safety-First*, 9.

10. For scholarship on early Las Vegas history, see Eugene P. Moehring and Michael S. Green, *Las Vegas: A Centennial History* (Reno: University of Nevada Press, 2005), 1–79; Stanley Paher, *Las Vegas, As it Began—As It Grew* (Las Vegas: Nevada Publications, 1971); Ralph Roske, *Las Vegas, NV: A Desert Paradise* (Tusla, OK: Continental Heritage, 1986).

11. See William Managam, *The Clarks: An American Phenomenon* (New York: Silver Bow Press, 1941); Michael P. Malone, "Midas of the West: The Incredible Career of William Andrews Clark," *Montana: The Magazine of Western History* 33, no. 4 (Autumn, 1983): 2–17, for scholarship on Senator William Clark. See also Twain, "Senator Clark of Montana (Monday, January 28, 1907)," in *Autobiography of Mark Twain*, Vol. 2: *The Complete and Authoritative Edition*, ed. Benjamin Griffin and Harriet E. Smith (Berkeley: University of California Press, 2013), 387–89, for Twain's opinion of Senator Clark (incl. "rotten a human," 388).

12. For a history of the LA&SL and the UPRR at the turn of the century, see John R. Signor, *The Los Angeles and Salt Lake Railroad Company* (San Marino, CA: Golden West Books, 1988); Klein, *Birth of a Railroad*; Klein, *The Rebirth*.

13. Signor, *Los Angeles and Salt Lake Railroad Company*, 28, 30, 38; Klein, *Rebirth*, 116; "Battle Royal Between Railroads," *Los Angeles Times* [hereafter *LA Times*], Apr. 10, 1901; "Talking Up Clark's Road," *LA Times*, May 2, 1903; "Clark First from the Lake," *LA Times*, Jan. 14, 1905; "First Train Through," *LA Times*, Feb. 13, 1905; "Salt Lake in

Two Months," *LA Times*, Feb. 23, 1905; "Earnings of Clark's Road," *New York Times*, Mar. 21, 1907.

14. Eugene P. Moehring, *Resort City in the Sunbelt, 1930–2000* (Reno: University of Nevada Press, 2000), 4–6; Signor, *Los Angeles and Salt Lake Railroad Company,* 441.

15. Separate from changes in technology was a dramatic change in the labor market. Labor turnover declined and there were fewer inexperienced employees. See Aldrich, *Death Rode the Rails*, 181–82; and "Railroad Slaughter," *Las Vegas Age,* Nov. 16, 1907.

16. Walker, *A Life's Review and Notes on the Development of Medicine in Nevada, From 1900 to 1944* (Reno: n.p., 1944) (incl. "The question arising," 28).

17. Part of the NIC's duties was to gather statistical data on industrial accidents in the state. See *Report of the Nevada Industrial Commission: Reviewing the Administration of the Nevada Industrial Insurance Act for the Period of Three Years—July 1, 1913 to June 30, 1916* (Carson City, NV: SPO, 1917), 40, 42, 44, 48–49, 60, 66–67; "Report of Inspector of Mines," *Appendix*, 26th Sess., Vol. 1 (Carson City, NV: SPO, 1913), 5–12; *Second Biennial Report from the Commissioner of Labor, 1917–1918* (Carson City, NV: SPO, 1919), 45.

18. See Joseph Melling, "The Risks of Working and the Risks of Not Working: Trade Unions, Employers, and Responses to the Risk of Occupational Illness in British Industry, 1890–1940s," Discussion Paper 12, Centre of Analysis of Risk and Regulation (CARR), London School of Economics and Political Science, London (2003).

19. Moehring and Green, *Las Vegas*, 34–36 (incl. "swarthy sons" and "Judge Brennan," 35); "Murder, Not an Accident—Jury," *LA Times*, Nov. 28, 1912 (incl. "from ear to ear").

20. Witt, "The Federal Employers' Liability Act."

21. Aldrich, *Death Rode the Rails*, 198.

22. "Traffic Blocked by Serious Washouts: Extensive Damage to Union Pacific Track Blocks Road for Five Days," *Las Vegas Age*, Jan. 7, 1922; "Train Leaps Off Bridge: Wreck in Nevada Due to Flood," *LA Times*, Aug. 6, 1929.

23. Signor, *Los Angeles and Salt Lake Railroad Company* (incl. "topple into" and "all they could do," 69).

24. Walter Bracken to W. C. Hussey, memorandum, July 14, 1926; "Verdict in the Matter of the Inquisition into the Deaths of Five Persons found in Tourist Pullman Car #1642," June 16, 1926; both in UPRR Collection, LVL&W Co., Walter Bracken Files, Claims for Damages and Personal Injury, Box 15, File R-14, University of Nevada, Las Vegas [hereafter UNLV] Special Collections [hereafter SC].

25. Walter Bracken to W. H. Comstock, memorandum, July 8, 1918, UPRR Collection, LVL&W Co., Walter Bracken Files, Claims for Damages and Personal Injury, Box 15, File R-14, UNLV SC; "Railroad Employee Is Killed by Train, *Las Vegas Age*, Jan. 12, 1918 (incl. "delivered to" and "two open").

26. "Two Are Killed: Falling Crane Crushes Out Lives of Two Salt Lake Railroad Employees at Washout Near Alton Station," *Las Vegas Age*, Mar. 30, 1907; "Death Results," *Las Vegas Age*, July 13, 1907; "Mixer Crushes, Whirls, Kills: Friends Learn of Death at Las Vegas, NV," *LA Times*, Oct. 19, 1909; "Divorce Suit and Tragedy: Murder in the Desert—Seventy Men of Salt Lake Railroad Construction Force Quit," *LA Times*, Mar. 22, 1904.

27. "Wreck Due to Carelessness: Gang of Workmen Rushed into a Death Trap," *LA Times*, Mar. 2, 1907; "Deadly Crash: Salt Lake Train at Washout Collides with Tie Car," *Las Vegas Age*, Mar. 2, 1907 (incl. "horribly mangled others" and "thorough investigation").

28. "Cut to Pieces under the Wheels," *Las Vegas Age*, Oct. 20, 1917 (incl. all quotes).

29. Barbara Young Welke, *Recasting American Liberty: Gender, Race, Law, and the Railroad Revolution, 1865–1920* (New York: Cambridge University Press, 2001), 47–48; Aldrich, *Death Rode the Rails*, 213; "Human Lives the Safeguard: Salt Lake Issues Remarkable Report Showing Scarcity of Fatalities," *LA Times*, Nov. 22, 1914 (incl. "menace").

30. Aldrich, *Death Rode the Rails*, 213–14; Ed. E. Bennett to W. H. Guild, Nov. 11, 1938; Walter Bracken to Ed. E. Bennett, memorandum, Sept. 18, 1940; both in UPRR Collection, LVL&W Co., Walter Bracken Files, Claims for Damages and Personal Injury, Box 15, File R-14, UNLV SC.

31. Guy Louis Rocha, "Regulating Public Heath in Nevada: The Pioneering Efforts of Dr. Simeon Lemuel Lee," *Nevada Historical Society Quarterly* 29 (Fall 1986): 203–7; Annie Blachley, *Pestilence, Politics, and Pizzazz: The Story of Public Health in Las Vegas* (Reno: Greasewood Press, 2002), 31; "Report of the State Board of Health," *Appendix*, 26th Sess., Vol. 3, 37.

32. "Report of the Board of Health," *Appendix*, 25th Sess., Vol. 1, 5–6, 8, 15.

33. Michaeleen Doucleff, "What's in a Flu Name? H's and N's Tell the Tale," *National Public Radio* (May 7, 2013); Emily Ann Collin, "Influenza D. Virus: Investigation of the Newly Proposed Influenza Genus" (PhD diss., South Dakota State University, Brookings, 2015).

34. George Dehner, *Influenza: A Century of Science and Public Health Response* (Pittsburgh, PA: University of Pittsburgh Press, 2013), 23–27.

35. Ibid., 55–56; John M. Barry, *The Great Influenza: The Story of the Deadliest Pandemic in History* (New York: Penguin Books, 2005), 238–39; "Report of the State Board of Health," *Appendix*, 29th Sess., Vol. 2 (Carson City, NV: SPO, 1919) (incl. "scarcely," 22).

36. "Report of the State Board of Health," 1919 (incl. "fear should" and "fear and worry," 23).

37. "Doctor Commissioned for Military Service," *Las Vegas Age*, July 21, 1917; "Dr. Hal Hewetson," Cahlan Collection, Box 24, Folder 99, Nevada State Museum Archives, Las Vegas (hereafter NSMA); Philip I. Earl, "Spanish Flu Bugged Nevada in the Early 1900s," *Reno Gazette-Journal*, May 14, 2000.

38. Memorandum to Employees Concerning Spanish Flu Precautions, 1919, UPRR Collection, UPRR Law Department, Employees General, Box 58, File 50, UNLV SC.

39. Earl, "Spanish Flu."

40. "Biennial Report of the State Board of Health," *Appendix*, 31st Sess., Vol. 2 (Carson City, NV: SPO, 1923), 7; Blachley, *Pestilence*, 20–22.

41. See Sellers, *Hazards of the Job*, 8–11; Melling, "Risks."

42. See Aldrich, *Death Rode the Rails*, 186, for further discussion on the history of railroad safety legislation.

43. "Safety Diplomas Are Given to 506 Men," *Chicago Commerce 18*, no. 1 (June 10, 1922), 14.

44. Witt, *Accidental Republic*, 67; Aldrich, *Death Rode the Rails*, 190–91; Welke, *Recasting American Liberty*, 35–37, 38, 41, 59, 225.

45. "Salt Lake to Protect Men: Conservation of Lives Is the Watchword," *LA Times*, Oct. 26, 1913 (incl. "We are each" and "the causes of").

46. "Block Signal on Salt Lake: Railroad Officials Announce Plans to Spend Large Sum for Safety," *LA Times*, May 19, 1916; "Human Lives the Safeguard: Salt Lake Issues Remarkable Report Showing Scarcity of Fatalities," *LA Times*, Nov. 22, 1914.

47. F. H. Knickerbocker to E. E. Calvin, June 19, 1926, UPRR Collection, Union Pacific Engineering and Industrial Development, Safety Matters, Box 82, Files 21-21, Vols. 1–9, UNLV SC.

48. The ARA, an industry trade group founded in 1892 to represent railroads across the United States, created the baseball analogy. See ARA, "Committee on Education Safety Program, Schedule of Activities," July 1926, UPRR Collection, Union Pacific Engineering and Industrial Development, Safety Matters, Box 82, Files 21-21, Vols. 1–9, UNLV SC.

49. F. H. Knickerbocker to E. E. Calvin, June 19, 1926; F. H. Knickerbocker to UPRR, Dec. 10, 1926; both in UPRR Collection, Union Pacific Engineering and Industrial Development, Safety Matters, Box 82, Files 21-21, Vols. 1–9, UNLV SC; "Rail Safety Prize Given Local Unit," *LA Times*, May 10, 1928; "Union Pacific Wins Contest: Salt Lake Union Trophy Arrives Here," *LA Times*, May 31, 1928.

50. Memorandum on Rules and Regulations Governing Safety Banner Contests Year 1927; E. E. Calvin to A. S. Halsted, Nov. 5, 1923; A. S. Halsted to E. E. Calvin, Nov. 13, 1923 (incl. "great deal" and "fraud should"); W. H. Comstock to All Employees, Mar. 7, 1924; "Committee on Statistics Casualties to Employees—Six Months Ended June 30, 1929," memorandum, Jan. 20, 1930; all at UPRR Collection, Union Pacific Engineering and Industrial Development, Safety Matters, Box 82, Files 21-21, Vols. 1–9, UNLV SC.

51. F. H. Knickerbocker to W. R. Armstrong, J. F. Long, R. L. Adamson, and W. R. Spettigue, June 25, 1930 (incl. "passed the"); R. L. Adamson to A. R. White, C. B. Reynolds, F. Nicholson, and J. F. Gorham, June 26, 1930; both at UPRR Collection, Union Pacific Engineering and Industrial Development, Safety Matters, Box 82, Files 21-21, Vols. 1–9, UNLV SC.

52. Moehring and Green, *Las Vegas*, 12-16.

53. Moehring, *Resort City*, 4 (incl. "In a year").

54. Walter Bracken to W. C. Frazier, May 24, 1913 (incl. "of little"); President of the Chamber of Commerce to W. H. Comstock, A. S. Halsted, W. R. Bracken, and J. Ross Clark, Aug. 13, 1919; City of Las Vegas to Walter Bracken, Sept. 11, 1919; Bill for the City of Las Vegas to the Las Vegas Land & Water Company, Aug. 1, 1924; all in UPRR Collection, LVL&W Co., Walter Bracken Files, Fire Protection, Box 10, File W16-3, UNLV SC. See also Moehring and Green, *Las Vegas*, 12–16, 26–30.

55. H. E. Nutt to W. H. Bancroft and J. Ross Clark, Nov. 3, 1912, UPRR Collection, LVL&W Co., Walter Bracken Files, Employee Loans, Box 8, Folder W12-3, W12-3-6, UNLV SC (incl. "a more desirable").

56. Hewetson Deed, Dec. 14, 1914; Hewetson Lease Agreement, July 1, 1915; both in UPRR Collection, LVL&W Walter Bracken Files, Box 8, Folder W12-3, W12-3-6, UNLV SC. Walter Bracken to F. H. Knickerbocker, Nov. 3, 1912, UPRR Collection, LVL&W Co., Walter Bracken Files, Employee Loans, Box 8, Folder W12-3, W12-3-6, UNLV SC (incl. "most attractive" and "a very"). See also Moehring, *Resort City*, 7–8; and Moehring and Green, *Las Vegas*, 7–15.

57. Walter Bracken to E. H. Calvin, Feb. 2, 1923, UPRR Collection, LVL&W Co., Walter Bracken Files, Employee Welfare, Box 16, File R-31, UNLV SC (incl. all quotes).

58. Walter Bracken to W. C. Frazier, May 24, 1913; Chamber of Commerce to W. H. Comstock, A. S. Halsted, W. R. Bracken, and J. Ross Clark, Aug. 13, 1919; City of Las Vegas to Walter Bracken, Sept. 11, 1919; Bill for the City of Las Vegas to the Las Vegas Land & Water Company, Aug. 1, 1924; all in UPRR Collection, LVL&W Co., Walter Bracken Files, Fire Protection, Box 10, File W16-3, UNLV SC. See also Moehring and Green, *Las Vegas*, 30-32 (incl. "From 1905-1910," 32).

59. The UPRR acquired the remaining half of the stock and all but $41,000 of the bonds of the LA&SL. Effective January 1, 1922, the UPRR and the LA&SL became constituent companies. See *Union Pacific Company Twenty-Sixth Annual Report—Year Ended December 31, 1922* (Omaha, NE: Union Pacific Railroad Company, 1922).

60. Frank McNamee to A. B. Halsted, July 14, 1922 and Aug. 8, 1922; E. H. Calvin to W. H. Comstock and A. S. Halsted, telegram, July 14, 1922; News Release from the Railway Age, July 27, 1922; Frank McNamee to Governor Emmet D. Boyle, Aug. 8, 1922 (incl. all quotes); all in UPRR Collection, Union Pacific Law Department, Assaults, Riots, Strikes, Box 56, Files 10, 10-5-4, 10-5-4H, UNLV SC.

61. Moehring, *Resort City*, 11; "U.P. Employees Form Athletic and Welfare Club: New Organization Will Be Big Factor in Activities of Las Vegas," *Las Vegas Age*, Mar. 4, 1922; "U.P. Employees Athletic and Welfare Club to Meet," *Las Vegas Sun*, Apr. 8, 1922. See also Walter Bracken to E. G. Adams, Apr. 7, 1927 (incl. all quotes); H. S. Baldwin to Walter Bracken, Feb. 28, 1922; both in UPRR Collection, LVL&W Co., Walter Bracken Files, Employee Wellness, Box 16, File R-31, UNLV SC.

62. A. E. Cahlan, "From Where I Sit," *Evening Review-Journal*, Mar. 28, 1930, copied by Florence Lee Jones Cahlan (Oct. 8, 1974), Cahlan Collection, Box 24, Folder 99, NSMA. At the turn of the century, doctors treated pulmonary tuberculosis patients with bed rest, and considered a dry climate essential to recovery. Sanatoriums consequently popped up across the West at higher elevations. See Clare Woodbury, interview by Ralph Roske, Sept. 12, 1974, UNLV SC; "Hal Hewetson, Pioneer Vegas Passes in L.A.," *Evening Review-Journal*, Mar. 28, 1930, Cahlan Collection, Box 24, Folder 99, NSMA; Moehring and Green, *Las Vegas*, 11.

63. Mazie Martin Jones, interview by Jane P. Kowalewski, Nov. 3, 1978, UNLV SC; "Las Vegas Hospital," *Las Vegas Age*, Feb. 2, 1907.

64. See "Message of Governor John Sparks," and "Report of the Board of Health," *Appendix*, 23rd Sess., Vol. 1 (Carson City, NV: SPO, 1907) (incl. "nerve" and "hundreds," 10).

65. No comprehensive scholarship exists on railroad medical programs. The best coverage is Mark Aldrich, "Train Wrecks and Typhoid Fever: The Development of Railroad Medicine Organizations, 1850 to World War I," *Bulletin of the History of Medicine* 75, no. 2 (Summer 2001): 254–89. See also Emory Johnson, "Railway Relief Departments," DOL *Bulletin 8* (1987): 39–57; Ronald Numbers, "The Third Party: Health Insurance in America," in *The Therapeutic Revolution: Essays in the Social History of American Medicine*, ed. Morris J. Vogel and Charles E. Rosenberg, 177–200 (Philadelphia: University of Philadelphia Press, 1979).

66. Aldrich's article, "Train Wrecks and Typhoid Fever," 258, 261–62, provides a discussion of development of medical services offered by the railroad industry.

67. Ibid., 258–59, 264.

68. By the mid-1940s the Union Pacific Employees Hospital Association had taken over the medical department. While benefits remained the same, the association adopted a board of directors, and established a uniform, systemwide program that included subsidiary/affiliated companies. "UPRR Employees Hospital Association— Authority for Payroll Deductions," Jan. 1, 1948, UPRR Collection, LVL&W Co., Walter Bracken Files, Hospital Fund, Employees, Box 7, File W8-1, UNLV SC (incl. all quotes). See also Frank Strong to A. M. Folger, Nov. 3, 1947; C. C. Barry to F. H. Knickerbocker, Apr. 9, 1925; F. H. Knickerbocker to Officers and Employees, May 10, 1933; all in UPRR Collection, LVL&W Co., Walter Bracken Files, Hospital Fund, Employees, Box 7, File W8-1, UNLV SC.

69. John A. Fuller, "Medicine in Nevada Half Century Age," quoted in Blachley, *Pestilence*, 18; "Tremendous Expansion of Hospital Facilities in Clark County Noted During Five Decade Growing Period," *Review-Journal*, Aug. 15, 1948; Jones interview.

70. Fuller, "Medicine in Nevada," 17–18 (incl. all quotes).

71. Ibid., 17–18. See also Walter Bracken to K. E. Calvin, Feb. 29, 1924; Hal L. Hewetson to Walter Bracken, Apr. 9, 1924; Walter Bracken to Hal L. Hewetson, May 8, 1924; all in UPRR Collection, LVW&L, Walter Bracken Files, Hospital Union Pacific, Box 18, File R2-56, UNLV SC. Walter Bracken to F. H. Knickerbocker, C. C. Barry, Guy Cochrane, and C. H. Bloom, Jan.–Mar., 1925; "Martin Vetti Payable to The Hospital of the Good Samaritan," Feb. 13, 1925, Invoice; both in UPRR Collection, LVL&W Co., Walter Bracken Files, Employees Personal Injury, Box 5, File W5-6-5, UNLV SC.

72. "Las Vegas Hospital," *Las Vegas Age*, Feb. 2, 1907 (incl. "met the requirements"); "Can See Through Things Much Better Than Before," *Las Vegas Age*, Nov. 13, 1920.

73. Rigor mortis is caused by coagulation of muscle proteins after death, causing a progressive but temporary stiffening of the muscles. Fuller quoted in Blachley, *Pestilence*, 18.

74. In most states it was difficult to obtain a divorce because their laws required long separations or other barriers before divorce and subsequently remarriage was allowed. But that was not true in Nevada. By the mid-1920s, columnists began covering the state's lax laws regarding divorce and hundreds of women traveled to Reno to get "Reno-vated." The Nevada divorce trade continued to boom after Mexico and other jurisdictions relaxed their own laws. The Nevada legislature eventually reduced residency requirements to only three months in 1927 and six weeks in 1931, and celebrities, socialites, and dignitaries flocked to the state to dissolve their marriages. See James W. Hulse, *The Silver State: Nevada's Heritage Reinterpreted* (Reno: University of Nevada Press, 2004), 199–200; "New Physician for Las Vegas Hospital," *Las Vegas Age*, May 18, 1918 (incl. "middle aged"). See also Elizabeth Harrington, "Dr. Martin and the First Las Vegas Hospitals," *The Nevadan*, Suppl. of *Review-Journal*, Feb. 6, 1977.

75. Walter Bracken to K. E. Calvin, Feb. 29, 1924; Hal L. Hewetson to Walter Bracken, Apr. 9, 1924; Walter Bracken to Hal L. Hewetson, May 8, 1924; all in UPRR Collection, LVW&L Walter Bracken Files, Hospital Union Pacific, Box 18, File R2-56, UNLV SC.

76. See Witt, *Accidental Republic*, 59, 62, for a discussion of the emergence of personal injury lawyers during the late nineteenth century. Elon R. Brown, "Some Faults of Legal Administration," in New York State Bar Association, *Proceedings of the Thirty-First Annual Meeting Held at New York, Jan. 21, 24–25, 1908* (Albany, NY: Argus Company, 1908) (incl. "marked by," "speculative," and "haphazard," 142). Walter Bracken to W. H. Comstock, July 8, 1918, UPRR Collection, Claims for Damages and Personal Injury, Box 15, File R-14, UNLV SC (incl. "sharks"). For coverage of the history of accidental injury law, see Welke, *Recasting American Liberty*, 81–124.

77. McNamee & McNamee Biography, "Finding Aid," Las Vegas for MS-58 McNamee Collection, NSMA.

78. Gitterman's article also argued that the courts needed to create a coherent interpretation of accident laws and a system that did not exhaust the patience and resources of individuals bringing suit. See John M. Gitterman, "The Cruelties of Our Courts," *McClure's* (June 1910) (incl. "not a slave," 151, and "be compelled," 161).

79. Edwin A. Jaggard, *Hand-book for the Law of Torts* (St. Paul, MN: West Publishing, 1895) (incl. "No action," 199). See also Witt, *Accidental Republic*, 50–51.

80. Frank R. McNamee to Leo A. McNamee, Apr. 19, 1917 (incl. "dependent upon"

and "disobedience"); McNamee Legal Notes on Kuckenmeister v. Company, 1917; both in McNamee Collection, 1917 Legal File, Box 144, Folder 18, nsma.

81. Leo McNamee to Walter Bracken, Feb. 10, 1931, uprr Collection, lvl&w Co., Walter Bracken Files, Insurance, Employee Compensation Nevada, Box 7, File W9-2, W9-2-5, unlv sc; Memorandum to Employers and Employees, "Nevada Industrial Insurance Act, Effective July 1, 1925," uprr Collection, lvl&w Co., Walter Bracken Files, Hospital Fund, Employees, Box 7, File W8-1, unlv sc.

82. Leo McNamee to H. I. Bettis, June 9, 1909, uprr Collection, uprr Law Department, Employees General, Box 58, File 50, unlv sc (incl. "almost compulsory").

83. By 1923 the la&sl discontinued accident and health coverage, calling it burdensome and expensive. See uprr to Officers and Employees, Dec. 15, 1922, uprr Collection, lvl&w Co., Walter Bracken Files, Box 16, File R-29, unlv sc. See also Y. O. Yette to Dana T. Smith, Dec. 23, 1918; E. E. Malton to Dana T. Smith, Nov. 20, 1918; F. H. Knickerbocker to F. E. Pettit, Nov. 15, 1927; Fred E. Pettit Jr. to F. H. Knickerbocker, Nov. 17, 1927; all in uprr Collection, uprr Law Department, Employees General, Box 58, File 50, unlv sc. uprr Supplement to Announcement of May 2, 1933, June 9, 1933, uprr Collection, lvl&w Co., Walter Bracken Files, Insurance, Employee Compensation Nevada, Box 7, File W9-2, W9-2-5, unlv sc (incl. "very low cost").

84. By the 1930s and early 1940s federal judges had given up policing the boundary between interstate and intrastate commerce. The Supreme Court articulated in 1938 that there was "no point" in creating a "mathematical line" between interstate and intrastate commerce. See Witt, *Accidental Republic*, 189–90.

85. F. R. McNamee to W. C. Hussey, July 3, 1925, McNamee Collection, 1926 Legal File, Box 145, Folder 5, nsma (incl. "whether or not" and "the burden of").

86. Walter Bracken to F. H. Knickerbocker, Sept. 30, 1924, uprr Collection, lvl&w Co., Walter Bracken Files, Legal Matters, Box 15, File R-33, unlv sc. See also F. R. McNamee to W. C. Hussey, June 19, 1925; F. R. McNamee to W. C. Hussey, June 19, 1925; Fred E. Pettit Jr. to F. R. McNamee, Oct. 13, 1925; F. R. McNamee to F. W. Chiswell, Mar. 16, 1925 (incl. "deprived of"); W. C. Hussey to Leo A. McNamee, Apr. 5, 1926; Leo A. McNamee to W. C. Hussey, Apr. 8, 1926 (incl. "great"); all in McNamee Collection, 1926 Legal File, Box 145, Folder 5, nsma.

87. See Sellers, *Hazards of the Job*, for more on university laboratories studying workplace safety and industrial hygiene during the 1920s.

88. While the la&sl initially contracted with Balcom and Ferguson, they actively sought a permanent replacement. The company first appointed Dr. H. C. Vander Meulen, but became unhappy with his performance. The chief surgeon of Union Pacific, Dr. J. C. Landenberger, decided against appointing a local doctor because it would arouse envy among his associates. He decided on hiring Dr. Hale B. Slavin, a young surgeon from Salt Lake City, who accepted the position in 1934, eventually becoming the Clark County physician in 1939. Slavin rehabilitated the Hewetson Hospital building, with the la&sl covering all renovation costs. The railroad did not charge Slavin rent for the property, only requiring him to finance electricity and water expenses. See Walter Bracken to Dr. J. C. Landenberger, Apr. 20, 1933; J. C. Landenberger to Walter Bracken, letter, Apr. 24, 1933; Hale B. Slavin to Walter Bracken, letter, June 14, 1933; and Walter Bracken to J. C. Landenberger, memorandum, 1933; all in lvl&w Co., Walter Bracken Files, Hospital Fund, Box 7, File W8-1, unlv sc. See also F. H. Knickerbocker to Walter Bracken, July 24, 1933, lvl&w Co., Walter Bracken Files, Old Hospital Building, Box 16, File R-42, unlv sc.

89. "They Court Disaster," *Evening Review-Journal*, Feb. 11, 1930 (incl. "probably the most," "would not be permitted," and "courting disaster"). See also Gerald Markowitz and David Rosner, *"Slaves of the Depression": Workers' Letters About Life on the Job* (Ithaca, NY, and London: Cornell University Press, 1987), 3.

90. The Las Vegas Hospital Association eventually dissolved over a series of disagreements between the doctors. It was renamed the Las Vegas Hospital and Clinic and served the Las Vegas community until the 1970s. See Walter Bracken to Phillip Stephens, Sept. 23, 1929; Phillip Stephens to Walter Bracken, Nov. 11, 1929; both in UPRR Collection, LVL&W Co., Walter Bracken Files, Hospital Union Pacific, Box 18, File R2-56, UNLV SC. See also Application for Service Certificate to Guaranteed Medical Service, Inc. A. B. Mortensen to Walter Bracken, Dec. 16, 1929; both in UPRR Collection, LVL&W Co., Walter Bracken Files, Proposed Memorial Hospital, Box 8, File W121-6, UNLV SC. See also K. J. Evans, "Roy Martin," in *The First 100: Portraits of the Men and Women Who Shaped Las Vegas,* eds. A. D. Hopkins and K. J. Evans, 50–53 (Las Vegas: Huntington Press, 2000),52; "The Hospitals of Clark County: Development of Medicine in a Rapidly Growing Nevada Community," *Greasewood Tablettes* 7, no. 4 (Winter 1996–97), 1.

91. H. R. 10449—A Bill to Authorize the Erection of a Veterans Bureau Hospital in the State of Nevada, Jan. 23, 1931, George W. Malone Collection, UNLV SC.

92. Veterans Bureau Hospital for Nevada Area to Sub-Committee of World War Veterans Legislation, Jan. 23, 1931, Washington, DC, 1–3, 7–8, 11, George W. Malone Collection, UNLV SC; Leonard Blood to J. Dayton Smith, Apr. 11, 1931, UPRR Collection, LVL&W Walter Bracken Files, Proposed Veterans Hospital, Box 10, File W-16-3-10, UNLV SC.

93. American Legion Post No. 8 to Carl R. Gray, Mar. 24, 1931 (incl. "repaid from"); Wm. L. Scott to Carl R. Gray, Mar. 24, 1931; F. H. Knickerbocker to W. R. Bracken, Mar. 19, 1931; Walter Bracken to Carl R. Gray, Apr. 1, 1931; all in UPRR Collection, LVL&W Walter Bracken Files, Proposed Veterans Hospital, Box 10, File W-16-3-10, UNLV SC.

94. J. D. Smith to the Federal Board of Hospitalization, 1931; Ryland Taylor to J. D. Smith, Apr. 11, 1931, UPRR Collection, LVL&W, Walter Bracken Files, Proposed Veterans Hospital, Box 10, File W-16-3-10, UNLV SC; Leonard Blood to J. Dayton Smith, Apr. 11, 1931, Leonard Blood Collection, UNLV SC.

95. Smith to the Federal Board, 1931 (incl. all quotes).

96. Roy W. Martin to Whom It May Concern, 1931 (incl. "I am somewhat"); F. M. Ferguson to Whom it May Concern, 1931 (incl. "one-half," "very rare," "practically negligible," and "at all times of the year"); R. D. Balcom to Whom it May Concern, Apr. 7, 1931 (incl. "conducive"); F. R. Mildren to Commander of the American Legion, Apr. 11, 1931; J. R. McDaniel to Whom It May Concern; H. C. Vander Meulen to Whom It May Concern, Mar. 31, 1931 (incl. "resort and tourist" and "Already we are handicapped"); all in UPRR Collection, LVW&L Walter Bracken Files, Proposed Veterans Hospital, Box 10, File W-16-3-10, UNLV SC.

97. The establishment of the University of Nevada School of Medicine in Reno solidified the split, allocating only clinical programs and residencies to Las Vegas. Many physicians in Las Vegas resented Reno for housing the education and research, and cited that the decision significantly hurt Las Vegas's quality of health care. See Richard G. Pugh, *Serving Medicine: The Nevada State Association and the Politics of Medicine* (Reno: Greasewood Press, 2002), 40–57.

# 2

# THE DAM

With the exception of university-run laboratories, interest in industrial health waned during the 1920s. After the end of World War I production needs declined and unemployment rose, leading to a brief economic downturn. Playing off American fears of socialist, communist, and anarchist ideology, and of radical immigrants, the private sector partnered with the Harding, Coolidge, and Hoover administrations to repress labor, and remove economic regulations and workplace safety controls. Labor unions consequently experienced a sharp decline in membership and strike actions, as companies pushed open shop, the American plan, and Yellow Dog contracts, and acquired worker loyalty with profit sharing, bonuses, and company stock.[1] Some unions, such as the American Federation of Labor (AFL), managed to survive the 1920s, but only by partnering with business. In 1929 the United States plummeted into a more intense economic depression. Twenty-five percent of Americans were unemployed, eager to work at whatever the cost. At least initially, the docile workforce allowed employers free rein, offering dangerous, temporary jobs at insignificant pay. The public–private partnerships also continued, and the federal government actively encouraged and participated in industrial development that posed serious threats to American workers. To pull the nation out of the Great Depression, injuries and fatalities became an accepted risk. But unlike in previous decades, increased media coverage made it difficult to conceal health and safety issues, and workplace safety reemerged as a human rights issue. There was no more high-profile case of this than construction of the Hoover Dam.[2]

Death shrouded the project even before construction broke ground. In 1922 J. Gregory Tierney, a Bureau of Reclamation (Reclamation) driller surveying the region, slipped off a barge and drowned. In a bizarre twist of fate, his son Patrick, a Reclamation electrician, fell to his death from an intake tower thirteen years later to the day. Father and son were the first and last to die on the project. In December 1928 President Calvin Coolidge approved the Boulder Canyon Project Act and authorized the Secretary of the Interior to oversee construction of a dam and reservoir. It was an ambitious project. Hoover Dam would be the highest dam project in the world, towering seven hundred feet, and hold the largest reservoir in the world. Reclamation expected the dam would take six years to complete, slating construction to begin in 1931 and first units operating in 1935. To construct the dam efficiently and economically, Secretary of Interior Ray Lyman Wilbur determined that the dam site was a federal reservation.[3] Making the site a reservation afforded the federal government complete control, with limited interference from the states. Nevada initially complied, forfeiting authority and acquisition rights to the federal government, but later disputed its role in policing workplace safety and taxation. By the end of dam construction, the state and federal government put aside their differences and forged a lasting relationship, housing federal projects in Nevada throughout the twentieth century.[4]

On September 17, 1930, Wilbur attempted to drive a silver spike into the ground to mark the beginning of the project. He missed. A second, successful attempt launched the UPRR's 22.7-mile branch line to the future company town, officially beginning the project. Wilbur contracted with the private sector to handle construction. On December 16, 1930, Southern Sierras Power Company of California Edison began stringing a 90,000-volt power line from Victorville to Boulder City. On January 7, 1931, he opened bids to build an eight-mile gravel highway and a ten-and-a-half–mile railroad spur from Boulder City to the dam site, awarding them to Robert G. LeTourneau and Lewis Construction of Los Angeles accordingly. The main contract went to Six Companies Inc., a conglomerate of seven separate companies incorporated in February 1931: Bechtel (San Francisco, California), Kaiser (Oakland, California), MacDonald & Kahn (San Francisco, California), Morrison-Knudson Company (Boise, Idaho), Utah Construction Company (Salt Lake City, Utah), J. F. Shea (Portland, Oregon), and the Pacific Bridge Company (Portland, Oregon).[5] Wilbur granted smaller contracts to

Babcock & Wilcox Company, and the Allis–Chalmers Manufacturing and Newport News Shipbuilding and Dry Dock Companies. After securing the contract, Six Companies authorized engineer Frank T. Crowe, the nation's foremost dam builder, to hire workers to build a railroad to the site and a temporary camp, and engineers to outline plans to begin construction. The contractors provided employment through the U.S. Employment Service in cooperation with the State of Nevada, and Leonard Blood, the appointed superintendent in charge, established an employment office in Las Vegas.

Given the size of the job, there seemed ample opportunity for unemployed men to find work, and thousands flooded the Las Vegas area. The prospective workers were a colorful group of characters, varying from experienced construction workers to cowboys from the western range. But the largest group were inexperienced city folk, factory workers, mechanics, sales clerks, lawyers, bankers, and students, none of whom had ever experienced hard labor in the desert. As expected, the population influx created a public health crisis in Las Vegas, leading Dr. J. C. Landenberger to call it "probably the most unsanitary [town] in the country" and if not the worst, "a decidedly close race for honors." The *Evening Review-Journal* agreed, reporting the conditions "would not be permitted" elsewhere in the United States and declaring that Las Vegas was "courting disaster to the health of the community."[6]

While soup kitchens fed some men and their families, hundreds starved. The once neatly organized railroad town was starting to look more like a Hooverville. It was a distressing sight. The *Phoenix Arizona Republic* reported that the "bonanza days of the Old West [were] being reenacted [in Las Vegas as] one of the strangest [cities] in the country today, [with people] streaming in from everywhere."[7] There were not enough hotels and homes to accommodate them all, and local banks could not finance new home construction, so people lived in communities of tents and shacks. Journalist Edmund Wilson described Las Vegas in the *New Republic* as a "battlefield…thronged with wanderers looking for work" and the train station was "full of sleeping men."[8] Reporters assigned to cover the dam construction did not share the local physicians' opinion that the southern Nevada landscape offered innumerable health benefits. Theodore White wrote in *Harper's*

*Magazine* that the federal reservation was a "a bowl formed by unsympathetic mountains…a deadly desert place." Reporting for the *New York Times*, Duncan Aikman observed "furnace-like winds blowing alkali and gypsum dust through sheer sunlight of the desert give sand hills…[and] a curious look of incandescence."[9]

The situation became so dire that the Interior Department issued a statement that urged prospective workers to not seek employment in Las Vegas. Interior stressed that construction would not begin for another year and no one should travel to the area unless they were "financially able to tide over an uncertain period of unemployment." The warning did little to stop them. Thousands continued to travel to Las Vegas, resulting in a large number of idle men. As mobs swarmed the employment office, Blood struggled to maintain order. Within only a few months, he received twenty-four hundred applications and more than twelve thousand letters inquiring about employment.[10]

Although the conditions in Las Vegas were poor, working conditions at the dam were far worse. The Boulder Canyon Project began construction ahead of schedule to create jobs during the Great Depression, and the rush inevitably fostered hazardous working and living conditions.[11] The potential workers, however, were aware of the danger and still pursued employment. Unfortunately for them, Superintendent Blood turned most away, because he had authorization to hire only clerical and temporary workers. The core group of workers were Frank Crowe's trusted labor from previous dam projects, which included the construction of the Arrowdock Dam in Idaho during his tenure at Reclamation. To fill gaps, supervisors recruited other positions by word of mouth, finding employees that fit their needs, and bringing their appointments to the employment office. After strike agitation in August 1931, the U.S. Employment Office took over all aspects of employment, and eventually maintained a 47 percent veteran workforce. Out of twenty-two thousand men examined for work, 920 were rejected. Of the rejections, 33 percent had cardiovascular problems, 22 percent had hernias, and 20 percent had defective hearing. The rest had so-called manual deficiencies. Workers were represented from nearly every state, with California and Nevada providing the majority. Most were white and married, with a medium age of 31.6 during the summer and 35 during the winter.[12]

Six Companies hired few minorities. In fact, the Boulder Canyon Act specifically prohibited employing so-called Mongolians (a term used to refer to workers of Asian descent) and neither the Hoover or Roosevelt administrations promoted a diversified workforce.[13] In 1932 the National Association for the Advancement of Colored People (NAACP) and the National Urban League alleged that both Boulder Canyon and the Mississippi River Flood Control Projects either denied employment to blacks or abused those that worked there. An NAACP investigation confirmed the charges, forcing the contractor to hire ten black veterans. Still, minorities represented less than 1 percent of the workforce. Six Companies gave minorities the most arduous jobs, such as working in the gravel pits, a hot, remote area in the reservation; or brushing steel. The contractor also prohibited minorities from living in the company town, forcing them to travel thirty miles from the West Las Vegas slums to the dam site via the Interstate Transit Lines Bus, a subsidiary of the UPRR.[14]

The sheer number of employees tested the contractors' commitment to health and safety. In April 1931 construction began six months ahead of schedule. As the UPRR laid roadbed on the canyon rim to the future site of a company town, Boulder City, and to an aggregate plant upstream, Six Companies drove adits in the cliffs and excavated pioneer tunnels. But before heavy construction could begin, LeTourneau and Southern Sierras Power Company needed to complete the highway and power line. In the meantime, Crowe assembled three hundred men to lay heavy equipment, explosives, and timber along the riverbank at Hemingway Wash. Crowe's crew also built a temporary mess hall in Boulder City, and a River Camp downstream with a mess hall to house single men.[15] In May the workforce varied from 520 to 700 men, and by July the number had quadrupled. When tunneling began in early September, the number increased from eight hundred to three thousand men. After engineers diverted the Colorado River, Six Companies employed 5,128 workers in June 1934. During the project's duration, Reclamation and the various contractors employed an array of skilled and nonskilled labor, including engineers, miners, muckers, carpenters, plumbers, electricians, engineers, railroad employees, clerical force, commissary attendants, truck drivers, riggers, mechanics, chemists, steelworkers, cement workers, and other general laborers. Unskilled labor ranged from $0.50 to $1.00 per hour, working an average of eight hours per day. Skilled labor, including engineers, and inspectional and clerical staff earned $1,400 to $5,600 per annum.[16]

Reclamation and Six Companies initially established an insufficient health and safety program, leaving workers vulnerable to brutal conditions. The only housing option for men with families was a makeshift, ragtag community along the riverbank called Ragtown.[17] Residents lived in tents, shacks, cars, and trailers, and endured extreme heat, strong winds, thunderstorms, and flooding. At its height, the settlement accommodated more than 550 people. The River Camp included a seventy-five-bed bunkhouse, but the accommodations were no better there. Workers slept in an open room on cots with dirty blankets, and there was no running water or electricity. Most men preferred working than sleeping there. When temperatures rose in June, conditions became so unbearable that many could not lift their forks to feed themselves. The mess hall's cooling unit failed regularly: in early July 1931 a batch of rotten pork sandwiches sickened thirty men. One worker who spent five years employed at Panama Canal lasted only three days at the River Camp, succumbing to heat prostration. Both camps were ultimately "more difficult to maintain" than Six Companies anticipated, who attributed it to "higher heat conditions along the river [and] humidity due to the location near the water." Dr. John McDaniel made house calls to both sites, describing the temperature as "about 130 [during the day and it] did not cool down much" at night. Residents bathed and drew drinking water from the river that looked like "an opaque yellow-like coffee with too much ice cream" contaminated by pathogens, and disease-producing bacteria and viruses.[18] While no major epidemics occurred during the summer of 1931 this time, waterborne diseases such as viral and bacterial gastroenteritis and typhoid fever contaminated both the river and the drinking water tanks. McDaniel noted that the other problem was dysentery from spoiled meat and vegetables.[19]

Although Reclamation director Elwood Mead was aware of the brutal conditions, he did little to resolve them. Mead thought the workers could survive the first summer without great losses and move to Boulder City in the fall. He was wrong. On June 24, 1931, the *Review-Journal* reported that the dam site was 140 degrees Fahrenheit in the sun and 120 degrees Fahrenheit in the shade. The average temperature during the summer of 1931 was 119.9 degrees Fahrenheit. Intense sweating subjected the workers to heat dehydration, a condition then referred to as heat prostration. It resulted from a combination of thermal and cardiovascular strain, where workers experienced fatigue, dizziness, confusion, increased pulse and respiration rates, and dry skin. The condition often developed into heatstroke: the workers' body temperature was so elevated that they experienced convulsions, brain swelling, coma, and even death. Over the next five years, numerous workers passed out or died of heatstroke. Although no one knows how many suffered acutely from the heat, Six Companies' records indicate that seventeen workers died from so-called heat prostration in the summer of 1931. It is unknown how many family members died.

To its credit, the contractor recognized the problem and created a work schedule that limited exposure to the sun. Still, the desert heat made the labor situation difficult for them, increasing labor turnover and delaying construction progress. Besides heatstroke, workers experienced terrible burns on the skin from the sun and wind, leading many to believe they had caught a waterborne disease from the river. Although no epidemics occurred in 1931, there was an outbreak of spinal meningitis as well as several pneumonia cases. During the first year of construction, forty-six workers and family members died on or near the dam site. Since Six Companies and Reclamation document most fatalities as "accidents sustained on and off duty [as well as] heat prostration [and] natural causes," it is difficult to determine the actual causes of death.[20]

Problems in health and safety were inevitable during the project's first year. Because they started six months early, Reclamation officials and Six Companies did not have time to establish the foundation of an adequate occupational health regime. If either party had, fewer workers would have died during the first summer. In fact, those deaths might have been avoided had Wilbur honored his original industrial medicine contract.[21]

As a medical doctor, Wilbur knew that the project would pose considerable health risks. In January 1931 he cited that the remote work site, magnitude of operations, and severe weather conditions would challenge "the health, comfort, and general welfare" of the project's workforce.[22] He therefore commissioned the establishment of a company town and hospital system. As a federally funded project, Mead assumed that the PHS would provide medical care. He wrote to U.S. Surgeon General Dr. Hugh S. Cumming to ask if the PHS could staff and operate a hospital. However, after the agency's massive defunding during the 1920s, the PHS lacked the resources to undertake such a huge job. Consequently, the Interior Department and Reclamation jointly opened bids for the project's industrial medicine contract in March 1931.[23]

Dr. Roy Martin jumped at the opportunity. Since arriving in Nevada, Martin had contracted to local industries his medical services as the company physician for the Las Vegas and Tonopah Railroad and for mining communities. Under the Las Vegas Hospital Association, Martin, with Ferdinand Ferguson, R. D. Balcom, John McDaniel, and Clare Woodbury, submitted a bid. Since the Department of Interior originally slated Las Vegas as the central point of the project, Wilbur awarded the association the contract. After visiting the town, however, Wilbur became disgusted by its embracement of vice, and determined that the combination of gambling, drinking, and prostitution was not the proper environment to foster a productive workforce. He revoked the contract and ordered Six Companies to create a comprehensive industrial medicine program.[24]

Six Companies was not prepared for the task. It scrambled together informal assistance, developing a health plan with company physicians on the payroll. The medical team had two goals: first, to promote a healthy workforce to boost production and second, to protect their employer from liability lawsuits. The most visible practice of defensive medicine was preemployment examinations. In the 1930s the growing number of fraudulent liability cases led employers to institute physical examinations. Most required preemployment assessments and periodic physicals to screen for disabilities. The examinations could have helped diagnose industrial diseases, but the doctors were loyal to their employer, rarely reporting findings to workers, colleagues, or medical journals. Their job was to keep production on schedule, even if it meant concealing harmful industrial hygiene issues and reducing workmen's compensation obligations. As a result, workers during the 1930s often mistrusted physicians and nurses on the company payroll.[25]

Six Companies' preemployment examinations documented existing health conditions and the overall well-being of the prospective employee, a practice that proved useful in compensation hearings. The contractor required all new employees to sign a disclaimer relinquishing the right to sue their employer for the compensation of preexisting conditions.[26]

The men also needed to pass the preemployment examination. Six Companies initially hired John McDaniel to administer the exams, paying him $250 a month. Most workers, he recalled, were in "bad shape, starving pretty much before they got here" with high blood pressure. He attributed their poor condition to the heat, work, their hard lives, and worry about unemployment. From 1931 to 1933 McDaniel and other company physicians rejected 101 out of 2,000 men for preexisting ailments and disabilities.[27]

Besides physical examinations, Six Companies established a rudimentary first aid station in Boulder City in May 1931, placing Charles Christal, the medical director for the California State Compensation Insurance fund, in charge. Though Christal referred to it as a "first class aid station," his assistants told workers their only job was to examine them to "see if they can do a day's work before we give them a job."[28] Six Companies instructed the medical staff to never treat women or children. The contractor also announced plans to build a hospital and bought two ambulances to transport seriously injured workers to Las Vegas. Of course, the ambulance ride was not complimentary; the workers paid a biweekly deductible for all medical services and ambulance rides. Until Six Companies finished the Boulder City Hospital, it contracted out medical care to the Las Vegas Hospital Association. The hospital was inadequate for most dam construction trauma care, and Roy Martin sent the most serious cases to Los Angeles. As an added inconvenience, patients had to travel to Las Vegas to fill their prescriptions at White Cross Drug. The contractor also established first aid stations at the work site to administer immediate care, but had an ulterior motive to protect itself from liability suits. For example, Rosario Levesque, the head attendant at a first aid station for tunnel workers, also worked as an agent for the Six Companies' insurance department.[29]

During the summer of 1931 most attempts by organized labor failed to unite labor at the project. There were several reasons for this, the first being that it was during the Great Depression. No matter the hazardous conditions, workers felt lucky to have a job. A second explanation is that Reclamation officials actively worked alongside Six Companies to bar union presence in order to ensure the project moved along swiftly, a continuation of the cozy relationship between the federal government and business throughout the 1920s. In early May the AFL asked to meet with Six Companies to discuss union representation, citing its record working alongside business and on the Swing–Johnson bill. The contractor rejected the request and used Swing–Johnson as justification, calling unions unneeded because all "specifications governing labor" had been "indicated by contract between the United States Government" and itself. The International Brotherhood of Electrical Workers received similar resistance; Crowe barred representatives from the reservation after pressing him about wages, saying there was "nothing to discuss."[30] The radical Industrial Workers of the World (IWW), or Wobblies, union also attempted to revive itself after a decade of near inactivity. Under the direction of Frank Desmond Anderson, it placed organizers throughout Las Vegas and adopted the classic Wobbly strategy; purposely getting arrested for free publicity, after which workers organized a strike under their guidance. In August 1931 Anderson and several other Wobblies began protesting the project conditions on the streets of Las Vegas. One by one, the police arrested each of them, crowding the local jail. They were all eventually acquitted, planting the seed among workers to question their labor conditions.[31]

Six Companies knew they had a problem on their hands. The contractor took measures to rectify some health and safety issues, shipping clean drinking water from Las Vegas to the work site and installing a small water cooler at the Anderson mess hall. But one variable was out of its control: the unrelenting heat. The summer of 1931 was one of the hottest on record, with an average daily temperature of 119.9 degrees. The heat reached 128 degrees during the day and 103 degrees at night. On July 20 alone, heat prostration incapacitated five workers, and caused the death of a fifteen-year-old girl in Ragtown. Over the next few days additional Ragtown residents died and four workers were admitted to the hospital. The workers became increasingly more angry and frustrated. After their shifts, they returned to Ragtown only to learn about more deaths and hospitalizations. Then, the workers continued to fester in the heat at night, averaging 95 degrees Fahrenheit, and barely slept. Many started to contemplate organizing a strike. All they needed was a spark.

On August 7 Six Companies implemented a wage cut for all tunnel workers, lowering muckers salaries from $5 to $4 a day, cable tenders from $5.60 to $4 a day, and drivers from $5.60 to $5 a day. The announcement of the cut put the workers over the edge. Influenced by Wobbly rhetoric, the workers organized a strike outside the Anderson Brothers mess hall, elected a committee to prepare a list of demands, and sent out workers to spread the word. At 7:00 P.M. work completely shut down, the first break in construction since March. A joint workers' committee generated a list of seven demands and presented it to Six Companies. Within only a few hours, Crowe had publicly rejected it, suspended work, and laid off the entire workforce. At first it seemed as if Walter Young, Reclamation's construction engineer, might come to their defense. But in the end he was equally unsympathetic, closing Ragtown permanently for what he called a clean start.[32] The move ousted hundreds of workers and their families. On August 13 Six Companies agreed to four out of nine demands: to install lights, to install drinking fountains, to build changing rooms at the River Camp, and to accelerate work on the completion of Boulder City and its hospital. While the weather was out of Six Companies' control, Mother Nature cooperated as well, with the heat abating by mid-August. By August 15 Six Companies had rehired 750 workers involved in the strike and resumed construction. Blood assumed a greater role in the hiring process thereafter, under the close supervision of Six Companies.[33]

The 1931 strike solidified the contractor's firm command over their workforce for the project's duration. During the negotiation process, the president of Six Companies, William Wattis, stated that employees had "to work under our conditions or not at all." This statement embodied employment terms for the duration of the project. The event also revealed that Reclamation and Six Companies operated as a team, conducting work at the expense of health and safety. The end of the strike aligned with the completion of LeTourneau's gravel highway and Southern Sierras Power Company's electrical lines. Crews also built a wooden bridge over the Colorado River to travel from the Nevada side to the Arizona side. With an obedient workforce, heavy construction on the diversion tunnels began. Crowe's construction timeline was horribly aggressive; he would finish the dam two years ahead of schedule.[34]

The project's occupational health regime was formed at the onset of heavy construction in September 1931, and focused on the hazards associated with diverting the Colorado River, blasting the canyon, and pouring the concrete. According to a 1932 physical exam report, every day one hundred out of approximately three thousand employees received medical attention at the Boulder City Hospital or at the two on-site first aid stations. More than 5,200 injuries occurred, with an average of four to sixteen daily accidents requiring a physician's care. The report calculated that a fatal injury occurred every 13,620 hours worked.[35] Accidents began in May 1931, most of them a result of rocks falling on workers working on the canyon floor.

When construction began, the work site was chaotic. Three shifts of crews worked twenty-four hours a day for various contractors. On May 17, 1931, the first construction deaths occurred when rocks buried Six Companies employees Harry Large and Andrew Lang at the entrance of a diversion tunnel on the Arizona side. Henry Ludwig managed to escape, but was knocked unconscious. The accident shattered his leg, which doctors had to amputate. It took hours to find the bodies of Large and Lang under the debris. One day later Lewis Construction employee Fred Olsen died from a premature detonation. The deaths were the beginning of a string of construction mishaps under the direction of Frank Crowe, a supervisor famous for placing unrealistic expectations on workers to finish the job ahead of schedule. Six Companies blamed the high death toll on their employees, citing that it seemed evident that the high number of deaths were "due to a fundamental lack of vitality or induced overeating or some other ailment."[36]

But injuries were not confined to workers. The construction site of Hoover Dam quickly became a popular tourist destination. The UPRR capitalized on it, operating sightseeing excursions every Saturday night from Las Vegas. However, visiting an active industrial site was dangerous. Even though Six Companies stressed that visitors were not allowed to touch or ride the equipment—especially the cable ways, monkey slides, trains, or trucks—they did it anyways, suffering serious consequences. After several fatalities and countless injuries, Six Companies ordered the railroad to discontinue the trips and increased its liability insurance. Tourists still could make the trip, but could view the dam site only from afar at several viewing stations. Despite the precaution, they still managed to sustain injuries or die. On November 16, 1932, Theodore Wells, a soldier from Fort MacArthur, Los Angeles, ventured past the "Keep Out" signs at the Lookout Point and bumped the steel awning of a floodlight. The awning fell, hurling him a thousand feet to the canyon floor.[37]

Given the urgency of the project, Six Companies and Reclamation officials haphazardly assembled an industrial health program. The contractor went through the motions of protecting workers, posting Safety-First signs, holding weekly first aid classes, and distributing helmets, belts, goggles, and protective mechanical devices. Frank Crowe also hosted regular propaganda meetings called "Safety-First smokers" for his foremen and the press. Swayed by Crowe's rhetoric, the *Review-Journal* reported that the "welfare and well-being" of Crowe's employees were closest to his heart. At the same time, the Florence Nightingale Institute introduced a program that awarded six honorary fellowships to foremen with crews that showed the fewest number of fatal accidents. But like most Safety-First campaigns during the early 1930s, Six Companies was more concerned with portraying the image of workplace safety than actual enforcement. The goggles, safety belts, and helmets were rarely used by employees. Six Companies employee Marion Allen also remembered that Six Companies did not require attendance to the safety meetings: "Nobody attended unless they were forced to [because they] took up too much of what little leisure time you had."[38]

Without adequate safety mechanisms and given limited training, human error, including carelessness, was the leading cause of death. Failures in operating machinery and equipment, falling rocks or cave-ins, fatigue, lack of sleep, lack of experience, poor communication, intoxication, hunger, or inadequate risk perception caused most accidents. Crowe's need for speedy work was also a hazard, a problem in most Depression-era workplaces to maximize production.[39]

High-scalers had the most dramatic job, dangling on thin ropes along the mountainside, drilling holes in the rock with forty-pound jackhammers. The first crews had experience working at heights: most were former sailors, circus performers, and Indian tribesmen. Given the risk, high scalers received higher pay than workers on the canyon floor, but most felt it gambled too much with their lives. One employee commented that "a lot of workers were pretty hungry that came to work. But they weren't that hungry."[40] Dr. John McDaniel vividly remembered high scaler injuries, most of them due to falls, frayed ropes, faulty knots, falling objects, and slips; one even waved goodbye to him as he fell. The first high scaler death was Jack "Salty" Russell on September 21, 1931. As a crew transported drill rods on the canyon rim, one fell, plummeting down the canyon wall and striking Russell. He was hurled four hundred feet to his death, scattering body parts throughout the riverbank. Instead of shutting down operation, the crew covered up his mangled limbs with three sheets and continued working while the insurance division determined employer liability.[41]

Fatalities significantly increased at the onset of tunnel construction. Diverting the Colorado River necessitated the construction of four fifty-six-foot tunnels in the mountainside, two in Nevada and two in Arizona. A jumbo, which is a retrofitted, World War I–era International truck, was outfitted with thirty drills, allowing three teams of drillers to penetrate the rock with dynamite. After drilling line, trucks arrived with crates of dynamite. The crew turned off power, loaded the explosives, and retreated for detonation. After the blast, a Caterpillar bulldozer led more than a dozen dump trucks into the tunnels for muckers to haul away the debris. From September to November 1931 alone, thirty workers died in premature blasts, rock slides, falls, truck accidents, and cave-ins associated with tunnel work. The handling of explosives produced the most chance for harm. During the loading process, powder men shoved in the dynamite too hard with their sticks, causing a premature explosion. Missed holes, or dynamite that never detonated, and cave-ins were also a common occurrence. After each discharge, safety engineers inspected the perimeter for loose rock before allowing reentrance, but weak spots were sometimes difficult to detect in the darkness. On December 15, 1931, M. J. Sidmore and Frank Manning were the first tunnel fatalities when they were dismembered by a premature explosion. The blast blew their foreman, Forest Weathers, out of the tunnel and into the river.[42]

However, the use of gasoline-powered trucks underground created the biggest death trap and most potential for long-term bodily harm. Idling during the loading process, the vehicles emitted exhaust and high levels of carbon monoxide, which accumulated in the tunnels due to poor ventilation. While long-term exposure produced mild symptoms in some workers, others experienced lasting neurological effects. If the tunnel's electric lights turned blue, they quickly retreated. Many workers used an old mining technique of bringing along caged canaries to detect levels. Still, mass poisonings occurred regularly. Large carbon monoxide clouds formed, emitted by currents and rock niches. Entire shifts became unconscious and crews had to drag the workers out of the tunnels. During the duration of dam construction, Six Companies doctors did not record a single death as carbon monoxide exposure, but deaths from "pneumonia" surged. Thirty-seven workers died of such ailments, usually in clusters. In the first two weeks of December 1932, five died of "pneumonia" and two from "heart trouble." Six Companies blamed the outbreak on the overindulgence of bootleg liquor.[43]

When engineers diverted the Colorado River on the Arizona side on November 1, 1932, workers began the pouring phase of dam construction, placing the first concrete on the riverbed on June 5, 1933. While not at the danger level of tunnel excavation, injuries and deaths were still common. The men worked in tight quarters, on slippery surfaces, and at great heights, dodging heavy objects flying through the air on an intricate, high-line cable system. During the graveyard shift on October 1, 1933, a cable hoist unexpectedly dislodged several buckets, which fell to the canyon floor. One crushed James J. Jackman to death, a worker who had been on the project for only three days. Concreting the spillway inclines, known as "glory holes," was another risky endeavor. Eight-cubic-yard buckets released sixteen tons of wet concrete into wooden forms, and puddlers and finishers packed the material while keeping their balance on slick, 45-degree grades. On September 19, 1933, a form gave way, launching four workers down the incline. One man was flung off, grabbing a nearby cable while his coworkers yelled, "We're coming through!" The momentum hurled another man off, instantly shattering his spine. The final two crashed into the Colorado River, floating until a crew rescued them downstream. Six Companies also began transporting workers to the canyon floor via skip lines hoisted by movable crane towers. The men boarded cages at the canyon rim and steel cables lowered them to the work site. Certainly, the contractor took a risk with this method, especially if a cable frayed or broke. One group spent three hours suspended three hundred feet over the canyon when a hoist twisted, emitting smoke and sparks. A rescue team had to lay a new rail for an adjacent skip, unloading them to safety mid-air. After joking about their tardiness, foremen instructed the workers to begin their shift.[44]

In comparison to the hazards of the job, the workers and their families experienced fair public health, with only a few, minor disease outbreaks. From September 1931 to February 1932 Boulder City and Las Vegas reported spinal meningitis outbreaks, but it was not the epidemic type. A least one worker and three local children died. From 1933 to 1935, Boulder City residents endured several minor disease rashes, including multiple instances of influenza, scarlet fever, measles, typhoid fever, polio, tuberculosis, mumps, gonorrhea, diphtheria, whooping cough, chicken pox, and bronchitis. Airborne disease contributed to most of the epidemics, as did contaminants in the municipal water supply and pollutants produced by the project's unsanitary conditions.[45]

A small percentage of workers also contracted venereal diseases from the Block 16 prostitutes in Las Vegas. City health officers approached the problem with preventive medicine, administering workers and prostitutes alike with shots of Arsphenamine to treat syphilis. Boulder City manager Sims Ely did what he could to prevent workers from going to Las Vegas to drink, gamble, and pay for sex, but his efforts did little good.[46]

The dam's occupational health regime materialized after the August 1931 strike, and developed out of a joint effort by Six Companies and Reclamation to improve labor productivity. Reclamation first closed Ragtown to limit radicalism that can breed in unsupervised camps and ordered the cleanup of River Camp. Six Companies accelerated plans to build a hospital, and mapped out a company town, drafting a city plan that implemented federal recommendations pertaining to water supply, waste disposal, and public health.[47]

Construction crews built sewers, sewage treatment facilities, and water purification plants. Reclamation also ordered the construction of a pumping, filtration, and distribution system to divert and purify the muddy waters of the Colorado River for use in Boulder City. Completed in 1932, the sanitation system pumped 2 million gallons of water to the town daily. Water analysts rigidly monitored the bacterial and chemical levels to maintain decent drinking water supplies. Crews also erected a sludge digestion sewage plant to chemically treat the disposal of a half million gallons of waste daily; Las Vegans used the chemically treated sludge as lawn fertilizer.[48]

After a rash of food poisonings, Reclamation began monitoring food consumption as well. By 1932 officials were conducting regular inspections at all establishments on the Boulder City reservation that sold, handled, or served food and drinks. In cooperation with the State Board of Health, Reclamation also inspected private and public bathrooms and toilets. On May 11, 1932, the State Board of Health inspected the River Camp facilities and reported that conditions had changed dramatically since the previous summer. No flies were present in the mess hall, and all facilities had installed heat, ventilation, and cooling units. The board also determined the nearby first aid station to be adequate, equipped with modern medical instruments, two cots, a surgical table, hot and cold water, and all necessary drugs.[49] The Anderson Brothers Supply Company, a catering firm known for feeding Hollywood location crews in Southern California, also increased its sanitization efforts in the mess hall. The company developed a state-of-the-art system for transporting milk from their 160-acre dairy farm in Logandale, Nevada via refrigerated trucks, and equipped its farm with a water and sewerage system, refrigeration plant, and steam plant. After the summer of 1931 no cases of milk-borne infections occurred in Boulder City, with the exception of one instance of typhoid, which authorities traced to the homemade butter brought in by an Idaho family. The sanitary practices pushed by Reclamation officials greatly improved conditions on the project, foreshadowing a growing federal role in health and safety throughout the 1930s.[50]

With these regulations Boulder City was designed to tightly regulate the health, safety, and lives of its white employees; the few minority workers were strictly prohibited from living in town. Urban planner Saco Rienk DeBoer originally had mapped out Boulder City as an egalitarian landscape promoting moral and civic uplift, with a forest belt, recreation fields, residential playgrounds, and secondary schools. With only $2 million allocated to the project, Mead and Young determined his plan was too expensive, and the town that was built better reflected the social stratification between labor and management. Reclamation managers and engineers ranked supreme on the project, with homes located near the Reclamation Administration Building, the highest, and coolest, point of town. Reclamation families picked out their lots, designing stucco homes with double walls and attics to absorb heat, and decorative features such as window boxes and front lawns. On the other side of Boulder City, Six Companies employees with families lived in the Avenues (A–F) in temporary bungalows with unfinished floors and no insulation. The homes had outhouses, but no running water, telephones, or refrigerators. One-bedroom homes rented for $15 a month, two-bedroom homes for $30 a month. For an extra $4 a month, workers could add a living room.

Six Companies separated unmarried men from families, housing construction workers and office employees in separate dormitories.[51]

City manager Sims Ely controlled every aspect of Boulder City life. The town functioned like the nineteenth-century Pullman company town, establishing strict behavioral standards. Technically, it allowed no liquor or gambling, although some exceptions occurred after the repeal of Prohibition. Public intoxication prompted immediate dismissal from the city. Six Companies hired Bud Bodell as its chief ranger, directing a squad of ten rangers. Very little violence occurred in town. For the most part the rangers tackled bootleg liquor violations and the threat of labor organizing, regularly interrogating and expelling suspected agitators. Ely licensed 113 commercial businesses, a nondenominational and Episcopal church, and eventually, an elementary school for the town's young children. Reclamation and Six Companies families rarely mingled with one another, shopping at different stores and joining separate social groups. Like the LA&SL railroad before it at the Las Vegas townsite, an additional goal of Six Companies and Reclamation was the promotion of healthy extracurricular activities in Boulder City. In 1933 a small library opened in the basement of the administration building with three thousand books on loan from the Library of Congress. A large number of Six Companies employees were college educated, which, along with poor radio reception, encouraged a huge demand for reading materials. The library program was very popular, with most workers requesting nonfiction selections.[52]

Boulder City never slept, continuously churning out workers for their shift. Beginning at 5:40 A.M. the Anderson Brothers, whistle announced breakfast for upcoming shifts, three times a day. At the height of construction, twelve hundred workers crowded the mess hall, eating high-calorie meals to sustain their workday. A typical breakfast consisted of cream of wheat and all-bran cereals, sausage, bacon, omelets, fried potatoes, and hot biscuits. For lunch and dinner, workers ate veal, Irish stew, fried veal steak with country gravy, and chili con carne. The meals were available to nonemployees at $1 per sitting.[53] Afterward they picked out lunches, selecting from three menus posted on the wall or wrapped sandwiches for the night shift, and loaded an open bed of a dump truck to transport themselves to work. Recognizing the safety issue, Six Companies altered this method in 1932, retrofitting three trucks with seats for 150 men in double decks. The crew dubbed the contraption Big Berthas.[54]

One of the biggest components of the tightly regulated occupational health regime established by Reclamation and Six Companies was an advanced industrial medicine system. At an estimated cost of $52,420, the Six Companies Hospital opened on November 15, 1931, equipped with portable x-ray and fluoroscopic units, a diathermy machine, infrared and mercury quartz lamps, and a laboratory to process blood and urine tests; it also housed a pharmacy. According to the *Review-Journal,* it was "as well equipped as hospitals in a large city," with twenty beds, an orthopedic ward, and an eight-bed isolation ward for contagious diseases. Initially, Dr. Charles Christal headed the hospital. Dr. Wales Haas replaced him as chief surgeon in 1932, and Dr. Richard Schofield succeeded Haas after his death in 1933. The chief surgeons earned $750 per month and did not have a formal written contract with the contractor.[55] This was an important tactic designed by Six Companies, because it protected the contractor from medical malpractice liability.[56] By 1936 Six Companies had expanded the hospital into a sixty-bed facility, with a chief surgeon, four assistant surgeons, ten nurses, four orderlies, a radiographer/pharmacist, and management staff, including a full-time auditor, office secretary, and chef.[57]

Most workers did not remember Christal because he left the project shortly after the hospital's opening, but Haas and Schofield were regular fixtures in their lives. Haas was a World War I veteran and a large man, weighing more than three hundred pounds. Most workers described him as a good-natured and caring doctor. Haas concerned himself with treating his patients, and was not interested in the business functions of the hospital. In 1933 he developed appendicitis. As he was being readied for surgery, he requested that Six Companies retrieve his colleague, Schofield, to perform the surgery. The two surgeons had attended the same medical school and practiced together during the war. Unfortunately, Schofield did not make it in time and Haas died. When Schofield arrived, Six Companies officials offered him the job. In terms of management style and bedside manner, Schofield and Haas were opposites. Schofield restructured the Boulder City Hospital more like a business, and quickly garnered a bad reputation for telling workers they faked their symptoms. Needless to say, most despised him.[58]

Schofield remained as Six Companies' chief surgeon for the duration of the project. In a memoir, he wrote a glowing review of the Boulder Canyon Project's medical program, claiming that it was successful because industrial medicine and surgery were "intimately associated with the State of Nevada." Individualism, he cited, made it cutting-edge. Since the early mining days, surgeons had to solve perplexing problems in Nevada, because practicing in isolated places forced innovation. Schofield concluded that these activities fostered the development of groundbreaking methods in Nevada. At the Boulder Canyon Project, he described Six Companies as safety minded, blaming the high number of deaths on inadequacies, namely the extreme weather and "high pressure system of construction." Schofield's assessment is a sweeping generalization rather than a careful, evidence-based analysis of the program. There is no evidence that Nevada's mining industry influenced the project's health and safety. Clearly, any previous studies on heat and carbon monoxide did not affect Six Companies' safety protocol.[59]

Schofield had one point right. Considering the economic environment, the collaboration of Reclamation and Six Companies produced remarkably advanced medical recourses. The network eventually served as a prototype for future employee health programs. Henry J. Kaiser, a Six Companies contractor and founder of Kaiser Permanente, admired the project's medical facilities and coverage so much that he modeled similar establishments on it at his shipyards during World War II. The major difference between the programs was that the hospital in Boulder City limited care to dam employees. Officially, families and government representatives could not use the hospital facilities, although there were several instances where the hospital broke company rules and treated outside patients. Kaiser's later programs would include families, too.[60]

Six Companies afforded their employees this health care by paying health insurance, deducting a $1.50 monthly premium from paychecks.[61] Fifty cents per month covered industrial medicine, in accordance to the Statutes of Nevada and Arizona, and $1 covered nonindustrial medical. The coverage was hardly comprehensive and did not include care at other hospitals. Moreover, it covered only workplace injuries, excluding treatment for mental disorders, venereal diseases, pregnancies, alcoholism, suicide, tuberculosis, preexisting conditions, and infections or diseases contracted within seventy-two hours of employment. The distinction between workplace and off-site injuries became important in defining Six Companies' legal obligations. While the medical coverage certainly helped maintain worker health, it was also useful in workmen's compensation and employer liability suits. Six Companies' health insurance provisions also demonstrated its commitment to offering employees just enough coverage to keep federal regulators off its back. As a whole, building and maintaining a medical facility was a very lucrative venture. During its operation, the contractor reported a profit of more than $25,000.[62]

As an added bonus to workers, academic researchers from Harvard University augmented the project's occupational health regime. Since heat felled so many workers in the summer of 1931, a research team from the Harvard Fatigue Laboratory traveled to Boulder City to study the relationship between the physical performance and heart rate of the human body, and external temperature. The researchers included Dr. David Bruce Dill, later of the Desert Research Institute (DRI) in Las Vegas. According to Dill, the Laboratory "quite naturally was devoted to fatigue," focusing on the physiological and applied physiological and sociological components of the human body.[63]

Prior to the construction of Hoover Dam, the Harvard Fatigue Laboratory had conducted studies at the Panama Canal and in Leadville, Colorado, studying tropical heat and high altitudes. Both studies tested working conditions, heat and humidity, and the reduction of efficiency. After learning that thirteen workers died from heat complications in 1931, Dill persuaded his colleagues to begin a new study focusing on high and dry temperatures, contacting Wilbur to make the necessary arrangements. During graduate school, Dill befriended

Wilbur, using the relationship "as an opening" to conduct the study. His connection paid off. After gaining approval from Mead, Wilbur authorized the research venture.[64]

Ten researchers arrived in June 1932 and set up shop in the municipal building basement in Boulder City. Reclamation assigned each a cabin, army cot, and stove for cooking, and instructed them to eat meals in the Anderson mess hall, paying $0.35 a day for boarding and meals. The team consisted of clinical investigators and doctors, one of which was Dr. J. H. Talbott. Talbott established a close relationship with Wales Haas, studying heat cramps among admitted workers at the hospital and conducting experiments on workers, dogs, and himself. The researchers were primarily interested in the effects of consuming large amounts of water, and the process of adapting to the desert climate. They concluded that the hard labor, high external temperatures, and sweating produced fatigue, and that the first three days of work were a crucial period of acclimation. In "Physiological Responses to High Environmental Temperature," published by the *American Journal of Tropical Medicine*, the researchers cited that workers with "physical deficiencies" and "poor mental stamina" typically quit the project. Those who survived usually continued indefinitely because their individual cardiovascular system could withstand the heat. Deaths occurred when workers lacked a "balance of electrolytes, particularly the loss of sodium chloride," which their body could not replace.[65]

After the researchers' arrival, a medic named Cornelius Van Zwalenburg discovered that administering salt supplements prevented heat exhaustion. Dill was credited for the discovery, but he denied discovering the breakthrough. By the early 1930s, most academic medical centers recognized that human beings needed to consume salt to endure high temperatures. But the practice was not common in American industry. In Europe, it was empirically known: German mill workers had added salt to their beer for generations. They drank a lot of beer, so heat-related deaths were rare. Arriving in Boulder City, the researchers came "fully prepared to look for salt deficiency," according to Dill. They found that heat exhaustion occurred not because of lost body fluids, but rather due to salt excretion in sweat. After confirming the findings, the researchers told Haas to instruct workers to consume a half tablespoon of salt daily. In the mess hall, the doctor posed a sign reading: "THE DOCTOR SAYS TO DRINK PLENTY OF WATER." Dill remembered Talbott writing underneath it: "AND PUT PLENTY OF SALT ON YOUR FOOD." Haas also directed workers to acclimate their bodies to the environment prior to beginning work. Six Companies obliged with the new recommendations, placing salt dispensers and sanitized water stations throughout the site. The Anderson Brothers also began adding more salt to its food.[66]

The changes drastically reduced deaths and hospitalizations during the summer of 1932. The researchers found that salt and a good night's sleep led to improved worker health, and concluded that heat cramps fell into three general categories. First, most workers were not properly acclimated to the environment, and salt concentrations decreased in those who had experience working in the desert. Second, many participated in weekend binges and did a lot of drinking and not eating in Las Vegas, depriving themselves of electrolytes. Third, some people naturally excrete more salt than others. The improved living conditions, sanitized drinking water, and acclimation to the desert climate were all crucial to the reduction of heat-related illnesses. But the real reason the heat did not produce worker deaths in 1932 was milder temperatures than the previous summer. A smaller turnover rate also helped Six Companies retain workers in good cardiovascular shape and acclimated to the environment.[67]

Over the following decade, these findings went far toward protecting American workers. Even though the idea of administering salt supplements was not unique to the project, the Harvard Fatigue Laboratory published its findings, informing the entire industrial medicine and hygiene community. The research appeared in several medical and scientific journals, including the *American Journal of Tropical Study* and the *Journal of Clinical Investigation*. It is also noteworthy that despite the initial apathy of Six Companies and Reclamation to health and safety, the Boulder Canyon Project managed, through scientific research, medical expertise, and a public–private partnership, to drastically improve industrial hygiene conditions within a year.

After Franklin D. Roosevelt assumed the presidency in 1933, his New Deal augmented the occupational health regime. Unlike his predecessor, Secretary of Interior Harold Ickes had no affection for Six Companies. He actively supported a federal investigation into the contractor's adherence to the eight-hour-day provision of their contract, eventually assigning a penalty for $100,000.[68]

Under the direction of Francis Perkins, the DOL also expanded federal involvement in the project's labor standards. However, it did not mandate universal labor standards for all American industries. DOL activity during the 1930s provided standards to clarify its role as an advocate for workers but did not assume control, seeking to promote action at the state level. In 1935 it evaluated safety at the dam, concluding what was well known about the project. Six Companies made little use of organized accident prevention, investigation, analysis, and effective safety programs. The DOL report recommended that the contractor keep detailed reports and investigate major disabling accidents, appoint a full-time safety engineer, and enforce the eight-hour law better. The DOL ultimately determined that deaths and accidents on the project were considerably higher than justified, but noted that no major catastrophes or serious failures occurred after 1932.[69]

Of course, Six Companies' health and safety program cannot take sole credit for the decrease in large-scale disasters. The year 1932 also corresponded with finishing the diversion tunnels and starting the pour of concrete, a considerably less hazardous phase of work.

In the end, New Deal regulations ironed out the project's remaining safety issues. Most importantly, the political environment fostered new interpretations of the law favoring employees in workmen's compensation and employer liability suits. Employee lawsuits against Six Companies met limited success until 1935. Even though workmen's compensation provided workers with compensation regardless of fault, the system continued to display flaws. Courts continued to deny damages to workers to compensate for their injuries, and premium incentives were not enough to force employers to enforce adequate safety improvements. Most employers also actively evaded liability payments to compensate for falling profits.[70]

Six Companies aggressively challenged employer liability on the project, scrutinizing each compensation hearing to pay the least amount possible to workers. The contractor provided workmen's compensation through the NIC and the Arizona Industrial Commission (AIC) funds, which covered injuries occurring on the Nevada and Arizona sides of the dam site, respectively. It also purchased an Employers' Liability Assurance Corporation policy, protecting against worker and third-party injuries on the federal reservation, and covering malpractice claims. For example, when an intoxicated worker struck a pedestrian while driving a company car in 1934, the Employers' Liability Assurance Corporation provided death benefits to the deceased man's family. Many workers also purchased supplemental workmen's compensation policies from aggressive private insurance salesmen who sold policies on the streets of Boulder City and Las Vegas.[71]

The AIC employed a full-time inspector to make safety inspections and represent the state in compensation hearings. The NIC did not provide an investigator until the final year of the project and then only because the DOL required it. In 1934 the AIC and NIC had settled numerous minor compensation cases, with Nevada paying workers seven days after an accident, depending on its seriousness, and Arizona fifteen days. Since Arizona compensated with higher premiums than Nevada, most workers fought hard to claim their injuries happened on the Arizona side. The line between states was often so blurred that crews had to measure it. Six Companies miner Altus "Tex" Nunley recalled such an incident. After a worker died mucking out the center of the dam, it was unclear where the accident happened. Nunley's foreman gave him a tape to measure the location, whispering, "Tex, make it Arizona." He determined that the man died in Arizona, barely.[72]

It did not take long for Six Companies to notice a discrepancy in the figures. Since most of the dam site was within Nevada's borders, the numbers did not add up. The Board of Directors first discussed the problem in 1931, determining a simple solution; it would henceforth employ only single men in Arizona to deter dependent payments. However, the foremen failed to pressure workers to accurately report injuries, and most continued to experience injuries on the Arizona side. As a result, Six Companies' Arizona costs soared. Men regularly dragged a coworker's injured or lifeless body from Nevada to Arizona. Eventually, AIC officials recognized the tactic and refused to approve payments, forcing workers to contest all decisions in court.[73]

Like Six Companies' health insurance plan, workmen's compensation covered only injuries occurring on the dam site. The distinctions between "on-site" and "off-site" injuries, and "at-fault" or "accidental/natural causes" deaths became important to define the contractor's legal obligations. The exact location determined compensation. Six Companies did not cover any off-site injuries or deaths by natural causes. In fact, dependents received benefits for natural causes only if a worker had purchased a private insurance policy. This policy infuriated workers. Most believed that Wales Haas and Richard Schofield listed natural causes to release Six Companies of its legal responsibility. In one case, a worker experienced a blow to the head on the job and died. At the hospital, Schofield listed the cause of death as "complications of spinal meningitis," a non-job-related illness and not compensable. His coworkers were outraged. Suspicious of Schofield's allegiance, they demanded that Clark County coronary officials investigate the death. An autopsy confirmed his findings. Afterward, Schofield issued a statement calling the investigation a vindication, saying that it "finally proved the thoroughness and integrity of the Boulder City Hospital, which in the past has been in question." Still, the workers mistrusted him, certain that he assisted Six Companies in denying damages.[74]

Of course, the contractor was not the only party that resisted compensation. While eager to sell the policies, private insurance carriers rarely compensated workers and their families without a fight. The Mutual Benefit Health and Accident Association regularly contested distributing benefits, citing a violation of contract. The policies contained the clause, "If application has been falsified, the company will only be responsible to return of the premium."[75] This denied coverage to numerous workers. In 1933 Frederick Kassel, a jackhammer operator, purchased a standard form 60W contract from the Mutual Benefit Health and Accident Association. The insurance company considered his occupation standard because he drilled holes for excavation. However, there was one provision. His policy did not cover hazardous operations, including handling explosives or underground mining. When Kassel died during a dynamite accident, insurance agents rejected his family's claim, citing that he misrepresented his profession.

As his widow fought for compensation, she gained an ally: Six Companies and Sims Ely. Eager to not front all the death benefits, Ely and the contractor's insurance department assisted her. Ely charged that it was a "matter of common knowledge" that jackhammers loaded dynamite. E. J. Brockman, manager of Six Companies' Insurance Department, alleged that the company was "willfully evading payment of a just claim," and the policy had been "grossly misrepresented." Six Companies and Ely ultimately helped her win the case; his widow received a death benefit settlement totaling $750.[76]

On a related front, dam workers began to extend the range of employer liability in once-hostile courts, using the carbon monoxide cases to establish a beachhead. As early as 1916 the PHS warned industries about the dangers of carbon monoxide and published guidelines to limit emissions. Several studies also confirmed that cumulative small doses killed or seriously injured humans. In 1921, Yale University's Yendell Henderson carried out scientific experiments in a chamber that gassed human volunteers to study the effects.[77]

In 1931 carbon monoxide was an easily identifiable cause of death, a fact that immediately put Six Companies on the defensive. Even though a Nevada mining law prohibited the operation of gasoline-powered motor vehicles underground, Six Companies used large trucks to haul rock out of the diversion tunnels. The trucks emitted carbon monoxide, which accumulated in the tunnels due to poor ventilation. The company contended that the operation was neither prohibited by Nevada law nor detrimental to workers' health.[78]

Out of the ordeal an ally came to the workers' aid. The state inspector of mines, Andy J. Stinson, knew that operating gasoline-powered trucks underground had deadly consequences.[79] Despite the project's location on Nevada soil, Stinson did not have authority to regulate workplace safety because Wilbur established the project as a federal reservation that was not required to follow state laws. This was an important distinction, because it established a blanket of federal protection for the contractor. Knowing the gravity of the issue, Stinson made his move. On March 25, 1931, legislators authorized him to monitor health and safety at the dam site's tunnels, drifts, and underground excavation. A month later, he inspected Black Canyon, issuing several citations to Six Companies and Reclamation. In most cases, both parties satisfied his recommendations. The gasoline-powered trucks were another story. The tunnels were in the predevelopment phase, but Stinson noticed glaring problems. Six Companies needed to improve ventilation as construction progressed and to provide sanitary water barrels for workers to survive the summer months. Six Companies complied with the requests. Stinson also ordered discontinuation of the plan to use gasoline-powered trucks to haul debris out of the tunnel. The contractor deliberately ignored him, avoiding the recommendation until the state filed formal charges in the fall. Nevada attorney general Gray Mashburn recognized that it was an added expense to the contractor, but it was his job to protect the health and lives of Nevada workers. The situation concerned other state officials as well. Frustrated with Nevada's lack of authority, Governor Fred Balzar vented to the state legislature that it was "impossible to enforce labor and safety laws [on the project and] no decision has been rendered on the matter." Likewise, the already high fatality rate troubled Senator Tasker Oddie, who blamed it on lack of supervision, safety inspections, and poor working conditions. Oddie found it absurd that the federal government would bar a state from enforcing health and safety within its borders. He too wanted to contest the decision, but knew the project would be completed before the courts rendered a decision.[80]

Despite these protests, Six Companies applied for a temporary restraining order against Stinson in November, allowing Crowe to continue constructing the tunnels. The contractor claimed that its contract with Washington, DC, stated that the site was under federal jurisdiction and not subject to state intervention. Nevada therefore lacked all authority to enforce safety laws.[81] Additionally, the statute authorizing Stinson's expanded role violated the Fourteenth Amendment of the U.S. Constitution. A state could not deprive a person of life, liberty, and property without the due process of the law. The statute in question deprived Six Companies of its gasoline-powered trucks without due process and denied equal protection under the law. The contractor argued there was no other "practical method of removing the dirt and rock [and] no reasonable relation" between the trucks and violations in public safety. It consequently requested a writ of injunction to restrain Stinson from enforcement.[82]

The court approved the temporary restraining order and set a trial date for spring 1932. As Crowe's men worked at a feverish pace to finish the tunnels, Six Companies and federal attorneys assembled their defense. The case was truly indicative of the history of industrial hazards in the United States. Very rarely were large-scale, workplace disasters solely caused by private sector wrongdoing. Most cases involved a public–private partnership in which the federal government encouraged and facilitated risky conditions. This was certainly the case at the Hoover Dam and, later, at the nuclear testing at the Nevada Test Site (NTS). Out of the immense pressure to finish the dam on time and provide unemployment relief, the Department of Interior and the Bureau of Reclamation fully supported Six Companies. The federal backing was very advantageous to the contractor. Wilbur and Mead were particularly instrumental, providing important assistance to Six Companies' attorneys. Wilbur was a medical doctor himself, but was ambivalent about the threat of carbon monoxide, citing that any intervention would "hamper the work." He personally contacted the U.S. attorney general William D. Mitchell for help, requesting that he "take…measures [to ensure] the protection of interests of the United States." Mitchell agreed to the job, rendering all possible assistance to Six Companies attorneys. Both Reclamation and U.S. attorneys ultimately served on Six Companies' counsel. While the federal government could not directly interfere with the pending suits, its attorneys appeared amicus curiae, establishing clear boundaries. "It would not be advisable [to the federal counsel]," attorney H. H. Atkinson warned, "to become antagonistic towards the state, [causing] a real [federal versus state] disagreement or dispute."[83] Along with Reclamation's attorney, Richard J. Coffey, Atkinson met with Six Companies' counsel and applied to appear amicus curiae in a statutory court.[84]

The judges granted permission. Next, the attorneys arranged an application for a preliminary injunction based on the following grounds:

1. That the defendants were acting and threatening to act under an unconstitutional statute of the state;
2. That the State of Nevada had ceded exclusive jurisdiction to the United States over the Boulder Canyon Project Federal Reservation;
3. That the United States could not be required to conform to State police regulations in the performance of its functions, and consequently the agents through which it functioned were also immune from state interference.[85]

Finally, the counsel gathered affidavits from expert witnesses. Six Companies' chief engineer, A. H. Ayers, estimated that safety recommendations would cost the company more than $1.5 million, delay work for several months, and force the dismissal of seven hundred workers. Other witnesses contended that the air conditions were clean in the tunnels and did not cause any adverse health effects.[86]

Both sides defended their case to a three-judge panel led by U.S. District Judge Frank Norcross. First, the panel needed to establish if the Department of the Interior created the federal reservation legally, and was subject to state and local taxation. If so, Nevada statutes did not apply. Second, Six Companies' legal team needed to prove that the tunnel conditions did not threaten human health. The contractor's attorneys presented numerous testimonies contending the tunnels were perfectly safe. Ayers presented the first affidavit, describing the tunnels as unusually large and reporting that the contractor exercised diligent care to ensure proper ventilation.[87]

Next, two chemical engineers, L. H. Duschak and Philip Samuel Williams, revealed the adequacy of the ventilating system and the volume of air moving in the tunnels. Both conducted extensive tests to determine if the truck operations were injurious to worker health. Duschak found two sources of carbon monoxide in the tunnels: motor exhaust and powder smoke from dynamite blasts. The degree of exposure varied based on air currents and a worker's location, however. Overall, he found a "natural circulation in the large tunnels" that introduced fresh air throughout the tunnel. Additionally, high temperatures forced the exhaust to rise to the "upper stream of the outgoing air" and naturally diffuse. Wind conditions and fans also improved ventilation. Out of fifty-eight tests, forty-eight revealed no carbon monoxide. Regarding the remaining ten, it was found that presence of the gas was due to a recent blast, but that the concentrations were "momentary." He concluded that the carbon monoxide exposure was "not sufficient" to harm human health and there was a "fair margin of safety."[88]

Williams's findings were similar; he found the ventilation to be "perfectly satisfactory" and there was "no physical reason why absolute safety from carbon monoxide 'poisoning' should not be maintained throughout the job." E. J. Brockman, head of the Six Companies insurance division, also testified that the contractor maintained a "fully equipped safety department" with the latest carbon monoxide detectors, and there were no past or present cases of carbon monoxide poisoning reported to their department. Finally, several employees working at various tunnel positions attested to the cleanliness of the tunnels. All of them stated they had never experienced injurious effects or discomfort from the presence of carbon monoxide. Six Companies' counsel concluded by acknowledging that carbon monoxide was a dangerous industrial hazard, but the tunnels did not contain enough concentrations to harm human health.[89]

The extensive case presented by the Six Companies legal team surprised Nevada's attorneys. They assumed that the hearing would cover only the facts set forth in the affidavits by the respective parties. The state scrambled to present a counterargument, offering several affidavits to contradict Six Companies' story. Led by Mashburn, Deputy Attorney W. T. Matthews, and District Attorney Harley Harmon of Clark County, the Nevada counsel contended that Six Companies had put themselves in this situation. Nevada's mining laws were well-known, enacted well before the project began. Still, the contractor purchased the trucks, "arbitrarily, if not contemptuously" ignoring the law. Since the temporary restraining order, it continued operating the trucks underground. The "great delay" ultimately risked the health of the workers. The state charged that Six Companies rushed to finish the tunnels to make safety "a moot question." Moreover, the statute was not unreasonable; it was a viable measure to protect workers that would cost only $150,000 to rectify. The counsel stressed that American law existed to safeguard the lives of its citizens, because corporations existed for profits. Finally, the existing ventilation system was not enough to protect workers from the deadly effects of carbon monoxide. The use of gasoline also increased the risk of fire and explosions. They alleged Six Companies failed to report dangerously high levels on "at least two occasions" and pointed out other inconsistencies in their case, stressing that even a few breaths of carbon monoxide could be "fatal, or at least, very dangerous to man." In fact, the American Engineering and Industrial Standards banned its use in all mining regulations, which prompted Nevada to enact the statute. Clearly, carbon monoxide fostered unsafe working conditions and it was imperative that the state intervene. Nevada wanted the Boulder Canyon Project to thrive, but it was at a terrible cost.[90]

The judges ultimately ruled in favor of Six Companies, stating that the Department of the Interior had legally established the federal reservation and that, under the terms of the injunction, Nevada could not enforce its labor laws or inspect site conditions. However, Six Companies agreed not to operate gasoline-powered trucks underground to a greater depth than 250 feet, satisfying provisions in the Nevada statute. Several months later, the judges ruled in favor of the contractor again, making the injunction permanent. They deemed that Nevada mining laws were not applicable to constructing a dam, but only in the mining industry. The judges also found parts of the Mining Inspector Act unconstitutional, ruling that the state had no jurisdiction over any aspect of the project. Stinson attempted to pass a rewritten bill in 1933, but legislators defeated it, deeming it a lost cause.[91]

Back at the dam site, Six Companies ensured it took every precaution to safeguard its employees' lives, claiming that the gas levels were similar to traffic tunnels like New York's Holland Tunnel. Crowe also publicly proclaimed that he "would rather take a loss of $100,000 than to hurt one man."[92]

But the tunnels were not safe, and hundreds of workers were dead, sick, and dying from carbon monoxide poisoning. Christopher Sellers and Joseph Melling have articulated that the worst hazards accumulate at the "neglected edges" of an industrial hazard regime, usually when "actors, actions and consequences [were] ignored or underestimated by authorities on a particular time and place."[93] In the case of Hoover Dam, the public–private partnership between Reclamation and Six Companies understood the risk of the summer heat in 1931 and operating gasoline-powered trucks underground, but considered the goals of Boulder Canyon Project more important than any potential loss of human life. Gambling with their employees' lives, both believed the majority could survive the heat without suffering great losses and could avoid a significant disaster if the tunnels were completed quickly.

This faulty reasoning caused the worst disaster on the project, but also helped force historic change. Because of labor militancy on the issue, laissez-faire eventually yielded to compensation and regulation for carbon monoxide victims; the workers felled by heat during the summer of 1931 would never be vindicated. But the process took time. By the mid-1930s employer liability had become increasingly easier to prove in the courts, especially among well-known workplace diseases like carbon monoxide poisoning and silicosis. At the same time, tighter government regulations during the New Deal facilitated successful employer liability lawsuits, and personal injury lawyers began to push judges to determine employer liability for ailments excluded from workers' compensation. In 1933 157 lawsuits sought $4 million in damages for silicosis victims involved in the Hawk's Nest tunnel disaster in Gauley Bridge, West Virginia. After jury tampering and fraud, the group ended up settling for only $130,000. But the workers continued to fight, taking a test case to the Supreme Court. They lost, settling for a fraction of the sum, but the Rinehart and Dennis Company's negligence garnered significant national attention. In 1936 a subcommittee of the U.S. House of Representatives held a hearing to investigate the disaster, prompting *Time* and *Newsweek* to publish numerous exposés on the incident. The subcommittee concluded that the contractor completed the tunnel with "grave and inhuman disregard of all consideration for the health, lives, and future of the employees" and that its "negligence was either willful or the result of inexcusable and indefensible ignorance." Regardless, little progress occurred to stop silicosis exposure in the American workplace. Congress denied funding to study the industrial disease, and punitive action was never taken against the Rinehart and Dennis Company.[94]

Unlike the Hawk's Nest victims, the carbon monoxide cases at Hoover Dam represented a victory for workers, and set a crucial precedent for future employer liability suits. In 1933 several Six Companies employees decided to sue for damages. Their attorney, Harry Austin, filed six personal injury lawsuits, seeking $77,186 in damages for permanent ailments. The cases sparked a media firestorm. Austin alleged that Six Companies failed to protect the health and safety of their employees, forcing them to inhale high concentrations of carbon monoxide and suffer significant bodily harm. *Ed F. Kraus v. Six Companies Inc.* was the first case to go to trial, involving Ed Kraus, a thirty-four-year-old truck driver who hauled debris from the tunnels. Kraus testified that he lost twenty-six pounds, and suffered from headaches, chills, and nausea while working in the tunnels. Since his time at work he experienced weakness, blurred vision, and loss of sexual desire. He described the exhaust fumes in the tunnels as so thick that he could not see the truck's electric lights. Other workers testified in his defense, describing a blue cloud of gas drifting out of the tunnels each afternoon. They testified that they regularly retreated because of gas-related nausea and dizziness. Instead of settling out of court, Six Companies decided make an example of him. It was the most sensational trial Las Vegas had ever seen. Six Companies' attorneys retained local attorneys Leo and Frank McNamee, and San Francisco-based trial lawyer Jerome White. The team argued that Kraus's symptoms were caused by extreme heat, preexisting conditions, and illicit lifestyle choices. They also interviewed workers that testified the air quality was acceptable to breathe and reached hazardous levels only a few times.[95]

The most telling parts of the trial were the physician testimonies regarding the origins of Kraus's health issues, revealing the changing role of medical professionals and their relationship with their employers and the law. In the early twentieth century doctors emerged as important expert witnesses in personal injury cases, facing no greater challenge to the Hippocratic Oath. Should doctors side with their employers, who pay their salary, or with their patients, who they swore to protect? The cases put them in an uncomfortable position. The law required objectivity, but it was difficult for doctors to give fair medical testimonies without prejudice. Of course, claims of neutrality were also self-serving. While it is impossible to know if employers influenced their company doctor's diagnosis, the high number of workers complaining of dishonesty suggests the practice was very common.[96]

Two points were clear about Six Companies' physicians. First, Wales Haas and Richard Schofield fostered a legal environment conducive to out-of-court settlements. The settlements were in the best interest of their patients, because Depression-era workers rarely won large settlements. Most received nothing at all. Second, most company physicians struggled to define their professional role in the framework of conflicting obligations to employers and patients. The logical outcome was to diagnose fraud. This was the case with Six Companies' physicians. Schofield described the medico-legal aspect of industrial medicine as the foreground of his job, and said that it played an intimate role in blocking the workers' attempts to establish a legal claim. His job proved that disabilities were not connected with employment, and the best defense of a company was to maintain detailed records, documenting the workers' schedules, first aid visits, medication, hospital entries, and other data. Schofield called the reports "a necessary part of the original industrial medical set-up." At the end of the project, he compiled the data and studied them, analyzing them for any "interesting facts, figures, and statistics" for future jobs.[97]

Most likely Haas and Schofield concealed cases of carbon monoxide poisoning out of the effort to diagnose fraud for their employer, a key part of their job description. As shown by Mark Aldrich, physicians struggled to define their professional role in the framework of conflicting obligations to patients and employers during this period of occupational health history. The logical outcome for company doctors was to focus on diagnosing fraud for their employer in exchange for a paycheck. Employers during the 1930s hired medical experts for two reasons, both of which saved them money. In the short term, diagnosing fraud was advantageous to employers in liability suits. In the long term, company doctors helped reduce labor turnover, eventually maintaining a healthy, productive workforce.[98]

Since dam construction took up to five years, Six Companies instructed its doctors to prioritize diagnosing fraud. Out of the effort to protect their employer, it is possible that Haas and Schofield purposely misdiagnosed patients as having pneumonia or tuberculosis instead of carbon monoxide poisoning. Indeed, the diseases displayed similar symptoms. During the Stinson trial, Haas testified that J. C. Bowles, a tunnel shovel operator, had the "long-standing disease tuberculosis" that he had contracted prior to employment. Haas denied that carbon monoxide caused or exasperated his symptoms. Bowles's ailments resulted from "a germ," he said, and nothing more. But Haas also testified that Bowles had "irritated tissues of the lungs," a symptom of carbon monoxide poisoning. When Nevada attorneys asked why his preemployment exam did not reveal the disease, Haas presumed that Bowles falsified his medical history. Physical examinations by company doctors, he insisted, were sensory, "based upon the statement of the applicant himself" describing health conditions and past history. It would "not be likely" that an examining physician would discover tuberculosis unless a patient directed attention to it. Haas suspected that Bowles lied about his tuberculosis to gain employment. With 100 percent medical certainty, Haas concluded that Bowles did not suffer from carbon monoxide poisoning.[99]

Convinced that Haas purposely diagnosed their respiratory problems as "pneumonia" or "tuberculosis" to protect their employer, the workers harbored a considerable amount of bitterness toward the company medical staff. The Boulder City Hospital became a hot topic of discussion among residents, commenting that workers were dying of pneumonia and nothing else. Tex Nunley said that "if they ever got you in the hospital, [the doctors recorded that] you didn't get killed on the job, you just died." The IWW's *Industrial Worker* even publicly accused Haas of purposely diagnosing carbon monoxide poisoning cases as "influenza" and listing "pneumonia" as the cause of death.[100] As explained by the wife of a tunnel inspector, "If you said they died of gasses in the tunnels, they were obligated to compensate you, to compensate the family. They'd say just 'pneumonia' and they'd get by with that. We never felt that was fair."[101]

Of course, there was no way to prove Haas and later Schofield were guilty of wrongdoing. During the Kraus trial the medical expert witnesses disagreed over the cause of his ailments. Dr. H. M. Behneman, a prominent physician from San Francisco, testified that abdominal ptosis, a sagging of internal organs, caused his conditions because of his build, which was tall and angular. Conversely, Drs. Walter Koebig of Los Angeles and J. N. Van Meter of Las Vegas determined that his symptoms were very consistent with extreme carbon monoxide poisoning. Six Companies' counsel ultimately employed unethical techniques to win the case, appointing Bud Bodell to uncover incriminating evidence on Kraus. Bodell hired a petty criminal, Jim Moretti, to lure Kraus to debauchery, drinking, and carousing with women, and engaging in various criminal acts. The testimony did not paint the picture of an ailing man. After spending three months with Kraus, Moretti explained Kraus's great health, his multiple sexual encounters with a prostitute named Merle, his use of counterfeit money, and his engagement in blackmail, robbery, and production of bootleg whiskey. Most importantly, Kraus admitted to Moretti that working in the tunnels had not impaired him and that he could "look pretty sick for $76,000." With this testimony, a jury declared the case a mistrial.[102]

The following year Austin took another case to court, *Jack Norman v. Six Companies Inc.* Like Kraus, Norman claimed that carbon monoxide poisoning from the tunnels left him physically impaired. But compared to Kraus, Norman was an honorable family man and was not corruptible. Six Companies' counsel bribed at least three jurors, forcing another mistrial. Even though Austin lost both, he continued to file suits. The cases mounted until August 1935, with forty-eight plaintiffs seeking $4.6 million in damages pending in Nevada courts. Due to the growing number of cases and the project nearing completion, Six Companies finally accepted defeat. In January 1936 Austin settled out of court and the contractor distributed an undisclosed amount to fifty plaintiffs.[103]

The civil trials were a huge embarrassment for Reclamation. When Austin requested tunnel inspection reports from September 1931 to

October 1932, officials worried about the implications. If there was "just cause for criticism of the working conditions," R. F. Walter wrote to Elwood Mead, they "must share the blame." In the effort to save their reputation, Reclamation decided to deny the request, writing, "While not admitting that such was one, [we risk exposing the records] to the scrutiny of partisan attorneys." In the end, the dam's carbon monoxide cases were a significant milestone for labor, exposing that it was much cheaper for the public and private sector to embrace health and safety in the workplace. While it took several more decades for the notion of responsibility to solidify, it was progress nevertheless.[104]

Of course, not all suits brought by Six Companies' employees were successful, particularly those concerning medical malpractice. Like other legal issues, the American malpractice phenomenon reflected the nation's political, social, cultural, and professional trends. Medicolegal writings rarely referred to malpractice during the nineteenth century; patients usually sued for breach of contract. Malpractice cases were also rare because the legal profession had not defined it yet. Most lawyers used William Blackstone's *Commentaries*, describing malpractice as an injury due to neglect or the poor management of the medical profession.[105]

After courts became willing to accredit malpractice decisions in the 1840s, the rate intensified. Technological advances in the medical profession also prompted newspapers to market malpractice suits as solutions to medical wrongdoing. By the turn of the century, the tenet of malpractice shifted from contract disputes to tortious liability actions. *Pike v. Honsinger* (1898) established a guideline for American physicians and medical liability, and decisions thereafter became founded on the legal definition of a standard of care.[106] The central definition remained consistent throughout the twentieth century. Other issues changed, including amendments of tort law, interpretations of joint liability, and general court procedures.[107]

During the 1930s public awareness of malpractice had dramatically increased. Knowing the risk, physicians and hospitals started purchasing a new form of insurance that gave them monetary protection from malpractice suits. Six Companies insured itself through the Employers' Liability Group, and Richard Schofield acquired a personalized plan to cover his practice. At the same time, medical journals began publishing information on how to avoid suits by improving record keeping. As such, defensive medicine and attempts to block suits brought the role of professional experts to the forefront of the profession. Still, suing for malpractice did not become a widespread tool to receive compensation for medical mishaps until the late 1960s. Throughout the 1930s and 1940s, major news organizations only occasionally covered malpractice suits. Malpractice did not garner public attention until the 1950s because Americans viewed the practice of medicine as one evolving clinical trial. To cure their conditions, patients simply had to accept the risk that medicine might fail.[108]

At the dam project, Haas and Schofield experienced their share of malpractice allegations, but they rarely went to trial. However, one case involving Oscar Allbritton, a sixty-six-year-old black steel worker, resulted in a malpractice legal battle that ended only after his death. The case highlights Six Companies' management of workers sustaining injuries off site and the treatment of minorities in its health-care system, as well as emerging interpretations of medical malpractice by physicians and the law. On March 13, 1935, Allbritton boarded the Interstate Transit Lines Bus to return to the West Las Vegas slums. While exiting the reservation, bus driver Hal Clements lost control of the steering wheel and overturned the bus, which hurled Allbritton from his seat. The impact crushed his skull, but he remained conscious until an ambulance arrived. As stated by Six Companies following the incident, "Under the circumstances surrounding the accident, the employer was not required to furnish medical attention."[109]

The bus overturned three miles from Boulder City and the employee health plan explicitly barred the coverage of off-site injuries. But paramedics could not take them to Las Vegas because, one, the Las Vegas Hospital prohibited the treatment of minorities, and, two, they worried that some workers might not survive the trip to the short-staffed, underdeveloped county hospital. Therefore, the ambulance headed back to town, dropping the patients off at the Boulder City Hospital.[110]

Schofield examined "about twenty" injured workers. In Allbritton's chart, he noted that he was dazed, confused, and complained of a "terrible headache," determining that his patient suffered from shock. However, there were no major abrasions or swellings to his head, face, scalp, or neck. Allbritton also complained of pain in his left shoulder, but Schofield resolved that "no gross deformity [could be] seen nor noted though clothes were not removed." He decided to hospitalize him, assuming Allbritton "probably [had] a slight concussion." The next morning, Allbritton's headache was gone, but he had pain throughout body, back, left shoulder, knees, and feet. Still, Schofield decided to discharge him. In his chart, he wrote that his patient suffered from contusions, but no fractures, dislocations, or bone injuries. All concussion signs also disappeared and were "only subjective immediately after injury." Although Allbritton was not satisfied with the diagnosis, Schofield determined that it was "the effects of nervous reaction or mild shock" and uneasiness due to "negro characteristics." After discharging him, Schofield advised to seek additional treatment with Dr. Hale Slavin at the county hospital.[111]

Allbritton pleaded with the doctor to look further into his condition, but Schofield sent him away. He left the hospital in "excruciating pain and agony" and sought out Slavin. Slavin immediately referred him to a specialist in Los Angeles, but he could not get an appointment until April 22. After the examination, Allbritton underwent emergency brain surgery. He never fully recovered. Partially blind, deaf, and paralyzed, Allbritton was convinced that Schofield unjustifiably discharged him, which aggravated his injuries. The accident and questionable medical care ultimately left him permanently disabled, unable to perform physical labor and support himself. Believing that the bus company, Six Companies, and Schofield had all wronged him, he hired a Los Angeles–based attorney, J. S. Manning, to sue for damages.

When Six Companies learned of the case, the board did not take it seriously. Their counsel watched as *Allbritton v. Union Pacific* pended in the U.S. District Court in Los Angeles, commenting that it was "quite likely" the case would "die of a natural death" and "no suit be filed." Under these circumstances, Six Companies decided to "close out the file under these circumstances without payment."[112] But the case did not disappear. In December 1935 a jury awarded $25,000 in damages to Allbritton against the Interstate Transit Lines, later dismissing the charges against the UPRR and bus driver. Since he needed $150,000 to cover his injuries, Allbritton's counsel decided to move forward with a malpractice claim against Six Companies and Schofield. On March 11, 1937, they filed a complaint against Six Companies, the Boulder City Hospital, and Schofield in the Eighth Judicial District Court of Nevada. The lawsuit alleged that the Boulder City Hospital handled Allbritton's case "negligently, carelessly, unskillfully, and unprofessionally," which left him "totally disabled." Allbritton sought $50,000 in damages.[113]

Six Companies' tone changed and it retained Leo McNamee to issue a demurrer challenging the case. During preparation, McNamee explored his options. He contemplated defaming Allbritton. The Employers' Liability Group, who insured Six Companies its malpractice insurance, found a local "negro woman named Mrs. Turner" that alleged Allbritton "did not sustain a serious injury" in the accident because he had "a previous injury to his head."[114] McNamee later dismissed the notion after determining the claim would not hold up in court. He ultimately argued that Allbritton's permanent injuries were a result of the accident, not Six Companies' negligence. Moreover, Schofield did not cause damages through malpractice, the complaint was ambiguous, and it merited immediate dismissal. McNamee also attempted to remove the case on the grounds of diversity of citizenship.[115] But since Allbritton and Schofield were both California residents, the judge determined that the case could not move to federal court.[116]

The case continued without resolution throughout the 1930s. In California an appellate court reversed the judgment against Interstate Transit Line, ordering a new trial. This stalled the malpractice case. McNamee attempted to terminate it under a Nevada statute, but the motion was denied. However, Allbritton did not give up. In 1942 he hired a new legal team and served an amended complaint. McNamee responded by filing another demurrer. One of the most interesting features of this case is that it reveals how Depression-era employers avoided medical liability and the ambitious, multifaceted role of retaining a company physician. When hiring Schofield, Six Companies purposely did not draft a formal contract. It was therefore unclear whether the doctor was an agent of the company or an independent contractor. Instead, Six Companies employed him under the verbal agreement that it would "furnish all insurances to him and the hospital." Schofield had personal malpractice insurance, but it did not cover his work at the Six Companies Hospital. The doctor was under the impression that Six Companies would "take care of it." Since Schofield was free to engage in private practice and treat nonemployees, McNamee argued that he was an independent contractor whose malpractice had no liability attached to the company.[117]

Another interesting aspect of the Allbritton case is that it defined the role of a company hospital during the 1930s. Was it a charitable enterprise or a for-profit? Company records indicated that the Boulder City Hospital was a for-profit; during its operations up to February 29, 1936, it showed an operating profit before income taxes of $25,321.26.[118] Therefore, McNamee argued that the hospital was ultra vires, or beyond the scope of Six Companies' corporate powers, due to the large number of deductions made from project employees.[119] Under this approach, the contractor's corporate charter issued by Reclamation had the limited purpose of furnishing heath care, but not managing it. Since the hospital was a for-profit, it was not technically part of the corporation. According to the original charter, it was "possible to distinguish the hospital corporation cases," because it was organized to secure "all necessary equipment and service for the treatment of patients." Since medical services were a "necessary incident," Six Companies was not liable. On the management side, Schofield claimed that he knew nothing about the hospital's financial condition; his duties included furnishing medical expertise, bookkeeping, and reporting expenses to Six Companies. The company paid the bills. He also stated that he had no knowledge of the deductions paid by employees toward hospitalization or medical treatment, or whether the hospital operated as a for-profit. The arrangement is indicative of early forms of company-run health-care programs. Until the 1950s corporations and company physicians could accept the benefits of a contract, and later refuse employer and malpractice liability on the grounds that it was ultra vires.[120]

The outcome of this case matched most allegations of company doctor malpractice during the 1930s and 1940s. Allbritton never received a settlement. Six Companies successfully delayed the case until his death in 1948. Upon hearing the news of Allbritton's death, McNamee contacted Allbritton's attorneys and prepared a motion to dismiss the $50,000 suit, citing a Nevada statute that trials needed to occur within five years after plaintiffs filed an action.[121]

In the end, the occupational health regime that coalesced at the Boulder Canyon Project had mixed results. Although a memorial plaque at the Hoover Dam sets the number of workers killed during its construction at ninety-six, the real figure was almost double that. An analysis of fatality records kept by Reclamation and Six Companies indicates that as many as 187 workers died working on the project, maybe more. The discrepancy exists because the reports did not account for "pneumonia" victims poisoned by carbon monoxide or fatalities of employees not "officially" working. It is also impossible to gauge how many workers died after the project was completed. The work left many men physically disabled the rest of their lives. Allbritton's death was due to complications of an off-site accident, twelve years after the fact. Of course, the statistics also omitted fatalities associated with disease outbreaks, including Eugene Schaver's questionable demise due to spinal meningitis, and the heat-related deaths of family members at Ragtown or oblivious tourists visiting the work site.[122]

While the Hoover Dam is known for its treacherous working conditions and high death count, one popular myth is inaccurate. There were no workers buried alive in the dam. The myth contends that workers fell into the cofferdams, and their coworkers, unable to stop the rapid concrete pour, watched as it submerged and suffocated them. This theory is untrue; the forms were too short to physically submerge a human body. While several men fell into the concrete and died on impact, they were immediately jackhammered out. According to Six Companies employee Bob Parker, there is a possibility that the remains of a man who drowned in the river ended up in the lower cofferdam before they laid concrete. There is no way to know if this is true. Despite firm denial by historians, Reclamation, and Six Companies, popular memory reinforces the story. Since the project's hazardous conditions have become folklore, it seems fitting for Hoover Dam to serve as a coffin of the workers who built it. In many ways, the myth is more compelling than historical fact.[123]

While the construction of Hoover Dam resulted in the loss of hundreds of lives and countless permanent disabilities, the project also represents significant advances in industrial health during the 1930s. Aside from its unrecognized value as a jobs program, bringing needed stimulus to the fledgling Las Vegas economy, and its status as one of the man-made wonders of the world, Hoover Dam set a crucial standard for future New Deal–era public works jobs. In this scenario, no reform movement forced the safety issue. As a high-profile project, bad publicity from 1931 to 1932 forced Reclamation and Six Companies to undertake health and safety reforms. The improvements would have been rejected in earlier decades and in less desolate locations. The actions provided momentum and support for a later generation of advocates seeking to convince Congress, the states, the judiciary, and a growing number of employers to prioritize safety in the workplace. In the rapidly changing environment of the Great Depression, Six Companies also had to endorse health and safety to enhance its corporate image and save money.[124]

One of the most significant features of the Boulder Canyon Project's occupational health regime is its impact on future New Deal–era programs. Throughout the 1930s, public works projects replicated Six Companies' industrial health program. After it completed Hoover Dam, the Six Companies conglomerate built Parker Dam, and several members went on to help construct the Golden Gate Bridge and the San Francisco–Oakland Bay Bridge. The contractors applied important lessons learned from Hoover Dam, such as organizing and controlling a large workforce in an isolated location, and providing a workplace safety and medical infrastructure to encourage an efficient and healthy workforce. When Roosevelt authorized the Bonneville, Grand Coulee, and Fort Peck Dams under the National Industrial Recovery Act, the contractors had little time to focus on design work, or on health and safety planning. The president stressed that they needed to provide jobs as soon as possible to unemployed Americans. Accordingly, some engineering designs were constructed from precedent and not innovation. At Fort Peck the rush job resulted in a partial collapse in 1938. But no dam project after Hoover Dam experienced major crises in health and safety. All contractors that built dams in remote locations provided workers with decent housing, food, hospital services, and health insurance. As a moral and monetarily costly cautionary tale, no contractor operated gasoline-powered trucks underground to construct its diversion tunnels. While some Fort Peck workers lived in shantytowns, the situation did not rival the arduous conditions of Ragtown and River Camp. As historians David Billington and Donald Jackson have shown, Hoover Dam is a symbol of the twentieth century just as the Brooklyn Bridge is for the nineteenth.[125] Hoover Dam played a crucial and important role in western growth by appropriating water and power resources to the region. However, the dam also symbolized a new approach to health and safety, marking the beginning of a transformation in notions of employer and government responsibility. By the end of the decade, most companies had voluntarily established industrial health programs, but the system was about to get challenged during an unprecedented, national effort to mobilize for war.[126]

## NOTES

1. During the 1920s most employers deemed unions un-American and adopted "the American plan," a strategy to deter union membership. An "open shop" referred to places of employment that did not require union membership, while a "yellow dog contract" was an oath between employer and employee in which an employee agreed to not remain in or join a union during employment.

2. Andrew Kolin, *Political Economy of Labor Repression in the United States* (Lanham, MD: Lexington Books, 2017).

3. Memorandum for the Solicitor, Dec. 14, 1931, RG 48 Records of the Department of Interior, Office of the Interior, Los Angeles, Boulder Canyon Project Files, Box 4, File 1.4.6.1 General: Legal: Litigation: Six Companies Inc. Suit 1930–31 Part I, National Archives and Records Administration [hereafter NARA], National Archives at Riverside.

4. See Michael Hiltzik, *Colossus: The Turbulent, Thrilling Saga of the Building of Hoover Dam* (New York: Free Press, 2010); and Joseph E. Stevens, *Hoover Dam: An American Adventure* (Norman and London: University of Oklahoma Press, 1988) for comprehensive coverage of Hoover Dam history. See also Guy Louis Rocha, "The I.W.W. and the Boulder Canyon Project: The Death Throes of American Syndicalism," in *At the Point of Production: The Local History of the I.W.W.*, ed. Joseph R. Conlin (Westport, CT: Greenwood Press, 1981), 214–17, 221–22; R. T. King, *Hoover Dam and Boulder City, 1931-1936: A Discussion Among Some Who Were There* (Reno: Oral History Project [hereafter OHP], University of Nevada, 1987); "Fatalities—Boulder Canyon Project: Accidental Deaths on the Job," Frank "Doc" Johnson Papers, 1 of 5, Boulder City Museum and Historical Association (hereafter BCMHA) SC; and Stevens, *Hoover Dam*, 249–50 for a discussion on the vagaries of fate.

5. The name "Six Companies" was an allusion to the Chinese Six Companies, a mutual coordination of six groups in San Francisco serving as an unofficial

government for Chinese immigrants. Since Six Companies employed the majority of workers and had the most obligations, all contractors will be referred to as Six Companies in this chapter unless otherwise specified. See "Certificate of Incorporation: Six Companies Incorporated," Feb. 18, 1931; Minutes of Adjourned Meeting of the Board of Directors, Feb. 25, 1931; Minutes of Special Meeting of the Board of Directors, Mar. 5, 1931; all in Six Companies Corporate Records, Vol. 1, Bancroft Library, University of California, Berkeley (hereafter Bancroft); Hiltzik, *Colossus*, 172–75.

6. Markowitz and Rosner, *"Slaves of the Depression,"* 3; "They Court Disaster," *Evening Review-Journal,* Feb. 11, 1930 (incl. "probably the most," "a decidedly close," and "courting disaster").

7. "Wide Open Las Vegas Recalls Hectic Scenes of Old West," *Phoenix Arizona Republic,* May 14, 1931 (incl. "bonanza days").

8. Wilson, "Hoover Dam," *New Republic,* Sept. 2, 1931 (incl. "battlefield").

9. Theodore White, "Building the Big Dam," *Harper's Magazine* 171 (June 1935) (incl. "a bowl," 115); Duncan Aikman, "A Wild West Town that is Born Tame," *New York Times Magazine* (Jul. 26, 1931) (incl. "furnace-like winds"). For more on the journalists' reaction to Las Vegas and the federal reservation in 1930-1931, see Stevens, *Hoover Dam,* 52–53; Six Companies Corporate Records, Vol. 7, Oversize Folder, Bancroft, which contains numerous newspaper clippings regarding the conditions in Las Vegas, the dam site, and other information pertaining to the project.

10. "Information to Applicants for Employment at Boulder Dam: Boulder Canyon Project," June 1, 1933, Cahlan Collection, Box 5, Folder 12, NSMA (incl. "financially able"); Stevens, *Hoover Dam,* 50–51.

11. The Great Depression expedited the Boulder Canyon Project. President Herbert Hoover and Secretary of Interior Ray Lyman Wilber pressed Elwood Mead, director of the Bureau of Reclamation, to start the project ahead of schedule. Engineers rushed to complete the project plans and construction began in the spring of 1931, well before Six Companies could build adequate housing for the workers and their families or develop a sufficient health and safety program.

12. "Report of the Commissioner of Labor," *Appendix,* 36th Sess., Vol. 1 (Carson City, NV: SPO, 1933), 12–15; Richard O. Schofield, "Industrial Medicine in Nevada as Practiced in the Construction of Boulder Dam," in Walker, *A Life's Review and Notes,* 89–90.

13. The New Deal brought little improvement for blacks at Hoover Dam. Although Secretary of Interior Harold Ickes was an outspoken advocate of rights of blacks, he could not alter Six Companies' hiring practices or force the contractor to allow minorities to live in Boulder City.

14. For the minority experience at the Boulder Canyon Project, see Roosevelt Fitzgerald, "Blacks and the Boulder Dam Project," *Nevada Historical Society Quarterly* 24 (Fall, 1981), 256; Stevens, *Hoover Dam,* 176–77; Andrew J. Dunbar and Dennis McBride, *Building Hoover Dam: An Oral History of the Great Depression* (Reno: University of Nevada Press, 1993), 140–44, 201, 239, 306–7.

15. Hiltzik, *Colossus,* 216.

16. Schofield, "Industrial Medicine," 91; "Progress Report-May 10 to May 31," Six Companies Corporate Records, Vol. 1, Bancroft; "Information to Applicants," June 1, 1933.

17. Ragtown was located on the floor of Black Canyon. From June to August 1931, the population ranged from 500 to 1,400 residents. After the completion of the dam, the town was submerged under Lake Mead.

18. Minutes of Regular Meeting of Board of Directors, July 20, 1931, Six Companies Corporate Records, Vol. 1, Bancroft (incl. "more difficult" and "higher heat"); John R. McDaniel interview, by Daniel Malloy, Oct. 24, 1974, UNLV SC (incl. "about 130"); Hiltzik, *Colossus*, 222 (incl. "an opaque yellow").

19. McDaniel interview; Hiltzik, *Colossus*, 216, 222; Rocha, "The I.W.W.," 216; Stevens, *Hoover Dam*, 54; Paul L. Kleinsorge, *The Boulder Canyon Project: Historical and Economic Aspects* (Palo Alto, CA: Stanford University Press, 1941), 206, 222.

20. The contractor revised the workers' schedules to shifts from 4 A.M. until noon and 4 P.M. until midnight, working with searchlights. Six Companies simply could not afford to lose any more workers to the afternoon heat. See Six Companies Inc., "Summary of Fatalities by Employers—Boulder Canyon Project—To and Including July 31, 1935," Frank "Doc" Jensen Papers, 1 of 5, BCMHA SC (incl. "accidents sustained"); "Second Victim of Heat Dies Here Last Eve," *Review-Journal*, June 29, 1931; King, *Hoover Dam and Boulder City*, 4; Minutes of Regular Meeting of Board of Directors, July 20, 1931, Six Companies Corporate Records, Vol. 1, Bancroft; "Meningitis Rumor At Dam Denied," *Review-Journal*, Sept. 28, 1931; "Dam Worker Has Spinal Meningitis," *Review-Journal*, Oct. 7, 1931; "Dam Worker Dies at Local Hospital," *Review-Journal*, Oct. 8, 1931; "Mahoney Meningitis," *Review-Journal*, Jan. 27, 1932. Six Companies and Reclamation's classification of fatalities sustained during the project found in "Summary of Fatalities."

21. For scholarship on health care at Hoover Dam, see Hiltzik, *Colossus*, 168-69, 260, 282, 285, 341-42; Stevens, *Hoover Dam*, 60-69, 103-7, 132-41, 157-58, 164-69, 200, 205-14; Dennis McBride, *In the Beginning: A History of Boulder City, Nevada* (Boulder City, NV: BCMHA, 1992), 36-39; Dunbar and McBride, *Building Hoover Dam*, 37, 129-34, 242-44, 261-64, 321; Rocha, "The I.W.W.," 214-17, 221-22; appropriate sections of King, *Hoover Dam and Boulder City*.

22. Ray Lyman Wilbur to Postmaster General, Jan. 21, 1931, letter, RG 48 Records of the Department of Interior, Office of the Interior, Los Angeles, Boulder Canyon Project Files, Box 4, File 1.4.6.1 General: Legal: Litigation: Six Companies Inc. Suit 1930-31 Part II, Holdings of the National Archives at Riverside (incl. "the health").

23. Elwood Mead to Surgeon General Hugh S. Cumming, Nov. 3, 1930, RG 48 Records of the Department of Interior, Office of the Interior, Los Angeles, Boulder Canyon Project Files, Box 4, File 1.4.6.1 General: Legal: Litigation: Six Companies Inc. Suit 1930-31 Part II, Holdings of the National Archives at Riverside.

24. Woodbury interview.

25. See Nugent, "Fit for Work"; Markowitz and Rosner, "Slaves of the Depression," 146-47; Aldrich, "Train Wrecks and Typhoid Fever," 273-76.

26. An original copy of the disclaimer is at the BCMHA SC.

27. McDaniel interview (incl. "bad shape"); "Report of the Commissioner of Labor," *Appendix*, 36th Sess., Vol. 1, 12-15; Dunbar and McBride, *Building Hoover Dam*, 36-37.

28. Quoted in King, *Hoover Dam and Boulder City*, 5.

29. Dunbar and McBride, *Building Hoover Dam*, 129; "50-Bed Hospital Planned," *Review-Journal*, May 21, 1931; "Here Are the Conditions Under Which Boulder City Hospital Aid Available," *Review-Journal*, Nov. 17, 1931; "First Aid Station for Tunnel Men," *Review-Journal*, May 23, 1931.

30. Six Companies and Crowe quoted in Hiltzik, *Colossus*, 230.

31. Ibid., 231-34.

32. Young quoted in ibid., 245.

33. For more on the 1931 strike, see Hiltzik, *Colossus*, 234–50, 263–64, 273, 283, 356; Rocha, "The I.W.W."; Minutes of Regular Meeting of Board of Directors, Aug. 17, 1931, Six Companies Corporate Records, Vol. 1, Bancroft.

34. Wattis quoted in Hiltzik, *Colossus,* 239.

35. "Boulder Canyon Project Employee Physical Exams, 1932," Six Companies Inc., Garnett, Box 66, Folder 1, BCMHA SC.

36. Hiltzik, *Colossus*, 217–19. Minutes of Regular Meeting of Board of Directors, July 20, 1931, Six Companies Corporate Records, Vol. 1, Bancroft (incl. "due to a fundamental").

37. Hiltzik, *Colossus*, 307–8. See also Minutes of Regular Meeting of Board of Directors, Apr. 15, 1934; Minutes of Regular Meeting of Board of Directors, May 21, 1934; both in Vol. 2, Bancroft. See also "Hoover Dam Site Becomes Major Lure," *Los Angeles California Express*, Nov. 14, 1931. See also Six Companies Corporate Records, Vol. 7, Oversize Folder, Bancroft for newspaper clippings on the topic.

38. In the 1930s the Safety-First campaign was marginally successful. It worked well in the railroad industry, but failed in steel production; accidents actually increased from 1927 to 1933. See Bureau of Labor Statistics, *Handbook of Labor Statistics* (Washington, DC: Government Printing Office [hereafter GPO], 1936), 6, 290; Markowitz and Rosner, *"Slaves of the Depression,"* 118–20; King, *Hoover Dam and Boulder City;* "Dam Safety Encouraged," *L.A. Examiner,* May 26, 1931; Hiltzik, *Colossus*, 338–40, for a discussion on how Six Companies did not strictly enforce safety; ibid., 339 (incl. "welfare and well-being" and "Nobody attended").

39. See Markowitz and Rosner, *"Slaves of the Depression,"* 111–14.

40. Hiltzik, *Colossus* (incl. "a lot of," 274).

41. Ibid., 273–74.

42. Ibid., 275, 280–84.

43. See McDaniel interview; Hiltzik, *Colossus*, 284–87.

44. Hiltzik, *Colossus*, 334–38.

45. "Dam Worker Has Spinal Meningitis," *Review-Journal,* Nov. 7, 1931; "Dam Worker Dies in Local Hospital," *Review-Journal,* Nov. 8, 1931; "Mahoney Child Contracts Meningitis," *Review-Journal,* Jan. 26, 1932; "Vegas Schools Will Reopen Next Monday," *Review-Journal,* Feb. 4, 1932; "Vegas, Boulder Schools Close," *Review-Journal,* Jan. 20, 1932; "Boulder Schools Close for a While," *Review-Journal,* Jan. 20, 1932; Ray Wilbur Jr., "Boulder City: A Survey of its Legal Background, Its City Plan and its Administration" (master's thesis, Harvard University, Cambridge, MA, 1935, BCMHA SC); McBride, *In the Beginning*, 36–39.

46. First synthesized in 1907, Arsphenamine (Salvarsan or compound 606) was the first effective treatment for syphilis and trypanosomiasis. An organoarsenic compound, it was the first modern chemotherapeutic agent. Dunbar and McBride, *Building Hoover Dam,* 242.

47. King, *Hoover Dam and Boulder City,* 4–5. In 1931 the PHS did not have the funding to build a hospital for Boulder City and could not be active in the project. The New Deal eventually brought changes to the PHS, allocating money to state and local departments to improve health conditions, sanitary engineering, tuberculosis control, laboratory research, and mental hygiene.

48. "Information to Applicants," June 1, 1933; Schofield, "Industrial Medicine," 87; Ray Wilbur Jr., "Boulder City: A Survey of Its Legal Background, Its City Plan and Its Administration" (master's thesis, Harvard University, 1935, SC, BCMHA).

49. "Report of the Secretary of the State Board of Health," in *Appendix*, 36th Sess., Vol. 1, 8–10.

50. "Peeling Studs for Three Thousand Hungry Men: The Job of Feeding a Peace Time Army at Hoover Dam," *LA Times*, Mar. 13, 1932; Schofield, "Industrial Medicine," 87.

51. Hiltzik, *Colossus*, 253–57.

52. Ibid., 261–65.

53. David Bruce Dill interview, by Lusie A. Soholt, Mar. 13, 1975, UNLV SC; "Medic Who Aided Dam Workers Dies," *Review-Journal*, July 25, 1935; Schofield, "Industrial Medicine," 89; "Anderson Brothers Menu," Cahlan Collection, Box 5, Folder 25, NSMA; Minutes of Regular Meeting of the Board of Directors, Apr. 16, 1934, Six Companies Corporate Records, Vol. 2, Bancroft.

54. Hiltzik, *Colossus*, 278.

55. "Estimate of Preparatory Expenses to Dec. 21, 1931," Six Companies Corporate Records, Vol. 2, Bancroft; "Equipment Put in for Opening of New $50,000 Plant on Sunday," *Review-Journal*, Nov. 14, 1931 (incl. "as well equipped"); McBride, *In the Beginning*, 36–39.

56. The absence of a formal written contract aided Six Companies in malpractice liability suits. If the doctor did not have a contract, he was not an official employee of the contractor and therefore it was more difficult to recover malpractice damages from Six Companies. See J. F. Reis to Leo McNamee, Apr. 28, 1942, McNamee Collection, Allbritton v. Six Companies, Box 18, Folder 5, NSMA.

57. "Estimate of Preparatory Expenses to Dec. 21, 1931," Six Companies Corporate Records, Vol. 2, Bancroft; "Equipment Put in for Opening of New $50,000 Plant on Sunday," *Review-Journal*, Nov. 14, 1931; McBride, *In the Beginning*, 36–39.

58. Dunbar and McBride, *Hoover Dam*, 131–34.

59. Schofield, "Industrial Medicine," 86–92 (incl. "intimately associated," 86, and "high pressure system," 88).

60. Six Companies medical insurance and Boulder City Hospital did not cover or see families for medical care; these individuals were expected to travel to Las Vegas for care. See "Hospital Permit Pleas for Dam City Are Asked," *Evening Review-Journal*, June 5, 1931; "Suicide Attempt Hinted in Plunge of Boulder Woman," *Las Vegas Age*, Aug. 19, 1932; Dunbar and McBride, *Building Hoover Dam*, 132–33; Ricky Hendricks, *A Model for National Healthcare: The History of Kaiser Permanente* (New Brunswick, NJ: Rutgers University Press, 1993), 1–40.

61. Six Companies matched the worker's contribution with $1.00, totaling $2.50 per month paid by Six Companies to the hospital fund. See Schofield, "Industrial Medicine," 91.

62. "Notice: To All Employees," Dec. 17, 1935, McNamee Collection, Allbritton v. Six Companies; "Here Are the Conditions."

63. David Bruce Dill, "The Harvard Fatigue Laboratory: Its Development, Contributions, and Demise," David Bruce Dill/Harvard Fatigue Laboratory Collection, Box 5, Folder 55, Mandeville SC Library, Geisel Library, University of California, San Diego (hereafter Geisel). David Bruce Dill interview, by R. C. Turner, May 4, 1976, UNLV SC (incl. "quite naturally"). See also "Boulder Chosen for Science Work," *Review-Journal*, Feb. 4, 1932.

64. Dill interview, Mar. 13, 1975; Dr. A. V. Bock and D. B. Dill, "A Resume of Some Physiological Reactions to High External Temperature," Aug. 21, 1933, David Bruce Dill/Harvard Fatigue Laboratory Collection, Box 1, Folder 42, Mandeville SC Library, Geisel.

65. Dill interview, May 4, 1976; D. B. Dill, A. V. Bock, and H. T. Edwards, "Mechanisms for Dissipating Heat in Man and Dog," reprinted in the *American Journal of Physiology* 104, no. 1, Apr. 1933, David Bruce Dill/Harvard Fatigue Laboratory Collection, Box 1, Folder 37, Mandeville SC Library, Geisel; J. H. Talbott, H. T. Edwyas, D. B. Dill, and L. D. Rastich, "Physiological Responses to High Environmental Temperature," *American Journal of Tropical Medicine* 13, no. 4 (July 1933), David Bruce Dill/Harvard Fatigue Laboratory Collection, Box 1, Folder 41, Mandeville SC Library, Geisel (incl. all quotes).

66. Dill interview, Mar. 13, 1975 (incl. "fully prepared," "THE DOCTOR," and "AND PUT"); "Medic Who Aided Dam Workers Dies," *Review-Journal,* July 25, 1935; Schofield, "Industrial Medicine," 89; menu sample in "Anderson Brothers Menu," Cahlan Collection, Box 5, Folder 25, NSMA. See also Minutes of Regular Meeting of the Board of Directors, Apr. 16, 1934, Six Companies Corporate Records, Vol. 2, Bancroft.

67. Dill interview, May 4, 1976; Talbott et al., "Physiological Responses."

68. A disgruntled Six Companies auditor informed Harold Ickes that Six Companies violated several U.S. codes, including the eight-hour workday. He charged that the contractor kept two sets of books: one recorded "regular time" and the other, "emergency time." The auditor calculated that Six Companies owed $300,000 in penalties. Ickes dispatched an investigator to study the matter. The allegations outraged Six Companies. Henry Kaiser contended that the project was in continuous emergency and therefore not subject to such burdensome restrictions. He launched a vigorous media campaign against Ickes, conducting radio and newspaper interviews. In the end, Kaiser's campaign worked and Ickes agreed to a $100,000 penalty, two-thirds of the original penalty in 1936. See Stevens, *Hoover Dam,* 232–34.

69. Clara Beyer, "Division of Labor Standards: Its Functions and Organization" (1934), RG 100, Serial 1, 1934–37, Box 24, NARA, National Archives at Riverside; Markowitz and Rosner, "Research or Advocacy: Federal Occupational Safety and Health Problems during the New Deal," *Journal of Social History* 18, no. 3 (Mar. 1985): 365–81; Markowitz and Rosner, *"Slaves of the Depression,"* 191–94; Markowitz and Rosner, "More Than Economics: The Politics of Workers' Health and Safety, 1932–47," *Milbank Quarterly* 64 (Fall 1986): 331–51; Sidney J. Williams, "Safety at the Boulder Dam," Special Representative to the Division of Labor Standards, DOL, Jan. 29, 1935, MS 78, Morgan J. Sweeney Papers, BCMHA SC.

70. Markowitz and Rosner, *"Slaves of the Depression,"* 110–11.

71. "Biennial Report of the Nevada Industrial Commission," *Appendix,* 36th Sess., Vol. 2, 7. See letters at McNamee Collection, 1934 Legal File, Box 147, Folder 2, NSMA; John J. Haydon to Leo McNamee, Jan. 21, 1938; John J. Haydon to Leo McNamee, Jan. 21, 1938; Dan Costello to Ed Brockmann, Aug. 17, 1934; Leo McNamee to Employers' Liability Assurance Co., Aug. 3, 1934; John J. Haydon to McNamee & McNamee, July 27, 1934; Beament & Beament to Six Companies Inc., July 24, 1934; Leo McNamee to Employers' Liability Assurance Co., July 5, 1934. See also Allbritton v. Six Companies.

72. Williams, "Safety at the Boulder Dam," 12; Stevens, *Hoover Dam,* 166; Dunbar and McBride, *Building Hoover Dam,* 262 (incl. "Tex").

73. Some accidents did not even happen on the job. Leroy Burt indicated that a coworker, Denny Greenwood, broke his leg in a fight with his brother and went to the Arizona side to collect compensation. See Dunbar and McBride, *Building Hoover Dam,* 262–64; and Stevens, *Hoover Dam,* 164.

74. Notice to All Employees, Allbritton v. Six Companies, McNamee Collection, NSMA; Stevens, *Hoover Dam,* 237 (incl. "finally proved").

75. Ed C. Peterson to Brockmann Agencies, Dec. 29, 1933, McNamee Collection, 1934 Legal File, Box 146, Folder 2, NSMA (incl. "If application has").

76. F. S. Peterson to Dan Costello, Sept. 22, 1933, letter; Sims Ely to F. S. Peterson, Nov. 21, 1933, letter (incl. "matter of"); Ed Brockmann to Sims Ely, Nov. 10, 1933, letter (incl. "willfully evading" and "grossly misrepresented"); Leo McNamee to Mrs. F. B. Kassell, Mar. 31, 1934, letter; all in McNamee Collection, 1934 Legal File, Box 146, Folder 2, NSMA.

77. The results of the tests revealed what scientists already knew: exposure made the human subjects seriously ill. See Sellers, Hazards of the Job, 168.

78. Six Companies claimed it had a $300,000–$500,000 investment in the trucks as well. The contractor knew carbon monoxide was lethal, but honored its investment over the health of their workers. See "Higher Bond to Be Demanded in Big Six Dam Suit," Review-Journal, Nov. 18, 1931; and David P. Billington and Donald C. Jackson, Big Dams of the New Deal Era: A Confluence of Engineering and Politics (Norman: University of Oklahoma Press, 2006), 137–38.

79. As Nevada Inspector of Mines, Stinson began outlawing the use of gasoline-powered trucks underground in 1931. See Section 4229 of Nevada Complied Laws, Statutes Nevada 1931, c.167, 274; "Report of the Inspector of Mines," Appendix, 36th Sess., Vol. 1, 32.

80. "Application of State Laws Boulder Canyon Project," 9–10; "Message of Gov. F. B. Balzar to the Legislature of 1933" (incl. "impossible to enforce," 29); "Report of the Inspector of Mines," 39–43; both in Appendix, 36th Sess., Vol. 1.

81. Since the dam site was a federal reservation, Nevada could not tax personal property. It was thought that placing the site under federal jurisdiction would help facilitate construction. Local residents feared it would become a permanent tax-exempt reservation, attracting industries that otherwise would be located in taxable areas of Nevada. See "Application of State Laws Within Boulder Can Project Federal Reservation," Hearing Before the Committee on Irrigation and Reclamation, U.S. Senate, 72nd Cong., 1st Sess. on S. 2885: A Bill Providing for the Application of State Laws Within the Boulder Canyon Project Federal Reservation (Washington, DC: GPO, June 14, 1932).

82. "Temporary Restraining Order and Order to Show Cause," Six Companies Inc. v. A. J. Stinson, Gray Mashburn and Harley A. Harmon, complaint Filed in 8th Judicial District Court of Nevada, No. C–191, Nov. 13, 1931, RG 48 Records of the Department of Interior, Office of the Interior, Los Angeles, Boulder Canyon Project Files, Box 4, File 1.4.6.1 General: Legal: Litigation: Six Companies Inc. Suit 1930–31 Part I, NARA, National Archives at Riverside (incl. "practical method"); "Bill of Complaint in Equity," 2, 8–10; "Memorandum of Points and Authorities"; both in Six Companies Inc. v. Stinson et al.

83. Ray Lyman Wilbur to Fred B. Balzar, June 3, 1932, letter (incl. "hamper the work"); Ray Lyman Wilbur to The Honorable Attorney General, Nov. 23, 1931, letter (incl. "take…measures"); H. H. Atkinson to Richard J. Coffey, Dec. 7, 1931, letter (incl. "It would not be advisable"); all in RG 48 Records of the Department of Interior, Office of the Interior, Los Angeles, Boulder Canyon Project Files, Box 5, File 1.4.6.1 General: Legal: Litigation: Six Companies Inc. Suit 1930–31 Part I, NARA, National Archives at Riverside. See also Elwood Mead, Dec. 5, 1931, telegram, ibid.

84. "Amicus curiae" is Latin for "friend of the court." The federal attorneys volunteered to assist Six Companies in the case, but were not an official party.

85. Coffey to Commissioner, Jan. 11, 1932, RG 48 Records of the Department of Interior, Office of the Interior, Los Angeles, Boulder Canyon Project Files, Box 5, File 1.4.6.1

General: Legal: Litigation: Six Companies Inc. Suit 1930–31 Part I, NARA, National Archives at Riverside.

86. Atkinson to Coffey, Dec. 7, 1931; Coffey to Commissioner, Jan. 11, 1932; "Plaintiffs Opening Brief," Six Companies Inc. v. A. J. Stinson, Gray Mashburn and Harley A. Harmon, Complaint Filed in Eighth Judicial District Court of Nevada, In Equity No. G-191, 72–74; all in RG 48 Records of the Department of Interior, Office of the Interior, Los Angeles, Boulder Canyon Project Files, Box 5, Bound Booklet, General: Legal: Litigation: Six Companies Inc. Suit 1930-31 Part II, NARA, National Archives at Riverside.

87. "Plaintiffs Opening Brief"; and "Affidavit of A. H. Ayers"; both in Six Companies Inc. v. Stinson et al.

88. "Plaintiffs Opening Brief"; and "Affidavit of L. H. Duschak"; both in Six Companies Inc. v. Stinson et al. (incl. all quotes).

89. "Plaintiffs Opening Brief," 72–76, 80; "Affidavit of Philip Samuel Williams"; "Affidavit of E. J. Brockman"; all in Six Companies Inc. v. Stinson et al. (incl. all quotes).

90. "Plaintiffs Opening Brief," 78–79; "Defendants Reply Brief" (incl. all quotes); both in Six Companies Inc. v. Stinson et al. See also "Higher Bond to Be Demanded in Big Six Dam Suit," *Review-Journal,* Nov. 18, 1931; and Stevens, *Hoover Dam,* 101.

91. "Mashburn Hurls Monkey Wrench in Big 6 Plans," *Review-Journal,* Nov. 4, 1931; Six Companies Inc. v. Stinson et al., 2F. Supp., 689–92, Feb. 15, 1933; "Report of the Inspector of Mines," *Appendix,* 37th Sess., Vol. 1 (Carson City, NV: SPO, 1935), 6.

92. Norman S. Gallison, "Construction of the Hoover Dam: Details of the Driving of the Four Tunnels Which Will Divert the Colorado River Around the Dam Site," *Compressed Air* 37 (May 1932) (incl. "would rather take," 3810).

93. Sellers and Melling, *Dangerous Trade* (incl. "neglected edges" and "actors," 198).

94. See Markowitz and Rosner, *Deadly Dust*; and *Congressional Record: Proceedings and Debates of the Second Session of the Seventy-Fourth Congress*, Vol. 80, Part 5 (Apr. 1–21, 1936) (Washington, DC: GPO, 1936) (incl. all quotes, 4752).

95. See Stevens, *Hoover Dam,* 207–13, for a full description of the trials. When cross-examined by Austin, the workers admitted they experienced headaches and nausea, but that their employer had required them to testify. See "Workman on Dam Job File Suit," *LA Times,* Feb. 11, 1934; and Stevens, *Hoover Dam,* 208–10.

96. See James C. Mohr, *Doctors and the Law: Medical Jurisprudence in Nineteenth-Century America* (Baltimore and London: Johns Hopkins University Press, 1993); Aldrich, "Train Wrecks and Typhoid Fever," 269–70; and Welke, *Recasting American Liberty,* 77–80 for discussion of the complicated job of a medico-legal expert witness.

97. Aldrich, "Train Wrecks to Typhoid Fever," 269–70; Schofield, "Industrial Medicine" (incl. both quotes, 92).

98. Aldrich, "Train Wrecks to Typhoid Fever," 269–70.

99. Of course, Wales Haas's testimony was disputable considering he did not arrive at the project until 1932. Had the doctor examined Bowles prior to his sickness, his opinion might have held more validity. See "Affidavit of Wales Haas, M.D." (incl. "long-standing disease tuberculosis," "a germ," "irritated tissues," "based upon," and "not be likely"); "Affidavit of J. C. Bowles"; both in Six Companies Inc. v. Stinson et al.

100. "Eugene F. McCarthy Tunnel Man Passes," *Review-Journal,* Dec. 11, 1931; Hiltzik, *Colossus* (incl. "if they ever," 285); "Iron Heel Is Used to Stifle All Squawks," *Industrial Worker,* Jan. 26, 1932.

101. Hiltzik, *Colossus* (incl. "If you said," 286).

102. E. F. Kraus v. Six Companies, Inc., Frank Bryant and John Tacke, complaint Filed in 8th Judicial District Court of Nevada, No. 4499, Apr. 13, 1933 (incl. "look pretty sick").

103. Jack F. Norman v. Six Companies, Inc., Woody Williams, and Tom Regan, complaint Filed in 8th Judicial District Court of Nevada, No. 5256, May 24, 1934.

104. R. F. Walter to Commissioner, Jan. 7, 1934, RG 48 Records of the Department of Interior, Office of the Interior, Los Angeles, Box 4, File 1.4.6 Boulder Canyon Project Files, National Archives at Riverside (incl. "just cause" and "While not admitting").

105. William Blackstone, *Commentaries*, St. George Tucker, ed. (Philadelphia: William Birch Young and Abraham, 1803), 122–23.

106. In 1898 the New York State Court of Appeals decided Pike v. Honsinger, a case that established a standard of medical care and highlighted problems in medical practice. For the following five decades, courts cited Pike v. Honsinger in most malpractice disputes. It not only defined and standardized medical care and error, but also helped transition the practice of medicine from a local to a national profession. See Pike v. Honsinger, 155 NY 201 (1898).

107. See Kenneth Allen De Ville, *Medical Malpractice in Nineteenth-Century America: Origins and Legacy* (New York and London: New York University Press, 1990) for the emergence of nineteenth-century malpractice law. See Neal C. Hogan, *Unhealed Wounds: Medical Malpractice in the Twentieth Century* (New York: LFB Scholarly, 2003) for medical malpractice history in the twentieth century.

108. See Hogan, *Unhealed Wounds*, 33–95. *Time* published the first high-profile case of malpractice, "The Doctor Loses," *Time* 37 (May 26, 1941), 47.

109. Nevada Industrial Commission to McNamee & McNamee, Feb. 4, 1942, McNamee Collection, Allbritton v. Six Companies, NSMA (incl. "Under the circumstances").

110. Dr. Roy Martin always treated minorities in house calls, but the Las Vegas Hospital Association and the Ferguson-Balcom Hospital did not extend the same courtesy. Adele Baratz, a registered nurse who practiced in Las Vegas during the 1930s, described the city as having a "strong color barrier," especially with regard to its medical community. She referred to Las Vegas as "the South of the West." See Adele Baratz interview, by Steve McClenachan, Mar. 4, 1979, UNLV SC; Nevada Industrial Commission to McNamee & McNamee, Feb. 4, 1942, McNamee Collection, Allbritton v. Six Companies, NSMA.

111. As the railroad and county hospital physician, Slavin provided minorities with medical care. See W. M. White to Mr. R. A. Boyd, Re: O 32396-A Allbritton v. Six Companies, memorandum, Apr. 17, 1942, McNamee Collection, Allbritton v. Six Companies, NSMA. See also R. O. Schofield for Six Companies Inc. Hospital, Boulder City, Nevada, Re: O. B. Allbritton, Report, McNamee Collection, Allbritton v. Six Companies, NSMA (incl. all quotes).

112. C. Higgins Re: O 32396-A Allbritton v. Six Companies, memorandum, June 18, 1936, McNamee Collection, Allbritton v. Six Companies, NSMA (incl. all quotes).

113. E. J. Brockmann to Employers' Liability Assurance Corporation, Dec. 15, 1935; Leo McNamee to the Employers' Group, May 27, 1939; both in McNamee Collection, Allbritton v. Six Companies, NSMA. See also Oscar B. Allbritton v. Six Companies Inc., Boulder City Hospital, a Corporation, Dr. John Doe Schofield, Demurrer, Eighth Judicial District Court of Nevada, No. 7398, June 25, 1937 (incl. all quotes).

114. John J. Haydon to Leo McNamee, Re: O. B. Allbritton v. Six Companies, Inc., July 30, 1937, McNamee Collection, Allbritton v. Six Companies, NSMA (incl. "negro woman" and "did not sustain").

115. Diversity of citizenship or diversity jurisdiction refers to federal court exercising authority to hear a lawsuit. Cases involving state laws can be heard in federal

court if the parties are from different states. However, there must be complete diversity for the federal court to hear the case. If both plaintiff and defendant are residents of the same state, the state court must hear the case.

116. Allbritton v. Six Companies, Demurrer, June 25, 1937 (incl. "ambiguous"); McNamee Collection, Allbritton v. Six Companies, NSMA.

117. During the 1930s several cases attempted to define the role of the company doctor. Schneiger v. New York Telephone Co., 292 N.Y. Supp. 399 (Jan. 1937, Supreme Court, Appellate Division) determined that company doctors were not servants of their employers, but instead engaged in an independent calling. Employers therefore were not liable for malpractice. See also Irene H. Bennett v. Paramount Pictures, Inc., a corporation, H. J. Strathern, et al., Memorandum of Defendant Paramount Pictures, Inc. In Support of Demurrer, No. 413975, McNamee Collection, Allbritton v. Six Companies. See also W. M. White to R. A. Boyd, memorandum, May 1, 1942, Re: 0-32396-A Allbritton—Six Companies, McNamee Collection, Albritton v. Six Companies, NSMA (incl. both quotes).

118. J. F. Reis to Leo McNamee, Apr. 28, 1942, McNamee Collection, Allbritton v. Six Companies, NSMA.

119. Ultra vires in common law means beyond the powers. Its inverse, intra vires, means within the powers. McNamee cited two cases as precedent for this argument. In Bowman v. La Societe Francaise 71 Pac 516 (California), the defendant—a railroad corporation—maintained a hospital for the benefit of its employees, deducting a part of their monthly wages to cover their medical expenses. The plaintiff alleged negligence in treatment and sued the corporation. The court turned the decision on a question regarding whether the hospital was a charitable or for-profit organization. Since the hospital was considered for-profit, the jury held the corporation was liable. However, McNamee also noted that the authority could go the other way. In Nicholson v. At. Top. & Santa Fe RR Co (Kansas), a jury held that company hospitals were charitable enterprises and not liable for malpractice. See Memorandum: Allbritton v. Six Companies, McNamee Collection, Allbritton v. Six Companies, NSMA.

120. Allbritton v. Six Companies: Allbritton v. Six Companies Inc., McNamee Collection, Albritton v. Six Companies, NSMA (incl. all quotes).

121. Leo McNamee to The Employers Group, Re: 0-32396A Allbritton v. Six Companies Inc., Dec. 3, 1948; Oscar B. Allbritton v. Six Companies Inc., Boulder City Hospital, a corporation, Dr. Richard Schofield, Notice of Motion to Dismiss Filed at the Eighth Judicial District Court of Nevada, No. 7398, Dec. 4, 1948; both in McNamee Collection, Allbritton v. Six Companies, NSMA.

122. "Summary of Fatalities by Employers—Boulder Canyon Project—To and including July 31, 1935," Frank "Doc" Jensen Papers, 1 of 5, SC, BCMHA, Nevada.

123. See Dunbar and McBride, *Building Hoover Dam*, 106; Louis A. Chadburn and Debbie Endsley, interview, by Dennis McBride, May 18, 1999, BCMHA.

124. Billington and Jackson, *Big Dams of the New Deal Era*, 9.

125. Most historians agree that the Brooklyn Bridge helped convert New York City into a major commercial center. Likewise, Hoover Dam had a similar effect, dramatically transforming Southern California and the Southwest. See David McCullough, *The Great Bridge: The Epic Story of the Building of the Brooklyn Bridge* (New York: Simon & Schuster, 1972), 547-48; Billington and Jackson, *Big Dams of the New Deal Era*, 11, 218-19.

126. Stevens, *Hoover Dam*, 231; Billington and Jackson, *Big Dams of the New Deal Era*, 9-10, 156-57.

# 3

# THE PLANT

AT THE START OF World War II American industry was considerably safer than it had been a decade earlier. Improvements in technology and the institutionalization of safety programs in most large firms helped considerably, as well as New Deal legislation. The Civil Works Administration, a short-lived job creation program that established temporary construction work during the winter of 1933-34, urged the use of safety engineers, programs with protective requirements, first-aid training, and education. The Public Works Administration (PWA), Works Progress Administration (WPA), and the National Recovery Administration (NRA) created safety organizations as well, mandating contractors to follow specific codes. In 1934 the DOL established a committee to develop NRA standards, including machinery protection, physical examinations, and injury reporting. Other legislation benefitting workers included the Fair Labor Standards Act of 1938, the standardization of the eight-hour workday, the end of child labor in most factories, the National Labor Relations (Wagner) Act of 1935, and the Walsh–Healey Public Contracts Act of 1936. The latter barred companies with hazardous work sites from gaining federal contracts. In practice, it was limited in scope, overlooking most of the public and private sectors. While most New Deal programs were discontinued or brief, each helped encourage health and safety, producing real results. The Bureau of Labor Statistics estimated that during the year 1936 2,700 construction workers died, 15,400 received permanent injuries, and 265,000 were temporarily disabled. Two years later, construction deaths had been reduced by 25 percent, and permanent and temporary injuries had been reduced by 30 percent. In 1939 only 1,500 workplace-related deaths occurred nationally, the lowest number ever recorded. Several factors attributed to the drop. The institution of health and safety programs by the Roosevelt administration and the National Security Council certainly helped, but most programs provided only information to state agencies about prioritizing health and safety. There were therefore two key factors that contributed to the reduction of workplace injuries and fatalities by the late 1930s: a decrease in labor turnover in most industries coupled with Depression conditions that encouraged employers to fire inefficient workers who were prone to accidents.[1]

Mobilization for war postponed the progress. In 1940 alone the accident rate rose 20 percent: more than 1.41 million workers sustained injuries in American war plants, and seventeen thousand died.[2] The new job opportunities reduced the unemployment rate, but increased turnover and injuries. With skilled, male employees drafted into military service, employers recruited inexperienced labor with limited instruction in health and safety procedures. The conditions worsened when Roosevelt called for increased production, prompting companies to extend the workweek and institute speedups. American workers were exhausted, but volunteered for double shifts or overtime to support the cause. The highest disease and injury rates occurred in war plants engaged in manufacturing—iron and steel, ships, bombers, automobiles, concrete, slaughtering and meat packing, fertilizer, and leather. Likewise, the production of ammunition, chemicals, electric goods, plastics, and rubber contaminated work sites with pollutants, dusts, and acids. Even though benzene, toluene, asbestos, and silica were known industrial diseases, the public–private partnerships did little to protect workers from them. Eventually, the urgent need for war material forced the issue. Since accidents and injury-related absenteeism slowed production, health and safety became synonymous with mobilization, ushering in a new era of occupational health history after 1945.[3]

While applying the previous war and New Deal as models, World War II mobilization was a marked departure from the past. It was a less centralized public–private partnership supervised by a national war council composed of military officers and civilians. The military did not participate in civilian mobilization, benefitting from unchecked control over equipment and recruits. Several agencies, and not just one, determined production and controls. After the attack on Pearl Harbor Congress passed the War Powers Act, granting Roosevelt the power to reorganize the federal government, creating mobilizing agencies and awarding government contracts without competitive bidding. Despite various problems, the American economy expanded significantly from 1941 to 1945, pulling the nation out of economic depression. The gross national product (GNP) grew from $88.6 billion in 1939 to $135 billion in 1944. Defense production also increased from 2 percent of the GNP in 1939 to 40 percent in 1943.[4]

Mobilization dramatically transformed the United States, especially the West. Western states were the closest proximity to the Pacific theater of the war, so the federal government invested more than $40 billion in the states' military and industrial development. California received 10 percent of all federal funds. Historian Gerald D. Nash has shown that the New Deal ended the West's colonial relationship with eastern and international capitals, but World War II charted its future.[5] Federal spending shifted the region's alliance on mining and agriculture to manufacturing and science. The West was an ideal location for the defense industry. Since Japanese bombers threatened coastal city production, inland cities like Las Vegas, Pocatello, Salt Lake, Phoenix, and Albuquerque were ideal locations for war plants and military bases. The climatic conditions of most western cities also accommodated year-round training for pilots, gunners, and bombardiers.[6]

Nevada was the perfect spot to locate military facilities. Not far from the Pacific, it had plenty of federally owned land. The entire state thrived. The "extraordinary conditions brought about by the war" lifted the state out of economic depression, according to Governor Edward P. Carville, bringing "prosperity" to Nevada. In the north the War Department built air bases in Tonopah and Fallon, and accelerated the use of an ammunition storage facility in Hawthorne. In the south Las Vegas's support for Roosevelt, the New Deal, and cheap water and electricity from Hoover Dam encouraged the War Department to extensively use the region. In June 1940 the military constructed a marine auxiliary base and electrolytic manganese pilot plant in Boulder City.[7]

The Civil Aeronautics Authority also helped Las Vegas purchase and upgrade the Western Air Express airport in January 1941, located northeast of town, to strengthen the western air defenses. The city leased the airport to the Army Air Corps for $1 per year. In return, the Army invested $25 million in the property, constructing hangars, storage facilities, barracks, fuel tanks, and two runways. The War Department eventually turned it into the Las Vegas Air Gunnery School, a training school for pilots and gunners in airborne combat. In preparation for the Battles of Iwo Jima and Okinawa, the Army Air Corps continued to expand the training facility; by spring 1945 it employed approximately thirteen thousand workers.[8]

The new dams built in the West and South also positioned both U.S. regions to be prime locations for war plants. Defense contracts quickly became big business. As Secretary of War Henry Stimson explained, if you are going to war in a capitalist country, you have to let "business make money…or business won't work." The close relationship between the federal government, the private sector, and the armed forces during World War II established what President Dwight Eisenhower dubbed in 1961 "the military-industrial complex." American business grew quickly, with manufacturing and technology firms rapidly building shipyards, steel and aluminum mills, research facilities, and chemical plants.[9]

An important component in the war effort was manufacturing magnesium. Pure magnesium was weak and soft, but increased in strength when it was combined with aluminum. It was two-thirds as heavy as aluminum and one-fourth as heavy as steel. Consequently, the metal was used in manufacturing bullets, flares, bomb casings, and bombing parts. Additionally, it was highly explosive, so was used in incendiary bombs.[10]

During the war, the military used 5 percent of American magnesium in military pyrotechnics and savaging, and 95 percent in nonflammable alloys, most commonly in aviation. There were two methods to manufacture the metal. A German company, I. G. Farbenindustrie, developed the electrolytic process, which extracted the metal from magnesite ores. Henry Kaiser's Permanente Company also acquired the rights to the carbothermic process, which had been developed by Austrian scientist Fritz Johann Hansgirg. The latter method mixed oxide with carbon, then quickly heated and cooled it.[11]

During the 1930s Dow Chemical Inc. and Alcoa Aluminum held a monopoly on magnesium production in the United States. During that decade Dow was the nation's only magnesium producer, shipping its output to Alcoa to fabricate metal fittings, but wartime conditions ended the arrangement. In 1941 a federal grand jury indicted Dow–Alcoa, American Magnesium Corporation, Magnesium Development Corporation, and other companies for conspiring with Nazi-affiliated I. G. Farbenindustrie. The Justice Department found evidence of German influence that discouraged production in the United States, charging that the companies raised the price of magnesium and created a shortage. The firms pled no contest, paid a $140,000 fine, and made its patents available royalty free. The War Production Board (WPB) also authorized an enormous increase in magnesium production in 1942, calling for an output of 700 million pounds annually, 75 percent more than previously planned.[12]

These conditions brought magnesium to Nevada, prompting Basic Refractories Inc. (BRI), a small firm from Cleveland, Ohio, to enter the business.[13] In 1919 Howard Eells inherited BRI from his father, a company that sold firebrick to steel companies. BRI also held a patent for producing aluminum from refractory bricks. But in order to use it, the company needed raw materials. In 1933 Eells sent geologists to investigate magnesite claims in the West, and in 1936 purchased several claims in Nevada: magnesite and brucite deposits in the eastern slopes of the Paradise Mountains in Nye County and adjacent claims in Gabbs with extensive deposits of ore.[14]

The war eventually shifted Eells's objectives to magnesium production. In January 1941 he learned that Magnesium Elecktron, Ltd., a British magnesium firm, wanted to build a production facility in Canada. The company's president, Major John P. Ball, purchased the rights for the electrolytic process from I. G. Farbenindustrie and enlisted German technicians to build a plant in Manchester. But after the London blitz in 1940 and 1941, he needed both sanctuary from Nazi bombers and raw materials. Ball attempted to negotiate with the Canadian government to build a plant in Quebec, but the deal fell through. Eells reached out to him and proposed a solution: if Ball provided the expertise, he had the raw materials.[15]

Impressed with Eells's holdings, Ball agreed. They incorporated Basic Magnesium Inc. (BMI) in Nevada, with Eells sitting as president and Ball as vice president. Next, they chose a location for the plant. The logical choice was to transport the raw materials from Eells's mining claims to California, but Eells had another idea. Why not build in southern Nevada? The region seemed like the perfect location. With the abundance of federally owned land and close proximity to Hoover Dam, the real estate and electricity savings would offset transportation costs. It was the first time an industrialist expressed interest in southern Nevada. Since the dam's completion, local residents had aspired to promote the area as a haven for industry. But there was one major problem. In order to bring power and water to Las Vegas, a company had to spend an estimated $7 million to build a water line and power transmission system from Lake Mead and the dam. Eells had to secure federal funding.[16]

He had several influential supporters in Nevada's congressional seat. George Thatcher, western counsel for BRI, began discussing the possibility of opening a manufacturing plant in southern Nevada with Senator Key Pittman in May 1940. Six months later Pittman was dead, and Thatcher contacted Senator Pat McCarran and Representative James Scrugham on the subject. By the time Eells traveled to Washington, DC, in spring 1941 Nevada's representatives enthusiastically supported the project. McCarran was a crucial ally, personally convincing Roosevelt to fund the project and enlisting the help of former Nevada senator Charles B. Henderson, the chairman of the Reconstruction Finance Corporation (RFC). Henderson oversaw the authorization of federal loans and investments in programs that encouraged the production of essential war material. The relationship paid off well. On April 15, 1941, BMI presented its plan to the Office of Production Management. Over the next few months, Eells held meetings with the War Department and Industrial Planning Section of the Army Air Corps, and with the Defense Plant Corporation (DPC). In July 1941 he secured a $63 million contract for the construction of a plant that would manufacture 33.6 million pounds of magnesium every year. When the contract was finalized in August, the War Department expanded production to 112 million pounds a year. That increase would be a huge boost to mobilization. In 1940 the United States produced only six thousand tons of magnesium. In comparison, Germany's output was twelve thousand tons a year. The contract stated that the federal government owned all land, structures and equipment, and magnesium, and rights to approve all sales and stockpiling. Additionally, the U.S. Treasury compensated BMI for management services and paid employee salaries. Eells agreed to manage operations and receive a salary of $1 per ton of magnesium produced.[17]

With federal approval, the last component was transferring the blueprints and chemical formulas to the United States. But the task of crossing the Atlantic with the documents proved to be very difficult. The first attempt ended when a Nazi torpedo sank the ship carrying the documents. The technicians escaped, but lost the plans. Ball organized a creative second try. He transferred the plans to microfilm and sent them on a plane to Washington, DC. At the same time, his technicians boarded a decoy ship to trick Germany spies. It worked. But while the plans and technicians arrived safely in the United States, problems continued. The courier transported the microfilm from Washington, DC, to Las Vegas, but accidently left it on the plane. After being located in a Seattle airport, the plans finally arrived in Las Vegas. Given the code name of Plancor 201 for security, the BMI plant was born.[18]

Mobilization transformed southern Nevada. Like the dam before it, Las Vegas boomed from the federal spending. "World War II was essentially a boom for Las Vegas," Dr. Clare Woodbury remembered. As he recalls, tourism spiked and people with black market money "did not want to report their revenue," so they gambled and reported that their winnings came from the casinos. The divorce trade also thrived, in large part due to publicity garnered from the much-publicized Clark Gable–Rita Langham divorce in 1939. However, the Las Vegas Air Gunnery School and BMI plant provided the biggest boosts to the local economy.[19]

Indeed, many American cities boomed from defense contracts. In Detroit General Motors, Ford, and Chrysler, which together produced 90 percent of the nation's automobiles, cut their production of commercial vehicles to supply the war effort. Willow Run, a small creek west of Detroit, was a quiet area surrounded by woodlands and farmhouses in 1940. Two years later, Ford built an airfield and aircraft assembly plant in the area to manufacture four-motored consolidated bombers; the plant employed more than ninety thousand workers.[20]

As cited in *Time*, the Census Bureau estimated that from April 1, 1940 to May 1, 1942 the population of Detroit jumped 21 percent.[21] Likewise, in Mobile, Alabama, the federal government awarded a $26 million contract to convert the city's municipal airport into Brookley Field, a major Army Air Force supply depot and bomber modification center. Mobile emerged as a major war town that housed an Alcoa plant as well as numerous shipyard companies. The Brookley Field operation employed more than seventeen thousand men and women. Mobile became the second largest city in Alabama, as thousands of workers flooded the city to seek employment.[22]

As in Detroit and Mobile, the population of southern Nevada grew as a result of defense spending. Las Vegas's population rose from approximately eight thousand to fifty thousand residents. BMI was a far bigger job than the Hoover Dam had been. At its peak, the dam employed 5,128 workers. In July 1942 the BMI plant employed approximately thirteen thousand workers, with a weekly payroll that surpassed the dam's monthly payroll. Military services drafted workers to construct the plant or produce magnesium. Since dam employees vacated the region after the project's completion, BMI recruited its large workforce from neighboring states. Ragnald Fyhen, secretary-treasurer of the Central Labor Council of Clark County, observed "whole groups of men [brought by the] 'train-loads' from war recruiting centers, mostly from Los Angeles and San Diego."[23] The Employment Division of the Industrial Relations Division handled all recruitment and employment. One such employee was Jonreed Lauritzen, a western novelist. While working at the plant in 1943, he published *Arrows into the Sun* and wrote a short story, "Hellbent on Victory," about his time at BMI. Lauritzen, a chemical lab technician, described his experience: "We of the West know freedom. Our obligation is therefore the greater to help preserve it. They won't let me fight—but they will let me make magnesium. I consider that a privilege."[24]

As with most wartime industries, the BMI workforce included men too old for military service, minorities, and women. Thus far, gender has been omitted from this story of occupational health. This is not by design: only a very small percentage of women worked on the railroad or dam construction, usually in nursing or clerical positions. American women always worked, especially among lower-class whites and minorities. Prior to World War II, two factors hindered women from seeking employment in industries. Cultural divisions of labor situated men in the workplace and white middle-class women at home. Industries also rarely hired women because there were plenty of men. During the 1930s male labor shortages were unlikely, but Pearl Harbor changed everything. Employers could not save a man from the draft board, no matter his industrial skills. At first, companies had difficulty recruiting women, prompting the War Advertising Council to launch the Rosie the Riveter campaign. The fictional Rosie was the perfect working woman: attractive, reliable, competent, and patriotic. She even had a popular song, and in 1943 Norman Rockwell memorialized her image on the cover of the *Saturday Evening Post*. Later, the War Advertising Council issued Rockwell's image on a government-commissioned poster with the slogan, We Can Do It. Women responded overwhelmingly to the campaign, especially lower-class whites and minorities. In 1945 the number of working women had risen from 12 million to 18 million. While most worked in the service sector, more than 3 million secured war plant jobs. Certainly, patriotism motivated the women, but it was also the pay. In 1942 female college graduates earned an average of $25 a week. War workers started at $25 to $40 per week, and applicants needed no prior experience. After a training program of only two to six weeks, they could begin work.[25]

The plant's version of Rosie the Riveter had many names: Magnesium Maggie and Chlorine Kate were the most popular. In February 1943 the company hired sixteen women for a so-called experiment for the production line. The women were the first employed in American magnesium production. BMI quickly learned the benefits of hiring women. Their safety records far exceeded their male coworkers, with the women exhibiting greater finger dexterity, focus, and excellence in inspection work. They were also less likely to strike and responded well to speed-up campaigns. Of course, there were some drawbacks, because it was heavy industrial work. Women needed assistance lifting equipment, were prone to fatigue, and had shorter industrial lives than men. They were also more susceptible to small accidents because of their lack of experience with the complex machinery. Most importantly, absenteeism was highest among working mothers. As shown by Allison Helper, working mothers stayed directly connected to their families, which affected how they interacted with the workplace. If a family member became ill, a mother was more likely to miss work to care for them. Women did not ask for special favors, however, and endured the same workplace discomforts as men. These dual roles often contradicted one another in the wartime workplace.[26]

BMI women received equal pay for equal work, approximately $0.90 per hour, per federal requirements.[27] They assumed many positions, driving forklifts, wrapping magnesium ingots, manufacturing asbestos gloves, and repairing gas masks, among many others. The company newsletters, the *Big Job* and *Basic Bombardier*, enthusiastically highlighted its female contingent, describing the Hydrogen Women, their "splendid women workers [who appeared] as though they'd stepped out of a Superman plot...taking cell voltages and cleaning out the glass tubes." Chlorine Kate, an employee named Thelma Lindquist, operated a cell that made chlorine gas in a 130-degree room in the summer to freezing temperatures in the winter. She regularly crawled on top of the cells for warmth, which was hazardous and forbidden by safety regulations. While new to industrial work, many women tailored their domestic experience to the job. One woman remarked that working alongside molten metal was similar to cooking over a hot stove.[28]

Of course, men had mixed reactions to women in the workplace. According to *Time*, their position was a "mixture of nose-out-of-joint and gallantry," either leaving the women alone or being too helpful. Surely, the concept was difficult to get used to. While a woman posed for a photographer, one male worker commented, "I ran that machine [for] two years and nobody ever took my picture." Many companies wondered why they had never employed women before. Still, most tried to separate the sexes at work. When asked the reason, an executive in Detroit responded, "You know how men are." Certainly, some men enjoyed the idea of working alongside women. At a womanless aviation plant in Kansas City, male workers complained that "the promised blondes" never arrived. Some women reported inappropriate behavior from their male coworkers. Tired of the whistles and comments, female workers at the Douglas Aircraft Company in Santa Monica began imitating their male associates. One girl yelled, "Look at Tarzan." The other commented on "what a build that guy's got." Apparently, "the men could not take it" and stopped hassling them.[29] BMI women reported little unprofessional behavior in the workplace, although that does not mean it did not occur. One reason sexual harassment might have been low was that management deliberately separated the sexes. But while the majority of BMI women were already married, some met their future spouses on the job, indicating there was some level of interaction at the workplace.[30]

Besides women, BMI employed thousands of minority workers, most of them blacks and a small number of Native Americans.[31] In response to civil rights activist pressure, Franklin Roosevelt signed Executive Order 8802 on June 25, 1941, prohibiting racial discrimination in the defense industry. The Fair Employment Practices Committee (FEPC) was the first federal commission to support equal opportunity, barring discrimination at a federally funded workplace. Throughout the war, FEPC rules banned discriminatory employment practices based on race, faith, color, or nationality in all federal agencies and private companies involved in war-related work. In 1943 Roosevelt strengthened the FEPC with Executive Order 9346, requiring all government contracts to have nondiscrimination clauses.[32]

While the FEPC tried to prohibit discrimination in the North, the committee did not actively challenge segregation in the South or parts of the West.[33] In the summer of 1943 shifts in demography and workplace desegregation had serious consequences. Rioting among whites, blacks, and Latinos erupted across the nation. In particular, desegregation in the workplace provoked riots in the South. In May 1943 a riot erupted at the Alabama Dry Dock after FEPC officials forced the company to promote twelve black workers to skilled positions. The riot forced the FEPC to permit Jim Crow arrangements in job positions and segregate workplace activities. A few weeks later, false rape allegations triggered a similar riot at the Pennsylvania Shipyards in Beaumont, Texas.[34]

While there was not as dramatic opposition to black workers in the BMI workplace, discrimination certainly existed. The best description of the plant's minority experience was that the company employed racial tolerance, not equality. In 1940 only 664 blacks lived in southern Nevada; of Las Vegas's 8,422 residents, just 165 were black. Dr. Clare Woodbury remembered treating "very few blacks" during the 1930s, and those few were "mostly on the Westside." He described these patients as "coming from the West" and "very fine" when he made house calls and "delivered [their] babies." In 1942 BMI started recruiting black men from the South, including Mississippi, due to labor shortages. In 1943 more than three thousand blacks moved to the region, making up 60 percent of all production personnel on the plant.[35]

Woodbury provided conflicting accounts of Las Vegas's reception of the influx of minorities. He described the newcomers as having an "entirely different philosophy" and their arrival "began our troubles in a way." But it was also a "pretty harmonious relationship," especially when it came to "medical care, education, and the freely mingling of the people of Las Vegas." The doctor's reaction illustrates the uneasiness among local medicine insofar as treating minorities. Up until this point, Las Vegas and its medical facilities had been segregated, and some called the city the Mississippi of the West. Contending with the need for workers at BMI, wartime conditions forced racial tolerance, at least temporarily in some spaces. While most hospitals continued to treat minority patients after the war, the hospitality industry was a different story. The Las Vegas Strip would not achieve desegregation until 1960.[36]

The company newsletters maintained that management strongly discouraged racial discrimination, claiming that "segregation was completely rejected in the effort to staff the huge plant, and there are several Negro foremen on the payroll."[37] Still, BMI established separate housing and restrooms, and even sought complete segregation of the plant. The FEPC denied the request, citing that full segregation could cause labor unrest. On October 23, 1943, two hundred black workers assembled a walkout in protest of the separate washrooms and toilet facilities. A day later FEPC examiner John Burke arrived in Las Vegas to investigate the allegations. While it is unclear what happened to the strikers, the *Review-Journal* reported that several were offered employment at the Hawthorne Naval Depot.[38] BMI claimed it discouraged racial discrimination, but white workers earned higher pay. According to local union representative E. E. Ward, "Negro workers [were] being discriminated against with the support of management [even though they performed] identical work" as coworkers. Louis Stricklan, a jeep driver, attested that blacks made $0.50 less an hour than whites and had no opportunity for advancement. He claimed the company believed black workers' wages were too high, and they did not want "the colored fellows to get that chance [for advancement]."[39] The *Review-Journal* also reported that blacks earned an income ranging from $1,500 to $2,000, while whites received $1,500 to $3,000. Even so, racial tensions among plant employees were rare. Most minorities had issues with management, but not with their coworkers.[40]

Regardless of race, all workers contended with uncomfortable housing. While the situation from 1942–43 was not as dire as it had been in the summer of 1931 at Hoover Dam, thousands of people traveled to Las Vegas to work at BMI. How to accommodate them all was an afterthought by management, a situation eerily similar to the dam. Las Vegas was hardly unique; the entire nation experienced housing shortages. Detroit workers lived in tents, shacks, and trailers, prompting *Time* to call the situation "tragic, dirty confusion." The poor planning led to material shortages, flaring tempers, sit-downs, strikes, and a drop in war production. Despite the extensive rearmament program, the 1941 unemployment rate was still 9.9 percent, compared to 3.2 percent in 1929. As a result, Hoovervilles continued to exist, especially in isolated areas employing migrant workers.[41]

In Las Vegas, the Federal Housing Administration (FHA) approved the financing of three housing developments in Las Vegas—the Biltmore, Huntridge, and Mayfair neighborhoods—under Title VI, but BMI still needed housing.[42] At first, Eells did not want to build a company town because there was little profit in the endeavor. His original plans provided for a plant and for all personnel to commute from Six Companies' employee housing in Boulder City. But when military demands increased production, BMI needed to accommodate ten thousand additional workers and their families. Like Six Companies, Eells faced criticism for not providing suitable employee housing, but the situation was beyond his control. The federal government not only substantially increased the size of the project, but also had trouble deciding the town site's location, delaying its funding.

When Eells realized he needed to build a company town, he contacted the Emergency Housing Coordination (EHC) and the Federal Works Agency (FWA) for funding. Mobilization was a busy time for both agencies. Since there was a national demand for similar needs, both agencies suggested also filing an application with the War Department, emphasizing the importance of the Nevada project to the war effort. Eells made arrangements with the War Department and recruited Justin Hartzog, a Defense Housing Coordination planner, to collect information for his application.[43]

In July 1941 Hartzog arrived in Las Vegas with several federal representatives, touring locations for the plant and housing development. He identified twenty-eight hundred acres of unclaimed federally owned land for the plant location southeast of Las Vegas at Black Mountain. The site provided access to Hoover Dam and Lake Mead's power and water, and was a safe distance from the dam in case of an attack.[44]

Determining a housing location was another story. Hartzog quickly concluded that Boulder City, Las Vegas, and Paradise Valley were inadequate. Boulder City, he cited, was constructed to house dam employees and was never intended to accommodate the population of a large industrial enterprise. The town lacked sufficient electricity, water, sewerage, and schools. Likewise, he determined that Las Vegas needed infrastructure updates including a modernized sewerage system. Moreover, Hartzog considered the land value too high and location too far from the plant site, which would cost the company in transportation costs. But above all, the stigma of Las Vegas was too great. Hartzog worried about the "wide-open conditions...booze, gambling, and brothels." He stressed that BMI needed a regulated community to minimize Nevada influences. In fact, Hartzog determined that the only redeeming quality about Las Vegas was its medical infrastructure. He felt the hospitals could accommodate an industrial enterprise, with 182 beds between the county and private hospitals. Hartzog also considered Paradise Valley during his inquiry, a section of vacant land between the plant and Las Vegas, but concluded the location was undesirable because it had no infrastructure.[45]

It seemed the best spot for a company town was adjacent to the plant. The close proximity gave the project access to fundamental civic facilities and the likelihood that workers would show up on time for their shifts. After selecting a town site, BMI continued its search for funding. This was a difficult task. Since Eells's original contract did not include housing, the DPC handled the application. The DPC ultimately postponed selecting the location until September 20 and did not file the application until October 12. Upon receiving it, the FWA expressed anxiety over the cost, $6 million. After a month of deliberations, it finally allocated $3 million to the company town if the DPC covered the balance.[46] In turn, the DPC authorized $240,000 to McNeil Construction Company to begin construction. The construction company prepared to begin work, erecting tents for workers in the desert.[47]

The news that Las Vegas had been overlooked for the company town infuriated local residents. Many businessmen feared that it would lure dam-bound tourism away from Las Vegas and interfere with local politics. In December Las Vegas banded together in an anti-BMI town site campaign. The Taxpayers' Association called a meeting, enlisting the help of Senator Berkeley Bunker, a thirty-six-year-old politician who had been appointed to Senator Key Pittman's seat in 1940.[48]

Bunker was the first southern Nevada resident to hold a congressional seat. *Time* described him as a "serious Mormon ex-Bishop" who rarely spoke on the Senate floor. But during his short time in office, he made headlines on one subject: BMI. Unlike Senator McCarran, who considered BMI a permanent addition to the southern Nevada economy, Bunker thought Eells had engaged in war profiteering. On December 11 Bunker sent a letter to the DPC charging that the town site was motivated by Eells's personal financial profit. After an investigation, the DPC struck a compromise: BMI would build temporary housing intended to be removed after the war. In exchange, the federal government granted Las Vegas a thousand additional building permits, facilitating the construction of the Biltmore, Huntridge, and Mayfair developments.[49]

On December 23 the DPC finally authorized the construction of Victory Village, a town site of one thousand demountable homes, dormitories, Army tents, and trailers. DPC mandated that the village meet PHS standards, requiring streets, stores, sewerage, recreational facilities, power, water, and gas supplies. The additional regulations forced BMI to erect an entire town. Construction began on February 17, 1942. BMI commissioned Paul R. Williams, a famed architect, to design the development. His plan provided for homes, several schools, a grocery and meat market, a department store, beauty and barber shops, a recreation center, a mess hall, a drug store, and other amenities. In May the McNeil crew finished and released fifty-nine homes, but they were not enough. The workforce continued to grow faster than homes could be built.[50]

Since Victory Village was an all-white community, BMI also constructed Carver Park for black workers and their families, located east of the plant. Completed in 1943, Carver Park had 324 houses, a grammar school, a recreation hall, an athletic field, and a small business district. Another option was to live in the Westside, Las Vegas's black district, located across the railroad tracks from Fremont Street. Until the completion of Carver Park in 1943, most black workers and their families lived in Army tents near the plant. Arriving in 1942, Viola Johnson lived in a tent with seven family members. Her family rotated shifts during the day and night, and constant rainstorms and heat spells heightened the cramped conditions. Johnson's recollection of the experience was that "it was awful living there."[51]

While the plans for Victory Village and Carver Park seemed promising, both developments could not handle the high number of workers. In July 1942 the BMI project employed 11,009 construction workers and 1,490 plant laborers. The turnover rate was remarkably only 5 percent a week, most of them unskilled laborers. The numbers surprised L. G. McNeil, president of McNeil Construction, "considering the living conditions." The housing situation eventually attracted the attention of both union and political leaders. Congressmen Scrugham spoke to labor leaders about the "titanic struggle," acquiring raw materials and recruiting labor, that faced the nation. He stressed that BMI needed to improve its living conditions to attract new workers.[52]

But the poor conditions continued. In October only one thousand workers lived in permanent structures. Most lived in a tent city accommodating forty-eight hundred workers, stayed in the Anderson's Camp barracks, or squatted in the desert. The Saturday Evening Post described the chaotic situation in the Las Vegas desert: "Anything larger than a parasol is rated a house.... If it has lights, water and sewer it is a mansion, and anything beyond [that] is pure paradise." The Post went on to say the workers were in "picturesquely squalid discomfort, [living in] trailers and tents, abandoned mine shafts, or sleeping in cars scattered over twenty square miles of desert." Each tent housed four workers and provided a cot, chair, and writing table. The area had no power, running water, or toilets. The workers found it difficult to sleep during the hot summer nights. Some wrapped themselves in wet sheets and slept outside in the dirt. Others visited Fremont Street's clubs or the taverns that dotted Boulder Highway for refuge and a cold drink. Most tried to spend as little time in the tents as possible, often working double shifts or playing card games in the mess hall.[53]

Besides the tent city, the workers doubled up accommodations with families in Las Vegas and Boulder City, participating in Share Your Home programs with households with extra rooms. Others shared beds with coworkers on separate shifts. BMI also entered an agreement with the Boulder Dam Hotel and Hualapai Lodge to rent their hotel rooms. The workers, government officials, and military personnel overwhelmed both hotels. To provide more beds, the Boulder Dam Hotel turned the dining room into a dormitory. The workers also slept on the lobby couches and staircase landings. The conditions lasted until April 1943 when BMI finally rented out thirteen hundred homes and five hundred furnished apartments in Victory Village, although most workers continued to reside in Las Vegas and other places. After construction ended in early 1944, the remaining McNeil crew and BMI workers lived in the town site. That same year its post office opened and Victory Village earned the moniker Henderson.[54]

But the housing controversy did not end there. BMI profited immensely from the development, and Bunker continued to cry foul. All he needed was a spark. Conveniently, his opportunity appeared in the form of a fire. On the evening of March 6, 1942, BMI guards noticed smoke in the southwest of the plant's administration building. Word of the fire spread quickly, and three thousand workers helped evacuate the building. With a limited water supply, they attempted to extinguish the flames. Several men drove bulldozers into the blazing ruins. According to the *Review-Journal,* one of the operators was engulfed in flames as he tried to save an important McNeil vault containing the plant's blueprints. With high desert winds fanning the blaze, the building burned to the ground. Miraculously, the men recovered the blueprints and protected neighboring buildings, and there were no reported injuries. BMI resumed construction the next day, building temporary field offices.[55]

Rumors of sabotage spread immediately. McNeil speculated the fire was the result of saboteurs attempting to halt work on the important war project. A local investigation revealed that the fire had originated in the engineering department. Each afternoon, the building's gas and power sources were supposed to be disconnected, but investigators discovered that the valves had been left open. This confirmed their suspicions; it was likely arson. Someone had entered the room and ignited the gas.[56] It was all the evidence Berkeley Bunker needed. Believing that BMI deliberately set its administration building on fire, he charged that the company's corporate records were intentionally burned. Eells denied the allegations and welcomed an investigation. The Fire Companies Adjustment Bureau ultimately found no indication of arson. Still, the controversy came to the attention of Washington, DC.[57] Headed by Senator Harry S. Truman, the Special Senate Committee Investigating the National Defense Program paid Las Vegas a visit to examine Bunker's allegations.[58]

In March 1942 the Truman Committee began its investigation. After several days of testimonies, it called BMI "one of the most flagrant attempts at war profiteering" observed by the committee. The company received $280,000 in ore royalties, $560,000 for operating the plant annually, and $300,000 for construction and engineering services. The committee called the fees "tremendous" considering the "miserable progress" under current management. It criticized Eells personally, noting that he had "little or no construction experience."[59] Since magnesium was a critical war material needed to advance the aircraft industry, the committee recommended a crackdown on BMI practices. Several days later, Bunker attacked the company on the Senate floor, charging Secretary of Commerce Jesse Jones with committing fraud and entering an unethical partnership with Eells. Jones answered that the allegations were "without foundation," and "false and misleading." He also called Bunker "unworthy" of his Senate seat because the charges not only discredited honest people but also damaged public confidence in the government during a crucial time of national unity.[60]

Throughout the summer Bunker continued to scrutinize Eells, regularly addressing the Senate floor about BMI. The campaign did little to save his political career. He lost the Democratic nomination to James Scrugham, who was a staunch supporter of BMI. Coincidently, Eells's attachment to the plant ended the same year. His contract contained a clause that the DPC could discontinue their relationship after three years and a payout of $1 million. The contract also stated that the DPC could fire Eells if he dishonored the agreement or violated the plans, designs, specifications, or schedules. The DPC dismissed Eells with the latter clause. The plant lacked a coordinated engineering effort, and there were several errors in its construction design and layout. The DPC also charged Eells with overspending, and overvaluing the quality and quantity of his ore reserves. Receiving half the payout the DPC had promised him, Eells was forced to sell BMI. On October 27, 1942, the Anaconda Copper Company bought his management rights for $75,000. The DPC purchased his mining claims for only $450,000.[61]

The BMI project was enormous; at one time, it employed 10 percent of Nevada's population. McNeil Construction Company handled plant and town construction, and more than a dozen subcontractors constructed power transmission lines from Hoover Dam, a fourteen-mile water pipeline, and other architectural and engineering services. The MacDonald Engineering Company also built an oxide plant and housing development at Eells's mine holdings in Gabbs.[62]

Due to its success at Hoover Dam, BMI hired the Anderson Brothers Company to feed its workers. Opening in 1941, its mess hall operated continuously throughout the project; during peak construction, it served forty thousand meals daily. At its peak employment, 13,000 workers demanded a lot of food. At one time, they consumed seventy gallons of coffee and ninety dozen doughnuts each morning, seventy-five gallons of beef stew daily, and three tons of frankfurters a week. The Anderson Brothers also provided beverage services at the plant, stocking canteen and coffee stands to ensure workers remained hydrated and alert. The company estimated that each worker drank more than two gallons of water per shift.[63]

McNeil employed the largest contingent of workers. In September 1941 the construction company began leveling and grading the 2,800-acre site. BMI was a cellular manufacturing factory that involved the utilization of multiple "cells" connected in an assembly line. The product moved from one cell to the next, with each station completing portions of the manufacturing process. Within a year the McNeil crew had erected several cells; installed electrical, plumbing, and heating; and constructed roads, fencing, foundations, machinery support, drains, and sewers. The company also subcontracted with the Columbia Steel Company to fabricate ten chlorination buildings, ten electrolysis buildings, two chlorine buildings, and a preparation building. With electrical transmission lines embedded in subterranean tunnels, McNeil built 40 percent of the plant underground. The electrical equipment cost $12 million, with more than two hundred thousand yards of concrete. McNeil described the plant as a "complicated, veritable jigsaw puzzle" with "endless miles" of pipes, compressors, pumps, tanks, and heat exchangers resembling "a great pattern of lace." His workers "toiled through wind, sand, and heat" to build it and were very efficient, setting new records daily. The Fritz Ziebarth Company constructed the power line from Hoover Dam, finishing twenty-five days ahead of schedule, and Engineers Limited completed the fourteen-mile-long water system from Lake Mead on time.[64]

Construction began at the mines in Gabbs simultaneously. The MacDonald crew built an oxide plant and housing development, and a loading area to transport the raw materials south. The plant became operational in June 1942 and employed nine hundred workers. The *Big Job* described it as "a triumph of modern engineering" that processed raw magnesite into magnesium through "a maze" of conveyors and pipelines. The first shipment left the following week. At first, BMI transported the material from Gabbs to Salt Lake to Las Vegas on railroad freight cars. But the eleven-hundred-mile trip was expensive and the cost convinced the DPC to build a highway connecting Gabbs to Las Vegas. BMI hired Wells Inc. to drive trucks on 668-mile round-trips every twenty-eight hours. It was the biggest trucking operation in the nation, and the longest haul undertaken on a continuous basis.[65]

Although construction in Henderson did not end until October 1943, the chlorine plant started production in August. Chlorine was an essential wartime material, providing a base in chemical warfare and purified water. It also helped in production of magnesium. The first batch of liquid chlorine left the plant on August 9. By the end of the month, workers operated an entire section of the plant. Within six weeks, they loaded the first shipment of magnesium to Southern California to make aircraft and bomb parts. BMI had reached full production a year later. It was the largest metal producer in the world. When the plant closed in November 1944, it had operated continuously for 807 days. The production numbers were astounding. In 1938 the United States consumed 2,400 tons of magnesium and by 1941 the national output was 12,400 tons. During BMI's short tenure, it produced more than 83,000 tons of marketable, refined, or alloyed magnesium.[66]

Constructing a war plant and producing magnesium was hazardous work. As with most industries during World Wars I and II, war provided an exception for health and safety, certainly in terms of legislation and public acceptance of the risks involved. The war increased demands on production, introducing unskilled workers to new, untested manufacturing processes and greater exposures to chemical hazards. Working in mobilizing America was dangerous business. In fact, during the first three years of the war, more Americans died at the workplace than on the battlefield. Eventually, the Division of Labor Standards took a more active role in plant inspections, training, education, and industrial safety, but workers still fended for themselves.[67] In Nevada, state intervention concerning workplace safety virtually disappeared within all federally backed projects. The state learned an important lesson from the State Inspector of Mines Andy Stinson's attempt to protect tunnel workers from carbon monoxide at the Boulder Canyon Project. If Nevada wanted federal development, it had to relinquish most decisions on protecting employee health and safety in their workplaces. This arrangement prevailed at BMI and later federal undertakings on Nevada soil, notably the NTS.

Unlike the Boulder Canyon Project, the occupational health regime that formed around BMI was not particularly unique or innovative, borrowing from existing methods in the region and resembling most American war plants. Most deaths and injuries occurred due to human error, fatigue, poor communication, limited experience, and inadequate risk perception. McNeil's construction crew frequently reported falls while working; in July 1943 one worker suffered terminal head and chest injuries after falling fifty feet.[68] Driving on uneven ground, the construction workers also regularly tipped over the trucks and cranes, crushing or trapping themselves underneath. There were numerous automobile accidents as well; cars repeatedly struck workers who were walking to work. In fact, traffic accidents in and around industrial work was a widespread problem nationally. In 1943 *Time* reported that battlefronts abroad were safer than working in America's war plants. The newspaper reported that traffic accidents had killed 22,500 war workers since Pearl Harbor, while 16,913 soldiers had died in combat.[69] Another hazard at BMI were frequent fires. The March 1942 fire that sparked Bunker's attention burned the administration to the ground within an hour. Remarkably, the workers who heroically saved the plant blueprints sustained only minor injuries. Several months later, a fire erupted in the electrolysis building. Subsequent fires in the peat pits and sheet metal shop burned the structures to the ground, with an estimated cost of $85,000. The causes ranged from arson to natural coincidences, according to the *Review-Journal*.[70]

Since the Gabbs workers were experienced miners, injuries and deaths were relatively rare. The miners entered the deposit by drilling and blasting, achieving the greatest degree of selective mining. After extracting the mineral, a nearby manufacturing plant handled crushing, floating, and drying the raw material. Still, workers regularly inhaled dangerous levels of dust, and experienced burn wounds and crush-related accidents while operating heavy machinery in the ore pit. At first the crushing unit did not make provisions to eliminate dust, but BMI corrected the problem after the State Inspector of Mines issued a citation. This was one of the only instances when the state intervened in health and safety on the project. Overall, most accidents were incidental to the industry; casualness with safety protocol contributed to most injuries. When a large boulder struck a worker in the mining pit, an investigation determined carelessness caused the accident. Anxious to finish work at noon, the miners overlooked safety precautions, and their coworker died from a cerebral hemorrhage triggered by a fracture to his skull.[71]

Back in Henderson, the plant's biggest problems were labor turnover and fatigued workers. At first the summer heat, chronic inhalation of chlorine gas, and inadequate housing attributed to its high turnover rate. Under Executive Order 9301, the plant's maximum work hours were forty-eight hours over a six-day week, with eight-hour shifts. But manpower shortages and various emergency situations forced most employees to work seven days a week, ten-hour shifts. BMI paid double time for Sundays, provided an employee had worked the six preceding days. All shifts rotated to ensure twenty-four-hour production. To be sure, the manufacturing process was complicated and most employees had very limited industrial experience. After Gabbs miners converted the raw magnesite into magnesium oxide, plant workers mixed it with peat moss, coal dust, salt, potassium chloride, and calcium chloride. Next, they cemented the compound into bricks, melted it in kilns, and placed it in an electric furnace. A blast with chlorine transformed the compound into magnesium chloride bars. Workers then packed and shipped it to another war factory.[72]

Of course, this manufacturing process facilitated adverse health conditions for all employees involved. One by-product was the intense heat. Temperatures soared in the plant during the summer because of the desert environment, but BMI also had installed inadequate ventilation and cooling equipment. Besides the heat, workers regularly handled dangerous chemicals. An essential part of the process was chlorine gas, but it was highly toxic.[73] Chlorine or sulfur gassings occurred regularly. Exposed workers complained of chronic coughing, chills, and fever. The company allowed disability leaves for up to three weeks. Most workers were understandably concerned about its harmful short- and long-term effects, but BMI stressed that "chlorine gas positively [did] not result in tuberculosis" or lung trouble, with the exception of rare cases. The cure to their regular, workplace gassings was simply "a few minutes of fresh air after exposure."[74]

Still, BMI recognized that gassings were a threat. To limit liability, its health-care policy specified that it covered all gassing injuries without cost to the employee. But while workers protected themselves with safety gear, including masks, gloves, protective eyewear, and wooden shoes, accidents were frequent. High labor turnover and an unskilled workforce contributed to a very high number of gassings, especially in the electrical department. In fact, injuries were plentiful throughout BMI's short tenure, involving inhalation of dust and other particles, life-threatening burns from hot metals, and explosions splattering employees with molten magnesium. In 1943 Clark County reported 356 accidents, the second most in the state. White Pine County was the state's most dangerous county in which to work. In 1944 the figures were identical, with both counties reporting 724 accidents in one year.[75]

To make matters worse, the housing shortage made living conditions very uncomfortable, and the Anderson Brothers developed a reputation for its inadequate hygiene and food preparation. On one occasion, ptomaine and food poisoning sickened 123 workers after they ate in the mess hall. In another, dozens of workers ate moldy pies, sickening them. The State Board of Health investigated the incident, revealing the pies spoiled due to fluctuating temperatures and unsanitary habits in the mess hall. Besides issuing a complaint, the State Board of Health had little authority to fix the conditions. Employees also did not have healthy options to spend their time off from work.

Unlike the LA&SL and Six Companies company towns, Eells did not initially plan out healthy extracurricular activities. Wartime rationing virtually prohibited employees from leaving, so many drank alcohol on site. Some workers managed to get to clubs on Boulder Highway and Fremont Street, where they gambled heavily. Consequently, the quality of work at the plant suffered; there were numerous reports of workers showing up to their shifts drunk, late, or not at all. BMI recognized the problem and began promoting wholesome recreational activities for employee leisure time, hosting dances, arts and craft instruction, and chess games. The company also sponsored church groups, fraternal organizations, and athletic teams. While the programs helped somewhat, workers continued to overindulge, leading to high rates of absenteeism. In fact, BMI had the highest absentee rate of any defense plant in the nation during World War II. In the week of January 18, 1943, 3,041 out of 4,000 employees were absent, averaging four hundred per day. Of course, the rate was not only due to local vice. Working mothers frequently skipped shifts as well, contending with their often-conflicting roles as family caretaker and wage earner. Both company newsletters regularly condemned absenteeism, calling the practice "Old Man Absenteeism" and the "production enemy and ally of the Japanazi," and warning that absent workers killed American soldiers on the warfront.[76]

The conditions resulted in a high labor turnover rate at BMI, a common problem among American employers during World War II. During the plant's construction, the U.S. Employment Service recruited one thousand workers per month to compensate for turnover. While the rate declined when Victory Village and Carver Park construction completed, workers continued to quit. Many suffered dust or gas inhalation, and left because of health reasons. Union representative E. E. Ward testified to the Truman Committee that "hundreds of cases of workers" quit because "their lives [were] endangered" and they did not want to take "any further risk." Indeed, high labor turnover plagued the nation throughout the war. While Depression-era workers desperately sought employment, World War II employment was so plentiful that companies competed for labor. War workers frequently quit for better pay, because competition between employers produced an inequality of wages, housing, and transportation arrangements; and unhygienic and dangerous conditions. The War Manpower Board tried to fix the problem, issuing a freezing arrangement with employers and unions stating that no worker could seek new jobs without obtaining a certificate of separation. To solidify the agreement, the War Labor Board also raised mining wages. In theory, both arrangements prevented BMI workers, employees of the manganese plant in Boulder City, and miners in Goodsprings from terminating employment. However, there were exceptions made. Employers could leave in cases of gross misconduct or an inability to perform higher-skilled work, and workers could quit if they had compelling reasons or their wages were less favorable in comparison to the community. Since these conditions were often difficult to prove, BMI workers were denied discharge requests at the rate of 240 to 250 per day.[77]

In the end, the order failed and BMI continued its chronic labor shortage. Each department lacked enough employees to perform their assignments well. Some workers estimated their departments were short, some by more than fifteen men. *Basic Bombardier* projected that during the project's duration there were 21,022 terminations and 22,514 hires at the plant, excluding construction hires and quits. The plant experienced the highest turnover rate from 1943 to 1944, averaging 20 to 30 percent per month. As a last resort, BMI arranged a bargain with local courts. Judges in Lincoln Heights, Las Vegas, and Los Angeles began offering minor offenders and alcoholics the choice of jail time or employment at BMI. Petty criminals arrived by the busload, working long enough to draw their first pay and then quitting. While serving as a sheriff in Pittman, M. L. Reese remembered arresting a man who spent eighteen months in jail for driving drunk. After an all-night drinking bender, Reese arrested him again after finding him naked in broad daylight, taking a bath in a galvanized tub. Three days later, the man became a BMI employee, working in the mechanical maintenance department. Headhunters in Phoenix, Reno, Tucson, Barstow, San Diego, and Los Angles also began offering recruits $10 for getting on a bus headed for Las Vegas. The recruits often worked an hour and disappeared, while others lasted a week or two.[78]

The hiring practices did not foster a competent workforce, but management was partially to blame. E. A. Phaenuf, who had worked as an operator for BMI for over a year, told the Truman Committee in August 1943 that there was "no management" at the plant and his subordinate supervisors were "afraid to assume any responsibility." Under those conditions, it was very difficult to monitor health and safety. Moreover, Phaenuf attested that BMI's poor working conditions "very definitely" contributed to high labor turnover. Still, he testified that most employees were proud to work there. To help with the war effort, many men and women worked double shifts and overtime. He blamed the underlying problem on "incompetent management."[79]

The situation would have been worse if not for BMI's dedicated labor presence, which served as the strongest faction of the plant's occupational health regime. In the 1940s unions rose to prominence due to wartime labor shortages and a strong relationship with the Roosevelt administration, who legitimized their presence in the American workplace with the National Labor Relations (Wagner) Act in 1935. Union membership increased from 10 million workers in 1940 to nearly 15 million in 1945. Moreover, the portion of the labor enrolled in collective bargaining rose from 30 to 45 percent. Prior to World War II labor activists were at odds with employers, but the National War Labor Board arranged a compromise to agree to a nonbinding, no-strike pledge for the duration of the conflict. The arrangement did not end strike activity completely, but forged a generally harmonious relationship between the various parties. Most historians agree that unions reached a new level of maturity during World War II. Labor and management shared a common goal, and learned how to communicate and negotiate better under the direction of the federal government. Instead of advocating for structural economic reform or redistribution of wealth and power, unions started focusing on economic growth through increased consumption. In turn, the new relationship enhanced industrial stability and provided workers with enhanced job security, a pattern that continued into the postwar period.[80]

While often at odds, the AFL and the Congress of Industrial Organizations (CIO) both represented the BMI workers. Both unions played important roles in wartime production throughout the nation, and fought to control the labor market. The AFL initially had a stronghold on southern Nevada, securing a contract with BMI to oversee the operation. However, it was a union known for conservative leanings and refusal to represent minorities, and for maintaining a close relationship with management. When the AFL barred black workers from acquiring union membership at BMI, it provided an opening for the CIO. In December 1942 the International Union of Mine, Mill, and Smelter Workers (IUMMSW), a CIO affiliate, launched a campaign, printing newspaper ads directed toward employees to rethink their union representation.[81]

Eventually, the National Labor Relations Board (NLRB) had to intervene. According to the Wagner Act, employers were obligated to recognize a union chosen by the majority of its workers. But when BMI drafted its original AFL contract, it had no employees. The agency consequently ordered an election to determine whether employees would be represented by the CIO, AFL, or neither. The CIO won with a clear majority. Still, the AFL declared its contract was still valid, and filed an objection with the NLRB. In July 1943 the NLRB had established that the AFL had no merit and granted certification to the CIO. Even though the National War Labor Board did not accept jurisdiction in this case, the Truman Committee eventually had to intervene. It invited the AFL and CIO to testify about dealings and working conditions at BMI. After hearing both sides, the Truman Committee determined the absence of a decent labor-management relationship influenced not only production but also morale, significantly disrupting the work process at BMI. They called for a quick resolution. In the end, the struggle brought national attention to discrimination and unsatisfactory conditions at the plant, prompting the federal government to enforce tighter regulations. For the duration of the project, BMI employees enjoyed an improved workplace environment under CIO direction.[82]

One of the major benefits of the CIO securing an influence over operations was improved health and safety at the plant. Like the Boulder Canyon Project before it, the initial program was lackluster at first, but gradually improved. BMI management promoted safety, posting Safety Pays signs and requiring workers to attend training classes. Using methods established by the WPB, the target of the program was employing unskilled workers and acclimating them to production line jobs quickly. It was based on four instruction steps: preparation, presentations, job tryout, and follow-up.[83] Foremen, assistant foremen, or experienced workers trained 90 percent of the workers. Engineers oversaw the operation from the Safety Department, stressing that prevention is better than a cure, mandating that all employees wear protective hats, dust respirators, gas masks, goggles or plastic face shields, and rubber gloves. The department also provided decontamination showers, as well as first aid stations and oxygen treatment in the case of gassings.[84]

The Safety Department adapted different programs based on the individual work conducted in each division: Preparation, Electrolysis, Chlorination, Refinery, and Recovery Departments; and the Neutralization and Chlorine Plant. The Refinery Department provided face shields, respirators, asbestos gloves, asbestos aprons, and fire blankets if an employee's clothing caught fire. Foremen in the Chlorine Plant were instructed to tell workers to hold their breath and "walk unhurriedly away from the area into the wind" in the event of a gassing. If unable to do so, they were advised to "breathe shallow and short breaths to avoid coughing." Of course, BMI management also stressed to inform workers that chlorine gas was "not cumulative" and eventually wore off "without permanent after effects." In all the divisions, the Safety Department encouraged good housekeeping; prohibited smoking, drinking liquor, and all roughhousing; requested that workers report unsafe conditions; and punished negligent behavior. If workers were drunk, fell asleep, ignored safety requirements, or acted insubordinate, their actions were grounds for dismissal.[85]

Similar to the dam project, the NIC provided compensation benefits to injured workers. The BMI Legal Department established a division to assist with making claims for medical benefits and compensation. Disabled employees received 60 percent of their average earnings, up to $72 a month. Similar to Hoover Dam, the program was marginally successful. The NIC did not cover cases in which an employee refused or neglected to submit to medical attention, or chlorine gassings and dust inhalation. As outlined by union representative E. E. Ward, "If you get dust infection of the lungs or gas infection [while working at

BMI], the only way you get anything out of it is to die. If you are injured in your lungs by this dust and gas infection, there is no compensation for it—if you die the estate may benefit by a few dollars." To its credit, BMI attempted to cover the NIC exclusions, adopting a blanket insurance program. But while it provided accident and death benefits, and surgical and hospital care, the program did not meet all the needs of its employees.[86]

Another lacking program was the plant's medical facilities. Eells originally conceived the hospital as a temporary structure providing first aid care to construction workers and plant employees, with serious cases sent to Las Vegas or Los Angeles. But the lack of medical care in close proximity to the plant fostered a "drastic" situation in 1942, according to Eells. Knowing that heat contributed to high fatalities at the dam project, he recognized that the environmental conditions were "dangerous and critical," and that his medical facility could not accommodate the sheer number of workers and their families. He pleaded with the Truman Committee to provide funding for "proper care" with the "hot weather approaching." Still, hospital construction did not begin until the summer, and BMI had to ambulance injured workers to Las Vegas or transport them via rail to Los Angeles.[87]

The McNeil crew completed the facility in only two months. Located adjacent to the plant, BMI appointed Dr. F. E. Clough as chief surgeon, a specialist in industrial medicine and bone and joint surgery, to consult on its design. The *Big Job* recounted the job, describing the doctor as "busy as a tail gunner for months," checking the details of construction and expediting the technical apparatus. The design was hardly innovative, and borrowed from Clough's experience as the chief surgeon of the Homestake Mining Company in South Dakota. When he joined the project, Clough stressed the importance of health and safety: "The big and important about the new hospital is that it represents something relatively new in American industry. Embodied in its physical structure and the apparatus and equipment which it houses, the hospital is a monument to the insistence of modern industry that health and safety of employees is of vital importance." Clough called the hospital "relatively new in the industry." He sought to provide medical care "with the utmost expedition" and "wholehearted personal service" to workers, and to treat families when "space was available." Built according to the PHS code, the hospital had a sprinkling system for fire safety, an air-cooling and heating system, x-ray equipment, delivery and operating rooms, and an outpatient section. It also retained twenty-four-hour ambulance service with drivers trained in first aid, well-equipped with the "latest equipment" in medical science. According to Clough, BMI spared no expense, guaranteeing workers they had "the best," with three doctors on staff: Drs. Chauncey Baird, A. F. O'Conner, and Ned D. Miller, and twenty-five nurses. After a dedication ceremony, which Clough described as a mixture of "patriotism, medical ethics, and the concern for modern industry for the welfare of its employees," the hospital opened in October 1942.[88]

The swift construction led to multiple issues. Anaconda Copper Company's acquisition of BMI in October 1942 also disrupted the workers' health insurance coverage. Furthermore, the new company decided to discontinue their pay-deduction insurance plan, causing mass confusion among workers who did not understand the terms of their coverage. Even the doctors were confused. In December Clough finally received clarification from Anaconda and issued a statement. The plan covered injuries sustained on the job and service-connected cases such as chlorine gassings, without charge. Industrial diseases not covered under state laws were handled individually. For injuries and illnesses sustained off duty, workers paid out of pocket at reduced rates ranging from $5 to $6 a day. Operating and delivery room fees were $15. Clough believed the rates were reasonable and that they conformed to all accepted standards. By summer 1943, organizational and billing issues prompted Anaconda to adopt a blanket insurance plan. Thereafter, employees made hospital payments through payroll deductions if the NIC did not provide coverage. In cases of short-term disability, workers could not return to the plant until the medical division had cleared them.[89]

Problems also manifested on the hospital floor. With only fifty beds, the facility could not accommodate thousands of BMI employees. Workers complained of waiting hours or days to see a doctor. Overwhelmed with employee cases, the medical staff rarely treated families. Most workers expressed dissatisfaction with the quality of care, which contributed to the labor turnover. The hospital was also understaffed, a condition that affected the entire American hospital system during World War II. After Pearl Harbor, Washington, DC, required all male physicians under forty-five years of age to register for the draft. Those older than forty-five served in civilian roles. Until the war ended in 1945, military hospitals managed a ratio of 6.5 physicians per 1,000 soldiers, while civilian hospitals dropped to 1 physician per 1,500 civilians. In response, medical colleges accelerated their doctor of medicine (M.D.) programs from four to three years of training, and elderly physicians had to come out of retirement. Despite the efforts, all American hospitals during the war were short-staffed.[90]

Rural regions like southern Nevada, with limited prewar medical care, were particularly hard hit. Las Vegas tried to accommodate the influx of war workers, but the physician-to-patient ratio was highly disproportionate. In 1942 the Las Vegas Hospital and Clinic had to recruit doctors, such as state epidemiologist Dr. Gerald Sylvain, to ease the problem. Sylvain found Las Vegas's hospitals to be highly deficient, with the exception of the Las Vegas Hospital. As with preceding decades, surgeons performed few surgeries in town and sent the most serious cases to Los Angeles. The influx of military trainees and war workers from the Las Vegas Air Gunnery School and BMI made Sylvain's job very busy, a stark contrast from his quiet practice in Goldfield. "We were absolutely overworked in Las Vegas" and "short of doctors." "We did everything," he recalled. Sylvain worked long hours, seeing patients during the day and making house calls at night. While he rotated shifts, the schedule was often overwhelming. In 1944 Sylvain was drafted, and he entered military service. The doctor called it a "two-year vacation" compared to practicing in Las Vegas.[91]

Until the completion of the hospital, BMI transported injured employees to Las Vegas, not Boulder City. While the Boulder City Hospital prospered during the Boulder Canyon Project, Six Companies Inc. closed it in 1935. Boulder City residents traveled to Las Vegas for medical care, a long trip that sometimes proved fatal. In 1938 the National

Park Service acquired the hospital building, turning it into a museum, only to abandon it in 1941. In December 1943 the PHS reopened the hospital to treat wounded soldiers, but not locals.[92]

White employees and their families chose between two options in Las Vegas: the Las Vegas Hospital and Clinic and Clark County General Hospital. Black employees typically stuck to the latter, because it was more tolerant of race than the private hospital. Opening in 1931 the county hospital also accommodated indigents. In the 1940s doctors started to perform surgeries under the direction of Dr. Jack Cherry, the house physician and administrator. As the only public hospital in Las Vegas, however, it had great difficulty treating the population. In 1943 the Federal Works Administration assumed ownership and invested $447,000 in its modernization. But even with 146 beds, Army personnel and BMI employees continued to overwhelm the facility, often lining the hallways. As with most hospitals during times of war, the physician shortage forced nurses to play a bigger role in treatment. Registered nurse Mary Kennedy Rymer remembered that "there was nothing that was too big for [nurses]" at that time. They "tried it all," taking x-rays, delivering babies, and assisting in surgery. When the hospital opened at 3:00 A.M. to treat emergencies, she remembered the night shift attending to construction workers at BMI. Rymer described them as "rough and tough," regularly becoming drunk and crashing their cars or getting into fights. But unless the cases were "very tragic or very major," nurses treated the patients without the guidance of a doctor.[93]

Even when the BMI hospital opened in October 1941, the problems continued regarding quality and access to care. Overrun with patients, the medical staff complained of exhaustion, and worked multiple shifts for days at a time. With strict production deadlines, BMI also pressured them to get injured employees back to work as soon as possible. The practice often clashed with medical ethics, and sometimes cost doctors their jobs. When management requested that Dr. Arthur Miller clear an injured employee for work, he adamantly refused. The worker needed more recovery time, he attested. When management ordered him to sign the certificate regardless, Miller refused again.

He was subsequently discharged, which added to the problem of understaffing. Besides the exhausting hours, the company routinely discharged staff members that challenged company policy, but most doctors disliked working there and quit. Consequently, the hospital experienced a very high turnover rate. Even Cough eventually had enough, resigning in 1944; he was replaced by Dr. David E. Hemington. The hospital was so understaffed that Dr. Roy Martin came out of retirement to help out, administering physical examinations and delivering babies, until his death in 1943.[94]

Despite the poor living, working, and hospital conditions, southern Nevada maintained a fair health record during the war. As a whole, Clark County had a low mortality rate. According to the State Board of Health, the most pressing issues statewide were accident fatalities, not diseases. The high number of accidents in Nevada's industries indicated that it needed a widespread safety campaign that reached all Nevadans to make them accident conscious. Still, this recommendation was largely rhetoric, because the state had little authority to instill any real change in workplace safety. Besides accidents, degenerative conditions like heart disease and cancer steadily increased statewide, but health experts expected the increase since the general population was aging. To combat communicable diseases, the State Board of Health provided diphtheria, smallpox, and typhoid immunizations and regularly inspected labor camps and communities.

Although there were no major epidemics, Nevada reported one notable outbreak. The State Board of Health noticed a significant rise in venereal diseases, attributed to the state's increased military and industrial activities. In Nevada more people died per capita from venereal diseases than in any other state besides Wyoming. Indeed, venereal diseases were problematic nationally, hampering the war effort, leading Surgeon General Dr. Thomas Parran Jr. to refer to syphilis as a major threat to Americans during World War I.[95]

In 1943 Nevada reported 777 cases of syphilis and 351 cases of gonorrhea. The numbers remained steady throughout 1944, with 561 cases of syphilis and 460 cases of gonorrhea reported during the first ten months. The outbreak was particularly serious in Clark County, affecting numerous Army personnel and BMI employees. In April 1944 alone, the Clark County Health Department reported 176 cases.[96]

Since syphilis was painless and difficult to recognize, local doctors found the disease difficult to diagnose and treat. In the 1940s the medical profession understood the causes of syphilis and gonorrhea, and treatments were available. But until the mass production of penicillin in 1944, there was no speedy cure. To fight the outbreak, the Clark County Health Department established a venereal disease clinic completely devoted to the cause, and set controls for tuberculosis, food inspection and sanitation, school health, and other diseases. The clinic also applied advanced techniques to detect the diseases. Technicians examined slides of gonorrhea with a microscope and studied blood tests to diagnose syphilis. In cooperation with the military, the clinic also diagnosed gonorrhea by the culture method.[97]

Local residents also fought venereal diseases, focusing on prevention. The most visible campaign outlawed commercialized prostitution. In the early 1940s, Block 16's brothels still flourished on Fremont Street, but there was little regulation. The Clark County Health Department knew the brothels needed to be regulated or shut down. Dr. F. W. York, a public health officer, acknowledged that prostitution was "one of the main attractions to tourists," but it also heightened the threat of venereal diseases.[98] The Clark County Health Department pushed for tighter regulation, enacting policies requiring all prostitutes to receive physical examinations. If the women did not get a clean bill of health, they could not work. The program did little good, and syphilis and gonorrhea continued to spread. The social stigma and public health hazard eventually prompted a movement to end prostitution in Clark County. In November 1940 local attorney J. R. Lewis declared that "running, operating, and maintaining houses of assignation and prostitution" were "injurious to health." In mid-1941 the justice court cited four brothels for violating a statute that outlawed prostitution nearby a church.[99] By the time BMI construction began, federal authorities had stepped in. The stigma was far too great to the government to invest in a region that allowed prostitution. PHS surgeon Dr. F. T. Ford commented, "If we go to war, the red-light district [in Las Vegas] would [have to] be banned." While the federal authorities were primarily interested in the morality of prostitution, closing the brothels also would improve public health. At the end of 1942 Clark County outlawed prostitution and instituted a fine to individuals willingly transmitting venereal diseases.[100] One promiscuous local woman allegedly spread diseases to several Army personnel and BMI employees. When given the choice of a $500 fine or jail time, she chose the latter. Other plans included sex education programs in high schools and the disbursement of condoms. The legislature even discussed requiring couples to take premarital blood tests, which was a requirement in many states. Most programs instituted were unsuccessful, mainly due to the social stigma of discussing sex and the use of contraceptives, and opposition to the impediment of Nevada's hassle-free marriage industry.[101]

In the end, the occupational health regime that coalesced at BMI was fragmented and at times completely ineffective. The plant's accident rate was astonishingly high. During the first year of production, Clark County reported 356 accidents, with the majority at BMI. By the second year, high labor turnover and other factors drove the number to 723.[102]

In the national arena, 13,600 war workers were killed and 171,100 permanently injured from 1941 to 1945. As health and safety entered the national discussion, there was much debate regarding who to blame for injuries and fatalities in the workplace. Was it management's responsibility to protect their employees? Was it the fault of worker carelessness? Was America's need for production more important than human lives? *Forbes* acknowledged that war called for "stepped up production" involving "increased hazards," and "the hazards, if not controlled, [resulted] in accidents and lost manpower just when the loss may be disastrous." The magazine concluded that when management took the viewpoint that "production must be achieved at all costs—accidents [were] in the making." Most employers continued to refuse their responsibility to their employees, citing that wartime called for increased production, and that accident statistics were not accurate and did not account for the "personal factor." A March 1942 article in *Popular Mechanics* blamed the problem on "a blitzkrieg led by General Carelessness."[103]

Federal officials knew the importance of health and safety, and the staggeringly high fatalities and accidents during the first years of mobilization prompted action. In a letter to Frances Perkins, Roosevelt wrote, "Work accidents in 1940 cause an aggregate time loss of close to one and one half billion man hours lost." He also said that health and safety was mutually beneficial to all parties involved. Workplace accidents were a "heavy social burden inflicted upon workers and their families" as well as a "money loss" to employers and a "staggering wastage of effective manpower," slowing production. Under Perkins's direction, the DOL created the National Committee for the Conservation of Manpower in Defense Industries. The committee comprised labor, management, and federal officials, and led a public relations campaign outlining safety programs and minimum requirements for employers. In 1943 workplace accidents and deaths continued to mount, prompting the Roosevelt administration to found the Industrial Health and Safety Section of the Plant and Community Facilities Services Division of the Office of Labor Production in the WPB. Composed of the War Department, private organizations, and the CIO and AFL, it ultimately confronted a long-standing problem in American labor history. Despite the wartime conditions, neither management nor labor were prepared to change its view on health and safety. While most of the Service's campaigns never materialized, it helped create greater conformity in safety requirements in wartime federal contracts, and fostered improved dialogue and cooperation between labor and management. During the war, American workers also used their federal contracts as bargaining tools to improve conditions, and labor activists worked alongside the National Safety Council to help staff and support safety programs. The Council also convinced the National Committee for the Conservation of Manpower in War Industries to enlist the help of defense-related companies, and the Maritime Commission to promote health and safety at its shipyards.[104]

The significance of World War II in occupational health history is that it was the first time that the national stage seriously discussed the notion of employer and federal responsibility, laying important groundwork for its standardization in the following decades. Another visible benefit was that while accident rates soared, fatalities dropped.

In 1941 the National Safety Council reported eighteen thousand deaths in America's war plants. In 1945 sixteen thousand workers died, a drop of 11 percent. While high by modern standards, it was progress. At BMI there were considerably fewer permanently disabling injuries after 1943. From July 1942 to July 1943, seventy-five workers experienced permanent disabling injuries. The following year, the company reported only five. Moreover, there were very few fatalities in comparison to the Boulder Canyon Project. The number was less than twenty, with the majority occurring during construction. Finally, unlike the heat and carbon monoxide poisoning at the dam, there were no major disasters.[105]

One explanation for BMI's low fatality rate was its limited production time; the plant ran for only twenty-six months. This also explains why its occupational health regime never enjoyed much success. The plant was the largest magnesium producer in the world by 1943, manufacturing 25 percent of all American output. Yet despite its success, discussion regarding its future also began. In 1944 McCarran learned that the WPB planned to cut BMI production by 40 percent, arguing that there was an oversupply of magnesium and the nation needed to conserve energy. The senator launched a campaign to save the plant, charging that the federal government purposely built the plant with no postwar use in mind. He cited similar situations occurred across western and southern states, and charged that the WPB did not cut Dow Chemical's production or eliminate aluminum plants in Southern California despite surpluses. The fight to save BMI continued throughout the year. But with no need, the WPB ordered a nationwide reduction of magnesium in July. In September it announced the cut of all production, and the closing of BMI and International Minerals in Austin, Texas. Layoffs began immediately. In July 1944 the plant employed twenty-six hundred workers. In October that number was cut in half. On November 17, 1944, the plant closed shop.[106]

Despite the end of BMI, the plant site, community, and hospital evolved, eventually reorganizing its occupational health regime to support future industry at the site. In 1946 the RFC relinquished custody of the plant and arranged its sale. Determined to ensure the future of southern Nevada industry, the state purchased half the plant site and sold it to producers of titanium, alkali, and other chemicals. The new companies, and the expanded Las Vegas Air Gunnery School (renamed Nellis Air Force Base), attracted veterans to the region in search of employment after the war. The company town also grew into a booming community. Incorporated in 1953, Henderson became one of the fastest growing cities in the United States, with a population increase of over 100 percent in eighteen months.[107]

A key component of the community was the evolution of the company hospital, which remained open after the plant closed. Its future remained uncertain, however, until Reverend Peter Maran, a local pastor at St. Peter the Apostle Church, supported the cause. In 1946 he contacted the Adrian Dominican Sisters of Michigan to manage the hospital. They agreed, incorporating in the State of Nevada in 1947 after receiving endorsements from Clark County Medical Society and local doctors.[108]

The Sisters negotiated a deal with the RFC, signing a twenty-five-year lease of the land, buildings, hospital equipment, and supplies for $1 a year. The only stipulation was that they could not transfer ownership, and the hospital needed to provide twenty-four-hour medical and surgical treatment for lessees of the plant. The Sisters renamed the facility St. Rose de Lima Hospital, and staffed it with well-qualified nurses. Physicians were harder to recruit, a problem that continued throughout the century. But the hospital continued, playing a crucial role in supporting the health of the expanding community of Henderson.[109]

From August 1942 to November 1944, the plant produced 166,322,685 pounds of magnesium. The company newsletter boasted that "every drop of molten metal [was] on the first leg of its journey of destruction of Tokio [sic] and Berlin."[110] After leaving the plant, its alloy was used to construct bombs and fabricate bombers. Allied bombers dropped explosive incendiaries over Europe and the Pacific, dislocating the German and Japanese military, industrial, and economic system, and damaging morale. The most dramatic bombs came last: On July 26, 1945, the USS *Indianapolis* delivered a classified shipment to the Marianas. A Japanese submarine torpedoed the warship, but it had delivered its important cargo: a uranium-based atomic bomb. The Manhattan Project successfully tested its plutonium counterpart on July 16 at the Trinity Site in Alamogordo, New Mexico. On August 6, 1945, the *Enola Gay* dropped a bomb over Hiroshima. The nuclear explosion changed the world forever, ushering in a new period of occupational health history and an exceptionally risky line of work for American labor.

## NOTES

1. Aldrich, *Safety-First*, 156–57; Kersten, *Labor's Home Front*, 172–73.

2. Kersten, *Labor's Home Front*, 173.

3. Markowitz and Rosner, *"Slaves of the Depression,"* 166, 203–20, 271–72. See also David Brody, "The New Deal and World War II," in *The New Deal*, Vol. 1, *The National Level*, ed. John Braeman, Robert Bremner, and David Brody, 267–309 (Columbus: Ohio State University Press, 1975).

4. Paul Koistinen, *Arsenal of World War II: The Political Economy of American Warfare, 1940–1945* (Lawrence: University of Kansas Press, 2004), 502; Alan S. Milward, *War, Economy and Society, 1939–1945* (Berkeley: University of California Press, 1980), 63.

5. While some progressive reforms affected the West, the New Deal pioneered the connection between the region and the federal government, a connection that expanded during World War II. The New Deal restructured the region's social order by envisioning a new relationship between the people and land use, creating a legacy of constructive government accomplishments in conservation, public power, and natural resource use. It is questionable how well the federal government was able to sustain its achievements, leaving a mixed legacy in water management, land policies, and relations with Native Americans. In the end, World War II and not the New Deal revitalized the region. See Richard Lowitt, *The New Deal and the West* (Norman: University of Oklahoma Press, 1993); numerous works by Nash, including Nash, *The American West Transformed: The Impact of the Second World War* (Lincoln: University of Nebraska Press, 1985); Nash, *World War II and the West, Reshaping the Economy* (Lincoln: University of Nebraska Press, 1990); Nash, *The Crucial Era: The Great Depression and World War II, 1929–1945* (New York: St. Martin's Press, 1992). For historiography on the New Deal and the West, see Karen Merrill, "The New Deal's West," in *A Companion to the American West*, ed. William Deverell, 346–60 (Oxford, UK: Blackwell, 2004).

6. Moehring, *Resort City*, 31.

7. "Message of Governor E. P. Carville to the Legislature," *Appendix*, 41st Sess., Vol. 1 (Carson City, NV: SPO, 1943) (incl. "extraordinary conditions" and "prosperity," 3). See Hulse, *Nevada's Environmental Legacy*, 71–80, for a history of the ammunition depot and air bases in northern Nevada. See also "B. C. Manganese Pilot Plant OK," *Review-Journal*, Sept. 30, 1940; and "Science: Strategic Metal No. 1," *Time* (Oct. 13, 1941).

8. The Las Vegas Air Gunnery School was later renamed the Nellis Air Force Base. Moehring, *Resort City*, 31–32.

9. Richard Overy, *Why the Allies Won* (New York: W. W. Norton & Company, 1995) (incl. "business make," 198). President Dwight D. Eisenhower first used the term "military industrial complex" in his Farewell Address on January 17, 1961, to warn the nation about the policy and monetary relationship between the American military and Congress, and the arms industry.

10. There were two types of incendiary bombs used during World War II. One type had a mixture of magnesium and iron powders, and the other type was composed of petroleum. See "Science: Science of Fire Bombing," *Time* (Feb. 17, 1941); and Moehring, *Resort City*, 31.

11. Fritz Hansgirg's process differed from the electrolytic method by taking brucite clay (magnesium hydroxide) and baking it in rotary kilns to form magnesium oxide. The oxide was mixed with carbon and heated electrically into gas at 4,000 degrees Fahrenheit. The mixture was then cooled by cold natural gas. See "Metals: Magnesium—Lesson in Speed," *Time* (Mar. 3, 1941); U.S. Congress, House of Representatives, Charles H. Levy (D-WA), "Metallic Magnesium Production Possibilities in the Northwest," 77th Cong., 2nd Sess., Jan. 5, 1940, *Congressional Record*, Vol. 88 (Washington, DC: GPO, 1940), A661.

12. "Science: Revolution in Magnesium," *Time* (Nov. 17, 1941); "Government: Folklore of Magnesium," *Time* (Feb. 10, 1941); "Metals: Magnesium—Lesson in Speed," *Time* (Mar. 3, 1941); "Company to Build Magnesium Plants," *New York Times*, Aug. 14, 1941; William Dobbs, "Working at BMI: Reflections on Life and Labor at America's Largest World War II Magnesium Plant" (unpublished paper, 1984), 3–4; "Metals: More Magnesium," *Time* (Mar. 2, 1942).

13. There is limited scholarship on the history of BRI and its manufacture plant in southern Nevada, Basic Magnesium Inc. (BMI). Maryellen Sadovich, "Basic Magnesium, Incorporated and the Industrialization of Southern Nevada (master's thesis, UNLV, 1971) is the most comprehensive. See also William T. Dobbs, "Southern Nevada and the Legacy of Basic Magnesium, Incorporated," *Nevada Historical Society Quarterly* 34 (Spring 1991): 273–303; appropriate sections of Moehring, *Resort City*; and Hulse, *Nevada's Environmental Plunder*.

14. Eells began the undertaking in 1926, but did not acquire the claims until 1933. See A. P. Clark to M. W. S., letter, Feb. 10, 1965; Harley C. Lee to H. P. Ells, July 22, 1933, letter; both in Box 3, Folder 2, BMI Collection, UNLV SC.

15. Major John P. Ball first became interested in German magnesium production as a member of the Disarmament Commission after World War I, and began selling German-made magnesium in 1923. He would never have been able to manufacture magnesium in the United States if Congress had not lifted the patent rights. Magnesium Development Corporation, a 50 percent owner of Farbenindustrie and Alcoa, held the American patent, and American Magnesium had the fabrication patent. See Dobbs, "Working at BMI," 4; John Lowman to Howard P. Eells, Sept. 24, 1940, Box 1, Vol. 2, "Chronology of Basic Magnesium Inc. Supporting Data," Aug. 27, 1940-June 11, 1941, BMI Collection, UNLV SC (hereafter "Chronology").

16. BMI stock distributed 52.4 percent to BRI, 2.5 percent to George B. Thatcher, BRI's western counsel, and 45 percent to Magnesium Elektron. See Roy E. Thomas, "Factual History of Engineering, Basic Magnesium Inc., Henderson, Nevada," 1–2, Box 4, BMI Collection, UNLV SC.

17. "Company to Build Magnesium Plants," *New York Times*, Aug. 14, 1941; Moehring, *Resort City*, 34–35; Dobbs, "Working at BMI," 3.

18. See "Chronology," esp. Vols. 2–4. Eells and BMI management referred to Plancor 201 when referencing the plant. See also Sadovich, "Basic Magnesium," 7–8; and "Basic Magnesium Inc.," Cahlan Collection, Box 6, Folder 3, NSMA.

19. Woodbury interview (incl. both quotes); Moehring, *Resort City*, 29–30.

20. "Battle of Detroit," *Time* (Mar. 23, 1942).

21. Census Bureau statistics in "U.S. At War: War and Cities," *Time* (Dec. 14, 1942).

22. A helpful documentary to understand American war towns during the early to mid-1940s is *The War*, Sarah Botstein (producer), Ken Burns & Lynn Novick (director and producer), Florentine Films and WETA (Washington, DC).

23. Ragnald Fyhen, "Labor Notes," UNLV SC (incl. "whole groups," 15).

24. "Chronology," July 18, 1942; "The BMI Project Bigger Than Dam Job," *Big Job*, no. 6, July 30, 1942; Fyhen, "Labor Notes"; J. G. Platt, "Employee Union Membership and Hiring Procedure," Sept. 12, 1942, BMI Collection, Box 1, Vol. 4, "Chronology," Apr. 3, 1942–Sept. 20, 1942. Jonreed Lauritzen wrote numerous romantic novels about the Mormon experience in the West, including *Arrows in the Sun* (1943) and *Song Before Sunrise* (1948) as well as *The Rose and the Flame* (1951). He was unable to publish "Hellbent on Victory" because the manuscript was accidently burned. See "BMI Worker Is Novelist," *Big Job*, no. 29, Jan. 14, 1943; Sadovich, "Basic Magnesium" (incl. ""We of the West," 16).

25. See "Army and Navy—Manpower: Women & Machines," *Time* (May 11, 1942), for an informative article on women in the industrial workplace during World War II. See also Helper, *Women in Labor*, 67–82; and D'Ann Campbell, *Women at War with America: Private Lives in a Patriotic Era* (Cambridge, MA: Harvard University Press, 1984), 100. For literature on working women during World War II and Rosie the Riveter, see Karen Anderson, *Wartime Women: Sex Roles, Family Relations, and the Status of Women During World War II* (New York: Berkley Books, 2001); Campbell, *Women at War*; Melissa Dabakis, "Gendered Labor: Norman Rockwell's Rosie the Riveter and the Discourses of Wartime Womanhood," in *Gender and American History Since 1890*, ed. Barbara Melosh, 182–204 (London and New York: Routledge, 1993); Sherna Berger Gluck, *Rosie the Riveter Revisited: Women, the War, and Social Change* (Boston: Twayne Publishers, 1987); Chester Gregory, *Women in Defense Work during World War II: An Analysis of the Labor Problem and Women's Rights* (New York: Exposition Press, 1974); Susan M. Hartmann, *The Home Front and Beyond: American Women in the 1940s* (Boston: Twayne Publishers, 1982); Maureen Honey, *Bitter Fruit: African American Women in World War II* (Columbia: University of Missouri Press, 1999); Honey, *Creating Rosie the Riveter: Class, Gender, and Propaganda during World War II* (Amherst: University of Massachusetts Press, 1984); Leila J. Rupp, *Mobilizing Women for War: German and American Propaganda, 1939–1945* (Princeton, NJ: Princeton University Press, 1978); Emily Yellin, *Our Mother's War: American Women at Home and at the Front during World War II* (New York: Free Press, 2004).

26. See "First Women Are Put on Production Line at BMI Plant," *Review-Journal*, Feb. 13, 1943; "Army and Navy—Manpower"; Helper, *Women in Labor*, 67.

27. This was not always the case among female war workers on the national scale. A representative of the U.S. Women's Bureau found that a woman at a large war plant received 60 cents an hour to her male coworker's 70 cents. In most cases, men earned 10 cents more an hour than women, even though the jobs were the same. See Marguerite J. Fisher, "Equal Pay for Equal Work Legislation," *Industrial and Labor Relations Review* 2, no. 1 (Oct. 1948): 50–57.

28. BMI distributed the first issue of *Big Job* on June 26, 1942, published the bulletin weekly until 1943, and expanded the publication to a tabloid called *Basic Bombardier*. Editor-in-chief Guernsey Frazer published it every two weeks until November 17, 1944, recording the everyday activities of workers at BMI. See "Hydrogen Women," *Basic Bombardier* 1, no. 45 (May 21, 1943) (incl. "splendid women"). See also

A. D. Hopkins, "Magnesium Maggie," in *The First 100: Portraits of the Men and Women Who Shaped Las Vegas*, ed. A. D. Hopkins and K. J. Evans, 129–30 (Las Vegas: Huntington Press, 1999).

29. "Army and Navy—Manpower" (incl. all quotes).

30. Hopkins, "Magnesium Maggie," 130.

31. Most of the Native American workers lived near Boulder Highway next to the Pittman neighborhood in Henderson in huts and tents, and cooked meals over camp-fires. Many were also Zuni dancers that entertained in Las Vegas hotels and casinos during the weekend. See Sadovich, "Basic Magnesium," 16.

32. See William J. Collins, "Race, Roosevelt, and Wartime Production: Fair Employment in World War II in Labor Markets," *American Economic Review* 91, no. 1 (Mar. 2001): 272–86.

33. In the South, migrant workers moved to war towns like Mobile, Alabama, looking for employment. Like most Southern towns, Mobile observed strict Jim Crow segregation during the 1940s. Many black workers found jobs at the Pinto Island yard of the Alabama Dry Dock and Shipbuilding Company repairing and building ships for the U.S. Maritime Commission. The company employed nearly 18,500 employees, with 6,000 of them black. See Frederic C. Lane, *Ships for Victory: A History of Shipbuilding under the United States Maritime Commission in World War II* (Baltimore: Johns Hopkins University Press, 2001), 253.

34. Harvard Sitkoff, "African American Militancy in the World War II South: Another Perspective," in *Remaking Dixie: The Impact of World War II on the American South*, ed. Neil R. McMillen (Jackson: University Press of Mississippi, 1997), 70–92.

35. 16th Census of the United States, 1940, Vol. 2, *Characteristics of the Population* (Washington, DC: GPO, 1943), 721, 756; "200 Negro Workers Walk Off Jobs at BMI Plant Today," *Review-Journal*, Oct. 20, 1943; Woodbury interview (incl. all quotes).

36. Woodbury interview (incl. all quotes).

37. Sadovich, "Basic Magnesium" (incl. "segregation was," 15).

38. "200 Negro Workers Walk Off Jobs at BMI Plant Today," *Review-Journal*, Oct. 20, 1943; "Federal Agent Is Vegas to Sift Negro Walkout," *Review-Journal*, Oct. 21, 1943."

39. U.S. Senate, "Hearings Before a Special Committee Investigating the National Defense Program," 1st Sess., Pursuant to S. Res. 6, 78th Cong., Part 20, Aug. 19, 1943, 8247–8355, 8359–61 (incl. "Negro workers," 8349; and "the colored fellows," 8360). See also Sadovich, "Basic Magnesium," 15.

40. Dobbs, "Working at BMI" (incl. *Review-Journal* report, 17).

41. Alexander J. Field, "Technological Change and U.S. Productivity Growth in the Interwar Years," *Journal of Economic History* 66, no. 1 (Mar. 2006), 207; "MICHIGAN: Hitler or the U.S.," *Time* (Aug. 24, 1942) (incl. "tragic").

42. By 1940 Washington, DC, had begun allocating millions to defense housing. The programs gave financial support to cities to construct their own housing, and housing developments were built under federal jurisdiction. After Pearl Harbor, legislation approved additional funding for housing. The competing programs led to numerous setbacks and delays. To remedy the situation, the federal government consolidated all activities into the National Housing Agency (NHA) and Roosevelt amended the Housing Act of 1934 to create Title VI, authorizing the mass construction of FHA-financed homes in defense industry areas. See Paul F. Wendt, *Housing Policy—The Search for Solutions: A Comparison of United Kingdom, Sweden, West Germany, and the United States Since World War II* (Berkeley: University of California Press, 1963), 154; "Housing Relief

Hope Dim," *Review-Journal,* Aug. 24, 1945; "City Promises Cooperation in Vega Verde Improvements," *Review-Journal,* Aug. 7, 1947.

43. J. D. Platt, "Report on Permanent Housing Problem, Basic Magnesium Inc., Nevada Magnesium Project, D. P. C. Plancor 201," Dec. 12, 1941, BMI Collection, Box 1, Vol. 3; "Chronology," June 20, 1941–Mar. 30, 1942, 1–2.

44. As a main source of power and water for defense industries in the West, the federal government believed Hoover Dam could be targeted by saboteurs. See "Chronology," July 21–24, 1941.

45. J. D. Platt, "Report on Permanent Housing Problem" (incl. "wide open conditions," 3). See also Las Vegas Trip, memorandum, July 21 to July 24, Location Plant Site, Housing, BMI Collection, Box 1, Vol. 3; and "Chronology," June 20, 1941–Mar. 30, 1942, 1–3. Paradise Valley is located between Henderson and Las Vegas. The surveyors determined it had enough water and attractive surroundings, which they considered important to employee morale due to difficult conditions at the plant. They decided against the location though because it would be costly to build an infrastructure.

46. "Chronology," Sept. 13–20, 1941; and Moehring, *Resort City,* 35.

47. "Chronology," Nov. 17, 1941.

48. There has been much speculation about the circumstances surrounding Senator Key Pittman's death. One theory was that Democrats kept his corpse on ice in a bathtub at Reno's Riverside Hotel until his reelection. This theory has been disproven, although the Senator did suffer a heart attack before the election. Doctors determined he would eventually die, but Democratic leaders kept it a secret. Nevadans reelected Pittman on November 5, 1940, and he died at the Washoe General Hospital five days later. See "The Mysterious Demise of Key Pittman," *Nevada Magazine* (Oct. 1996), 83–88.

49. "The Congress: Rebirth," *Time* (Jan. 13, 1941); and "The Mood of the Statesmen," *Time* (Feb. 23, 1942). "Business: Anaconda Magnesium," *Time* (Oct. 12, 1942) (inc. "serious"). See Dobbs, "Working at BMI," 4; H. P. Eells to H. C. Mann, Dec. 16, 1941, BMI Collection, Box 1, Vol. 3; and "Chronology," June 20, 1941–Mar. 30, 1942.

50. Hobson to Sullivan, memorandum, Dec. 26, 1941; "Chronology," June 20, 1941–Mar. 30, 1942; Moehring, *Resort City,* 35–36.

51. U.S. Senate, "Hearings," Part 20, 8353; "Modern Business District for Carver Park Approved," *Basic Bombardier* 11, no. 12, Jan. 15, 1944; Jacqueline Jones, *Labor of Love, Labor of Sorrow: Black Women, Work, and the Family from Slavery to the Present* (New York: Basic Books, 2010), 207; and Viola Johnson interview, by Claytee White, Mar. 12, 1996, UNLV SC (incl. "it was").

52. Thomas, "Factual History," 81–82; "Chronology," July 28, 1942; McNeil, "BMI Labor Force Is at Peak, McNeil Reports Today," *Review-Journal,* Aug. 5, 1942 (incl. "considering").

53. Wesley Stout, "Nevada's New Reno," *Saturday Evening Post* (Oct. 31, 1942) (incl. all quotes); Moehring, *Resort City,* 37; Dobbs, "Working at BMI," 8.

54. The name "Henderson" honored the role RFC chairman Charles Henderson played in bringing the project to southern Nevada. See "Chronology," Sept. 1, 1941; "Nevada War Workers Are Housed in 7,301 New Units," *Review-Journal,* Sept. 11, 1944; Dennis McBride, *Midnight on Arizona Street: The Secret Life of the Boulder Dam Hotel* (Boulder City, NV: Boulder City–Hoover Dam Museum, 1993); and Dobbs, "Working at BMI," 9.

55. "BMI Blaze Sabotage: Investigation Reveals Definite Proof of Arson, Officials Say," *Review-Journal,* Mar. 7, 1942.

56. H. C. Mann to Howard Eells, memorandum, Mar. 7, 1942, "Chronology," June 20, 1941–Mar. 30, 1942; "Fire Razes Magnesium Plant Building Near Las Vegas," *LA Times*, Mar. 7, 1942; "Fire in Magnesium Plant," *New York Times*, Mar. 7, 1942; "Defense Pant Sabotage Hinted," *LA Times*, Mar. 8, 1942.

57. "The Facts About BMI's Company Town," *Review-Journal*, Apr. 10, 1942; H. C. Mann to Howard Eells, memorandum, Mar. 16, 1942, "Chronology," June 20, 1941–Mar. 30, 1942; "About the Fire At BMI," Berkeley Bunker Political Advertisement, "Chronology," Apr. 3–Sept. 30, 1942.

58. In early 1941 Senator Harry S. Truman heard rumors of mismanagement in America's defense industry. A preliminary investigation revealed the allegations were largely true. By March 1941 the Senate had created the Special Senate Committee Investigating the National Defense Program, dubbed the Truman Committee, by unanimous consent. From its founding until 1948 the committee revealed exploitation and mismanagement, abuses in cost-plus contracting, and faulty material production. Most historians agree the committee was a success, reportedly saving taxpayers more than $15 billion. See David McCullough, *Truman* (New York: Simon & Schuster, 1992), 304.

59. "Fraud Charged to Jones Unit in Plant Deal," *Chicago Daily Tribune*, Apr. 10, 1942 (incl. all quotes).

60. Bunker did not elaborate specifics, but the *Chicago Daily Tribune* speculated the "unusual political ramifications" were that Eells paid lobbyist Joseph B. Keenan a fee of $6,000 for so-called special services. See "RIP 'Flagrant' Profiteering in War Necessity," *Chicago Daily Tribune*, Apr. 3, 1942. See also Warren B. Francis, "Airplane Lag Laid to Poor Planning," *LA Times*, Apr. 3, 1942; Chesley Manly, "Rigid Profit Curb Favored," *LA Times*, Apr. 4, 1942; "Pact on Magnesium Hit; Jones Denies Charges," *LA Times*, Apr. 10, 1942; "Denies DPC Laxity Over Magnesium," *New York Times*, Apr. 24, 1942; "Jones Answers Bunker Charges against DPC," *Review-Journal*, Apr. 23, 1942 (incl. all quotes).

61. "About the Fire at BMI"; "Anaconda Deal with BMI Near Completion," *Review-Journal*, Sept. 29, 1942; Thomas, "Factual History," 4; "Anaconda Takes on BMI Plant Control," *Review-Journal*, Oct. 27, 1942; "Anaconda Buys Control of Big Magnesium Firm," *Chicago Daily Tribune*, Oct. 27, 1942.

62. See Thomas, "Factual History," 41–48, for a complete list of contractors on the project. McNeil Construction Company held the largest contract, tasked with leveling, grading, and draining the site; constructing all buildings; and installing power, lighting, plumbing, heating, ventilation, and housing. The Fritz Ziebarth Company built power lines connected to the Hoover Dam switch and telephone lines from Luning to the Oxide Plant at Gabbs. Engineers Limited provided the labor, material, and equipment to construct the water intake and booster pumping station at Lake Mead, the pipeline, and reservoir at the plant site. More than a dozen contractors contributed to the construction of the BMI plant, and the MacDonald Construction Company and five subcontractors built the Gabbs plant and facilities outside Luning.

63. The Anderson Brothers also operated sleeping facilities for workers, housing thirteen single men for $3.25 a week per person. See Florence Lee Jones, "Anderson's Is Biggest Concern for Food in State of Nevada," *Review-Journal*, Nov. 12, 1943; Moehring, *Resort City*, 36; and Stout, "Nevada's New Reno."

64. Thomas, "Factual History," 42–43; Sadovich, "Basic Magnesium," 23; McNeil, "First BMI Product Moves to Market by Rail Yesterday," *Review-Journal*, Aug. 10, 1942

(incl. all quotes); "Power System for BMI Completed," *Review-Journal,* May 19, 1942; Moehring, *Resort City,* 36.

65. "Magnesium Plant Contract Awarded," *LA Times,* Oct. 20, 1941; "To Build $3,000,000 Plant," *New York Times,* Oct. 20, 1941. See also Eells to Husbands, June 26, 1942; BMI Clippings, "BMI Gabbs Valley Plant Is Opened by Officials Today"; BMI Clippings, "BMI Gabbs Plant Operation Starts," June 27, 1942; all in "Chronology," Apr. 3, 1942–Sept. 30, 1942. See also "BMI Wheels at Gabbs Roll for Victory," *Big Job,* July 2, 1942 (incl. both quotes); Moehring, *Resort City,* 34; "Largest Truck Job in U.S. Will Start Here," *Review-Journal,* Nov. 12, 1943; and "Wells Inc.," *Basic Bombardier* 2, no. 10 (Dec. 17, 1943).

66. "McNeil Company Ends Construction Job at BMI Plant," *Review-Journal,* Oct. 11, 1943; "First BMI Product Moves to Market by Rail Yesterday," *Review-Journal,* Aug. 10, 1942; Ball to Eells, Sept. 1, 1942, Telegram, "Chronology," Apr. 3–Sept. 30, 1942; "BMI Plant Now World's Largest Metal Producer," *Review-Journal,* May 25, 1943; Sadovich, "Basic Magnesium, Incorporated," 26; "Government: Folklore of Magnesium," *Time* (Feb. 10, 1941).

67. Barth, George, and Hill, *Environmental Health and Safety,* 4.

68. For articles on the construction workers' deaths, see "Two Die of Hurts at BMI Plant," *Review-Journal,* Aug. 26, 1942; "Workman Dies of Injuries in Fall," *Review-Journal,* July 30, 1943. There are also numerous newspaper clippings located in the BMI Collection at UNLV SC that chronicle accidents, including those that resulted in fatalities.

69. "Battlefronts Are Safer," *Time* (Aug. 23, 1943).

70. "BMI Blaze Sabotage"; "Small Fire Hits BMI on Saturday," *Review-Journal,* June 23, 1942; "Chronology," July 11, 1942, Sept. 26, 1942; Mann to Snyder, July 14, 1942, "Chronology," Apr. 3–Sept. 30, 1942; "Fire in Peat Pits at BMI Brought Under Control Late Saturday Night," *Review-Journal,* July 13, 1942.

71. "Report of the Inspector of Mines," *Appendix,* 42nd Sess., Vol. 1 (Carson City, NV: SPO, 1945), 26, 113–14.

72. Drew Peterson, "Trouble Brewing in Las Vegas Merry-Go-Round, Author Says," *Review-Journal,* Nov. 1, 1943; BMI, "Company Policies—Hours," *Foreman Manual,* rev. June 30, 1943, BMI Collection, Box 4, UNLV SC (hereafter *Foreman Manual*); R. H. Ramsey, "The Why and How of Magnesium," *Engineering and Mining Journal,* Oct. 1943, UNLV SC; BMI, *Magnesium and You* (Las Vegas: BMI, 1943), 6–7, UNLV SC.

73. The use of chlorine marked the advent of chemical warfare during World War I as a choking gas. Chlorine was not used in combat during World War II, but was a major element in chemical and biological weapons, and produced magnesium.

74. BMI, *Magnesium and You,* 15 (incl. both quotes); Dobbs, "Working at BMI," 22; Eric A. Coddy, James J. Wirtz, and Jeffery A. Larsen, *Weapons of Mass Destruction: An Encyclopedia of Worldwide Policy, Technology, and History,* Vol. 1 (Santa Barbara, CA: ABC-CLIO, 2005), 102.

75. White Pine County was the leading mining producer in the state, with 59 percent of Nevada's five metals (gold, silver, copper, lead, and zinc), and was the first in output of copper and gold. By sheer volume, it edged Clark County out as the most dangerous county in the state. For a list of the various injuries experienced at the BMI plant, see reports of fatal and nonfatal accidents in "Report of the Inspector of Mines," 7–9, 35–74, 116–53. See also "Company Policies—Hospital," *Foreman Manual*; Dobbs, "Working at BMI," 22–23.

76. U.S. Senate, "Hearings," Part 20, 8355–56; "BMI Absentees," *Big Job*, no. 32 (Feb. 4, 1943); "Absenteeism Falling Off but Production Enemy Must Go Much Lower," *Basic Bombardier* (Aug. 13, 1943) (incl. "Old Man Absenteeism" and "production enemy"); "Magnesium Bombs Rain Fire on Berlin," *Big Job*, no. 40 (Apr. 1, 1943).

77. "Manpower: M-Day Is Around the Corner," *Time* (Oct. 5, 1942); "Vegas Defense Workers Are 'Frozen' On Jobs," *Review-Journal*, Sept. 8, 1942; U.S. Senate, "Hearings," Part 20 (incl. all quotes, 8352).

78. U.S. Senate, "Hearings," Part 20, 8351–52, 8354–57, 8361; Dobbs, "Working at BMI," 30–31.

79. E. A. Phaenuf quoted in U.S. Senate, "Hearings," Part 20, 8359.

80. See Kersten, *Labor's Home Front*; Nelson Lichtenstein, *Labor's War at Home: The CIO in World War II* (Cambridge, UK, and New York: Cambridge University Press, 1982); Alan Brinkley, *The End of Reform: New Deal Liberalism in Recession and War* (New York: Vintage Books, 1996); and Allan M. Winkler, *Home Front U.S.A.: America During World War II* (Wheeling, IL: Harlan Davidson, 2012).

81. Hal K. Rothman, *Nevada: The Making of Modern Nevada* (Reno: University of Nevada Press, 2010), 96–98; U.S. Senate, "Hearings," Part 20, 8346; "Labor, BMI Reach Agreement for Plant Operation," *Review-Journal*, Aug. 28, 1942.

82. U.S. Senate, "Hearings," Part 20, 8345–61; "Union Poll Ordered by NLRB for BMI," *Review-Journal*, Apr. 17, 1943; "Work Stoppage Hits BMI When AFL Holds Meet," *Review-Journal*, May 31, 1943; "CIO Is Certified Bargaining Agent by NLRB Ruling," *Review-Journal*, July 15, 1943.

83. Faced with the pressure to do overnight what Germany had done in nine years, and what Japan had planned for decades, the program was designed to get workers on the production line as soon as possible.

84. "Safety Engineer Is Hired By BMI," in *Review-Journal*, BMI Collection, Box 2, Folder 2, UNLV SC.

85. The *Foreman Manual* is an instructional manual that provides not only a view of industrial health and safety at the BMI plant, but also an explanation of the labor protocol. See "Explanation of Job Breakdowns," "How to Instruct a Man on the Job," "Preparation Department Safety Rules," "Safety Rules for Electrolysis Cell Room Operatives," "Chlorination Department Safety Rules," "Refinery Department Safety Rules," "Safety Rules for Recovery," "Neutralization Plant Safety Rules," and "Safety Rules for Chlorine Plant" (incl. all quotes); all in *Foreman Manual*. See also "Company Policies—Offense," *Foreman Manual*.

86. "Legislation," *Foreman Manual*, 6; U.S. Senate, "Hearings," Part 20 (incl. "If you get," 8350–51); "Blanket Insurance Plan at BMI Told," *Review-Journal*, July 17, 1943.

87. U.S. Senate, "Hearings," Part 13, 5623 (incl. all quotes).

88. "Hospital Opens for Community Service," *Big Job* 20 (Nov. 12, 1942); F. E. Clough, "Concerning B. M. I. Hospital at Las Vegas, NV: F. E. Clough, M.D., Formerly of San Bernardino, in Charge," *California and Western Medicine* 57, no. 6 (Dec. 1942) (incl. all quotes, 391); "Magnesium Plant Hospital Starts This Week," *Review-Journal*, May 25, 1942; "Basic Hospital Is Dedicated at Rites Yesterday," *Review-Journal*, Oct. 30, 1942.

89. "Hospital Procedure Clarified," *Big Job*, no. 23, Dec. 3, 1942; "Company Policies—Hospital," *Foreman Manual*.

90. Jonathan Engel, *Doctors and Reformers: Discussion and Debate Over Health Policy, 1925–1950* (Columbia: University of South Carolina Press, 2002), 189–91.

91. Annie Blachley, *Good Medicine: 4 Doctors and the Golden Age of Medicine* (Reno: Greasewood Press, 2000), 30–34 (incl. all quotes, 34).

92. McBride, *In the Beginning*, 38.

93. Mary Kennedy Rymer interview, May 4, 1977, by Mary Fitzgerald, UNLV SC (incl. all quotes); "History of Southern Nevada Memorial Hospital," *Southern Nevada Memorial Hospital News and Views* 3, no. 5 (Dec. 1968), 3; Sandra Klimek, "A History of Hospitals: Clark County, Nevada" (unpublished paper, 1985), 9; "The Hospitals of Clark County: Development of Medicine in a Rapidly Growing Nevada Community," *Greasewood Tablettes* 7, no. 4 (Winter 1996–97); Department of Pathology, Great Basin History of Medicine Division, University of Nevada School of Medicine, Reno, 1–2.

94. U.S. Senate, "Hearings," Part 20, 8351; Clippings on Clough's departure in BMI Collection, Box 2, Folder 6, UNLV SC. See esp. "New Head Now at Basic Hospital." See also Jones interview.

95. The problem was that most patients were unaware they were infected. If left untreated, the disease damaged their hearts, brains, eyes, and bones, and could be fatal. See "Health Department Providing Aid to Affected Persons in Clinic," *Review-Journal*, Apr. 27, 1944 (incl. "expanding military" and "the next great").

96. "Report of the Secretary of the State Board of Health," *Appendix*, 42nd Sess., Vol. 1, 11–10, 19–20, 29, 40; Betty Molignoni, "Nevada Has a Sorry, Alarming Record of Venereal Disease Mortality," *Review-Journal*, Jan. 15, 1945; "Rise in Social Diseases Told," *Review-Journal*, Apr. 27, 1944.

97. "Report of the Secretary of the State Board of Health," 19–20; Blachley, *Pestilence*, 44; Kevin Brown, *The Pox: The Life and Death of a Very Social Disease* (Stroud, UK: Sutton, 2006).

98. "Health Safeguard Drive Starts, Ends at Board Meeting," *Review-Journal*, Oct. 12, 1940 (incl. "one of").

99. "District Attorney Moves in upon Battle on Block 16 Sanitation," *Review-Journal*, Nov. 27, 1940 (incl. all quotes); "Abandonment of Houses on Block 16 Is Requested," *Review-Journal*, Apr. 10, 1941; "Four Block 16 Operators Are Haled [sic] to Court," *Review-Journal*, July 11, 1941.

100. "U.S. Health Clinic in Vegas," *Review-Journal*, Apr. 10, 1941; "Officials Move to Ban Prostitution," *Review-Journal*, May 28, 1942 (incl. all quotes).

101. Florence Lee Jones, "Nevada Has a Sorry, Alarming Record of Venereal Death Mortality," *Review-Journal*, Jan. 15, 1945; Blachley, *Pestilence*, 44–45.

102. "BMI Sets Record for Safety in Past 12 Months," *Review-Journal*, Aug. 17, 1944.

103. Aldrich, *Safety-First*, 271–72; Kersten, *Labor's Home Front* (incl. *Forbes* and *Popular Mechanics* quotes, 173–74).

104. Kersten, *Labor's Home Front*, 178–80 (incl. "Work accidents," "heavy social," "money loss," "staggering wastage," 178); Aldrich, *Safety-First*, 271–72.

105. Most likely the decrease in disabling injuries was because construction had ended. See "BMI Sets Record."

106. All producers were ordered to shut down production with the exception of Dow Chemical's Freeport plant. For more information on BMI's closure, see "BMI Plant Not to Be War Baby," *Review-Journal*, Apr. 6, 1943; "Permanency of BMI Is Sifted," *Review-Journal*, May 24, 1943; "McCarran Charges BMI Launched As 'Wartime Baby,'" *Review-Journal*, Feb. 14, 1944; "Plan to Curtail BMI Production Forestalled," *Review-Journal*, Feb. 28, 1944; Lorania Francis, "Power Bureau Called Foe of

Basic Magnesium," *LA Times*, Mar. 12, 1944; "Big Reductions in Magnesium Output Ordered," *Chicago Tribune*, July 30, 1944; "Government Cuts Magnesium Output," *New York Times*, July 30, 1944; "Basic Magnesium Gets WPB Curtailment Order," *Review-Journal*, Sept. 5, 1944; "Cut Magnesium Output 40 PCY; Close 2 Plants," *Chicago Daily Tribune*, Sept. 6, 1944; Dobbs, "Working at BMI," 32–33; Sadovich, "Basic Magnesium," 33.

107. R. Jackson Armstrong-Ingram, *Henderson* (Charleston, SC: Arcadia, 2002), 113; Sadovich, "Basic Magnesium," 35–36, 41; Hulse, *Nevada's Environmental Legacy*, 26.

108. "BMI Hospital to Remain Open," *Review-Journal*, Nov. 10, 1944; Mother Mary Gerald to Reverend Peter V. Moran, Jan. 6, 1947, McNamee Collection, Box 12, Folder 3, NSMA.

109. Sisters of Saint Dominic Trustees to the War Assets Administration, May 1947; "Quitclaim Deed," May 19, 1948; Mother Mary Gerald to Reverend Peter V. Moran; all in McNamee Collection, Box 12, Folder 3, NSMA.

110. "Magnesium Production Thrills Project," *Big Job*, no. 12, Sept. 10, 1942; "Magnesium Bombs Rain Fire on Berlin," *Big Job* 40 (Apr. 1, 1943) (incl. "every drop").

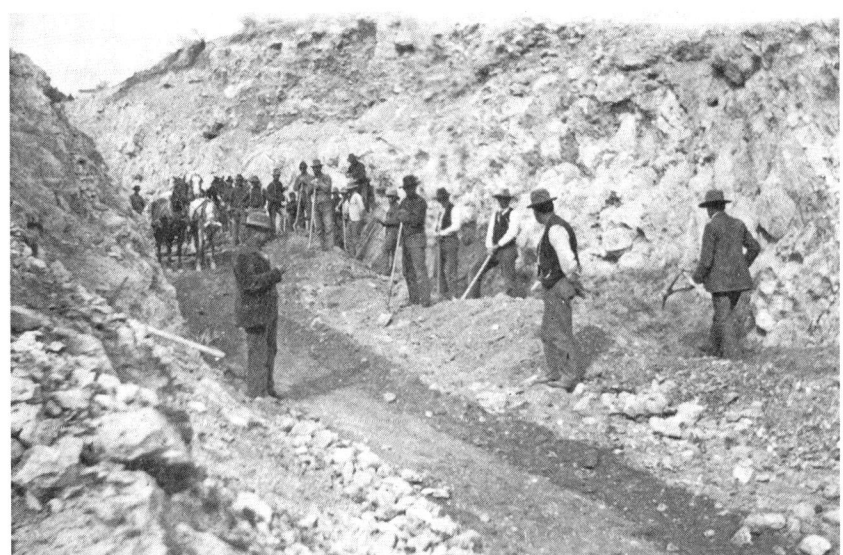

In 1900 Senator William Clark of Montana chartered the San Pedro, Los Angeles, & Salt Lake Railroad, organizing a construction company to build the line. The carrier founded a company town, Las Vegas, in 1905 as a half-way point between Salt Lake City and Los Angeles. Courtesy of Ferron-Bracken Photo Collection, UNLV Library Special Collections.

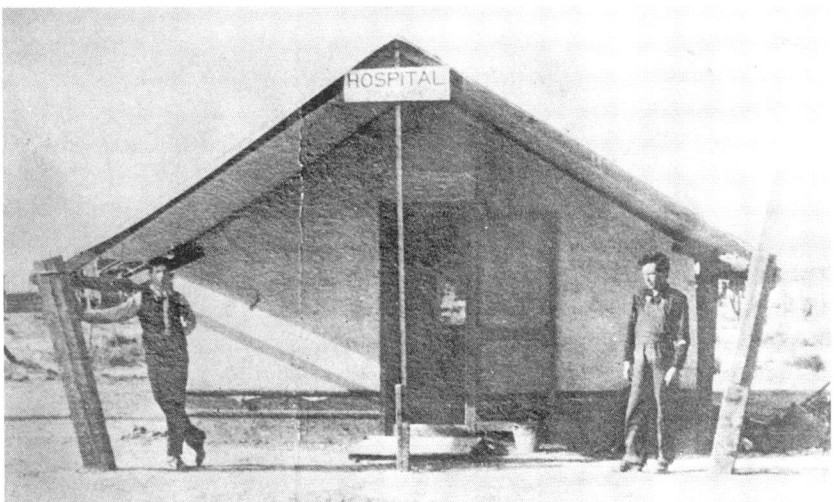

Faced with limited medical resources, western railroad carriers had to provide health care to maintain a productive and profitable workforce. The first hospital in Las Vegas, a tent in the railroad yard, was founded in 1904 by company physician Dr. Hal Hewetson. Courtesy of Doris Hancock Collection, UNLV Library Special Collections.

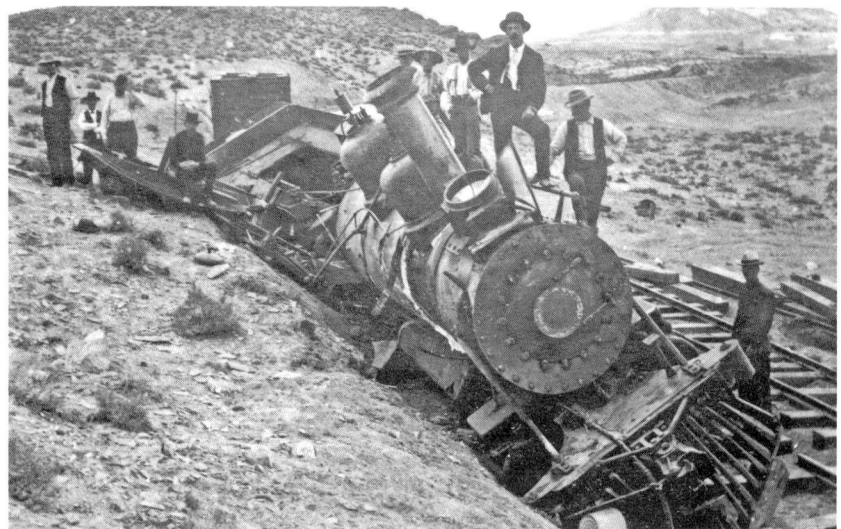

Southern Nevada's erratic desert storms caused the majority of derailments on the railroad, with heavy rain splintering the roadbed and causing wash-outs. This wreck in the early 1900s occurred on the Las Vegas and Tonopah Railroad near Desert Wells, west of Tonopah. Courtesy of Tonopah Goldfield Album, UNLV Library Special Collections.

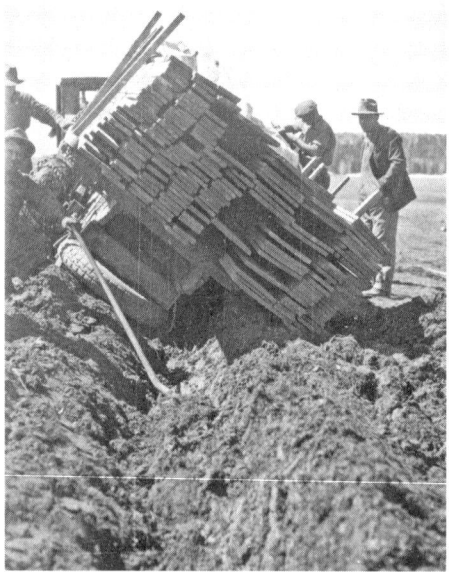

A Union Pacific Railroad truck filled with wooden planks tipped over outside Las Vegas, circa late 1920s to 1930s. Railroad management began the Safety-First program in 1913 to end "little accidents" like this, usually caused by inadequate risk assessment and other forms of human error. Courtesy of Squires Collection, UNLV Library Special Collections.

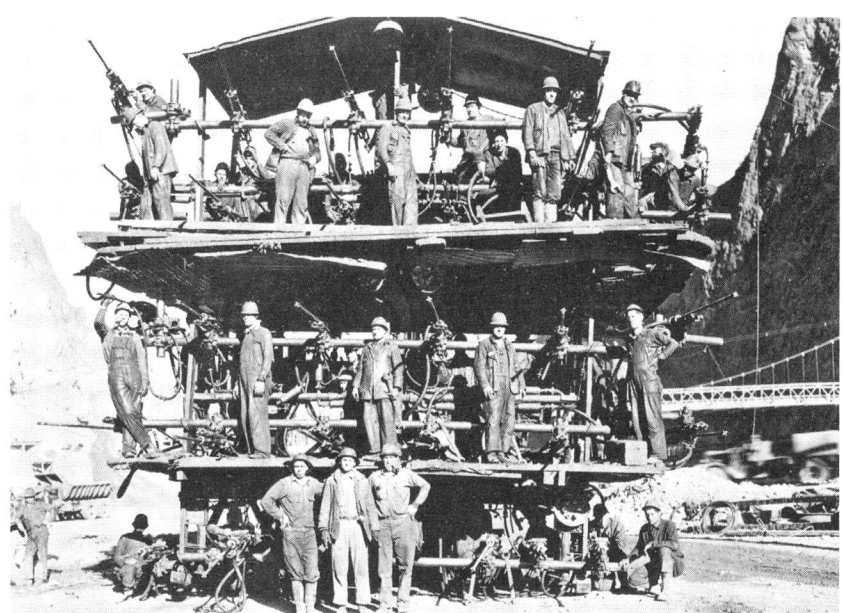

Diversion tunnel workers posing on a jumbo, a retrofitted World War I-era International truck with more than thirty drills, 1932. The construction of Hoover Dam began six months ahead of schedule without an industrial health program in place, leaving workers vulnerable to brutal conditions. Courtesy of Fred and Maurine Wilson Photo Collection, UNLV Library Special Collections.

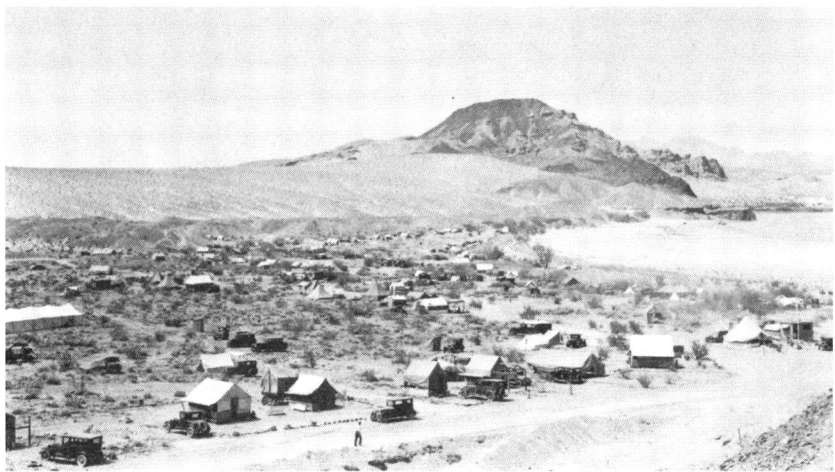

Before the completion of the company town, Boulder City, the only housing for dam workers with families was Ragtown, a makeshift, ragtag community along the Colorado River susceptible to extreme weather conditions and lacking clean drinking water. This photo circa 1931. Courtesy of Elton and Madelaine Garrett Photo Collection, UNLV Library Special Collections.

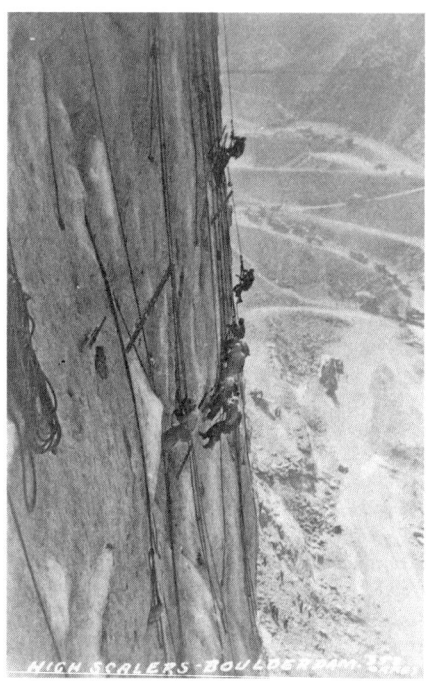

High scalers dangled on thin ropes along Black Canyon and drilled holes in the rock with forty-pound jackhammers, 1934. Accidents were very common, mostly due to falls, frayed ropes, faulty knots, and falling objects. Courtesy of Ferron-Bracken Photo Collection, UNLV Library Special Collections.

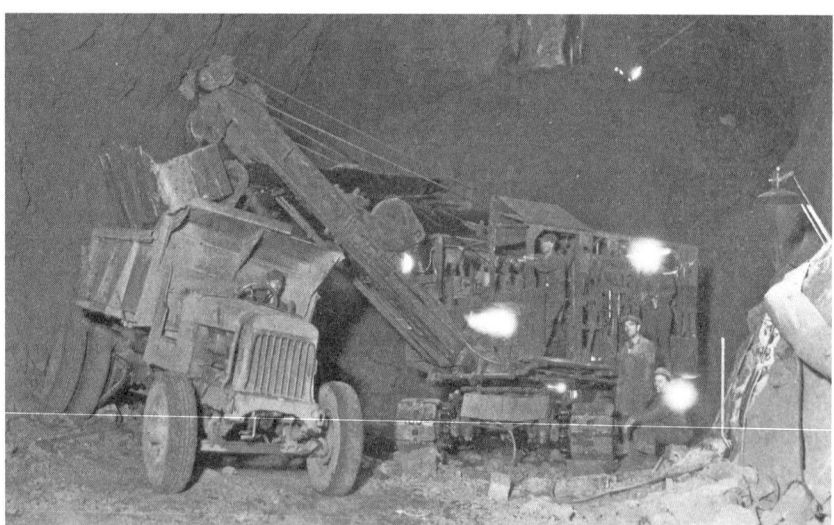

To haul away debris in the diversion tunnels, Six Companies Inc. authorized the use of gasoline-powered trucks underground, a practice prohibited by Nevada mining law. The vehicles emitted high levels of carbon monoxide, exposing workers to short- and long-term bodily harm. This photo circa 1932-1933. Courtesy of Manis Collection, UNLV Library Special Collections.

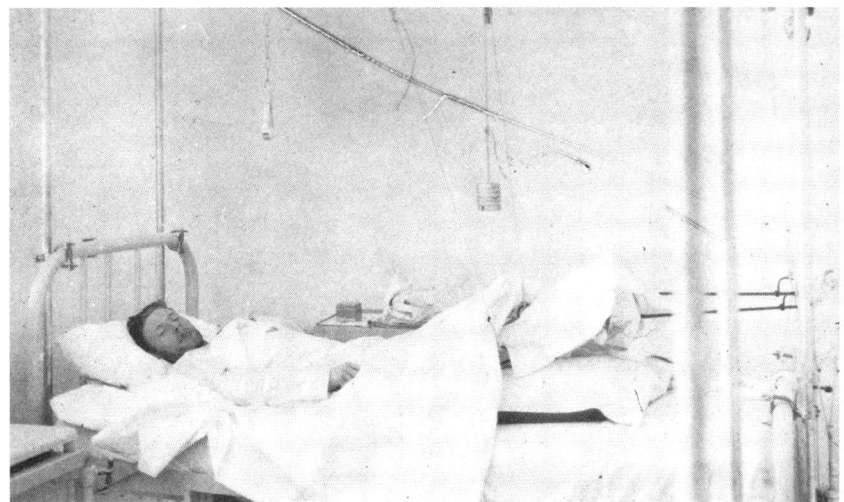

A worker recovering in the Boulder City Hospital, December 1, 1931. Despite initial setbacks, Six Companies Inc. and the Bureau of Reclamation eventually established an industrial health system that boosted subsequent New Deal–era programs. Courtesy of Bureau of Reclamation Collection, UNLV Library Special Collections.

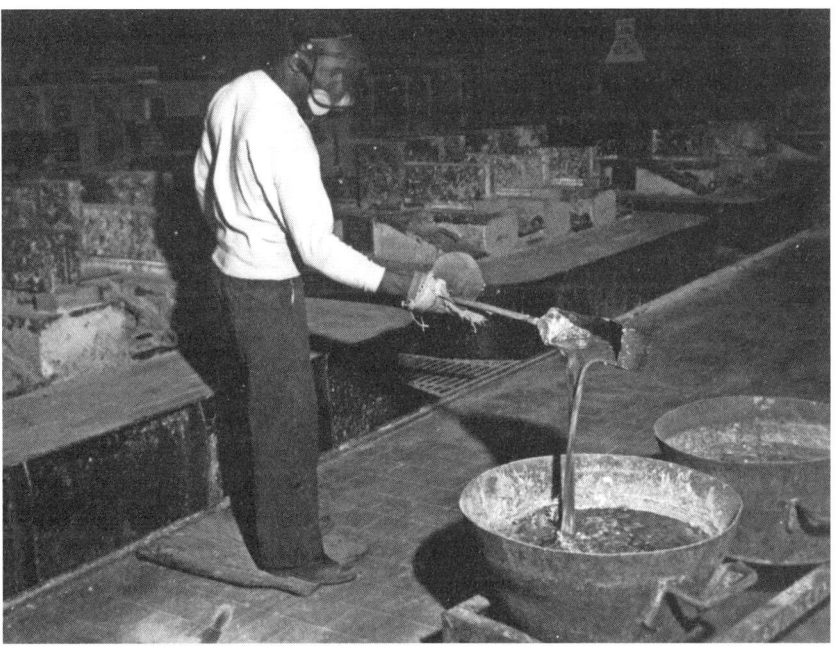

An employee of Basic Magnesium Inc. (BMI) in Henderson pouring liquid magnesium into a container, January 20, 1944. During World War II the plant was the largest producer of magnesium in the world, manufacturing 25 percent of all American output. Courtesy of Henderson Public Library Photograph Collection, UNLV Library Special Collections.

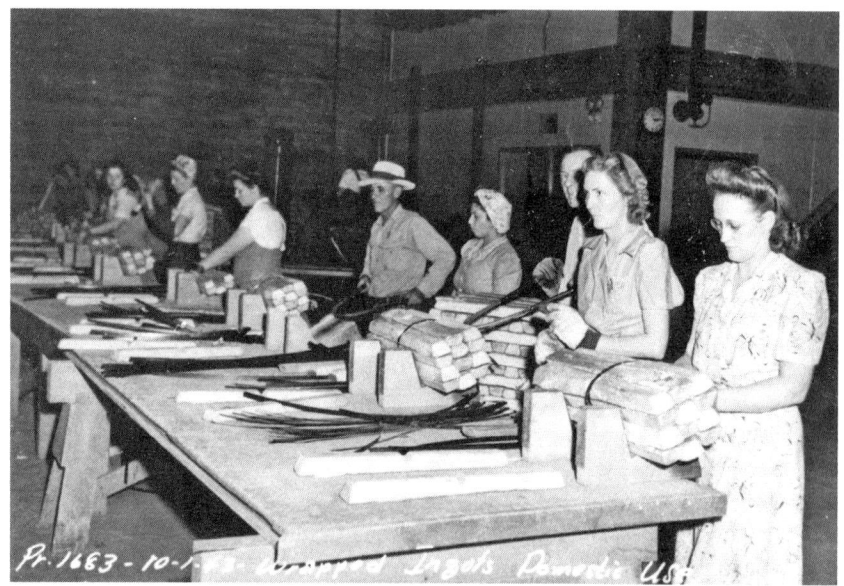

BMI's version of Rosie the Riveter had many names, including Magnesium Maggie and Chlorine Kate. Female employees' safety records far exceeded males', because they exhibited greater finger dexterity, focus, and excellence in inspection work. This photo circa early 1940s. Courtesy of Henderson Public Library Photograph Collection, UNLV Library Special Collections.

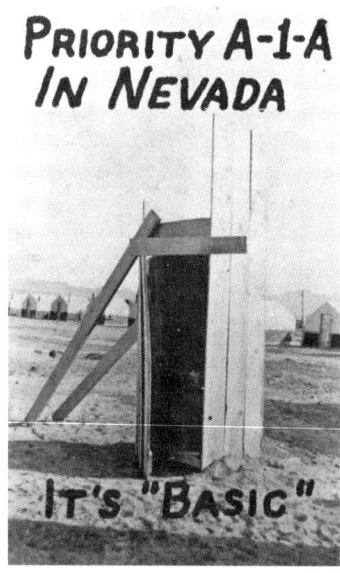

Postcard critiquing the poor housing conditions at BMI in 1942. With the company town still unfinished at the height of construction and operation, the majority of workers lived in a tent city with no power, running water, or toilets. Courtesy of Manis Collection, UNLV Library Special Collections.

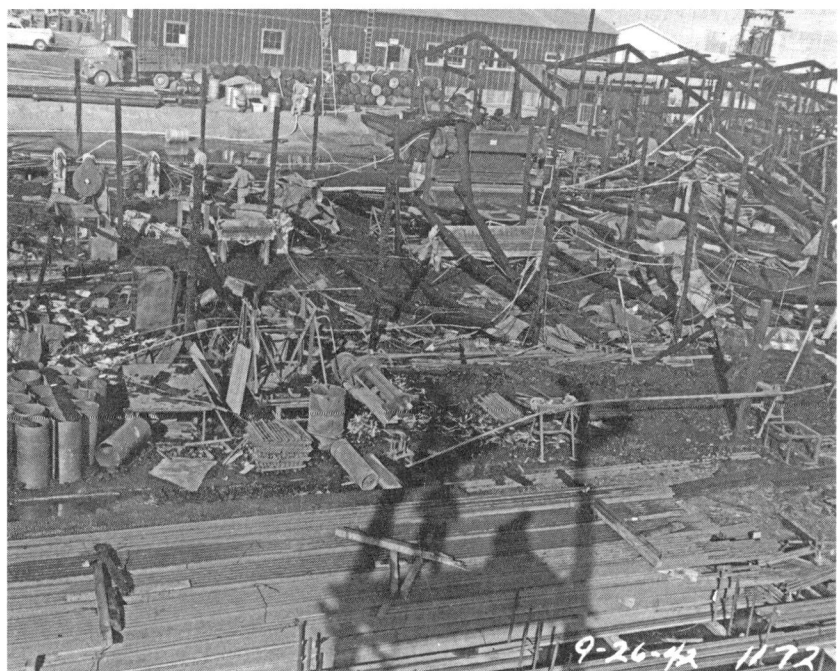

The BMI sheet metal shop after a fire, September 26, 1942. Fires regularly occurred during the plant's operation. Courtesy of Victor Kunkel Photograph Collection, UNLV Library Special Collections.

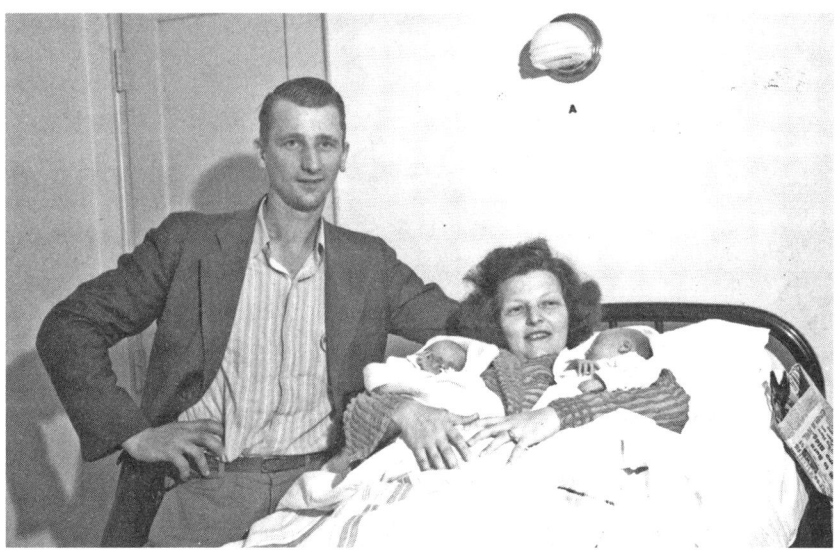

A worker, his wife, and their newborn twins at the BMI Hospital (later St. Rose de Lima), 1943. Most employees expressed dissatisfaction with the quality of care at the hospital, which contributed to high labor turnover at the plant. Courtesy of Henderson Public Library Photograph Collection, UNLV Library Special Collections.

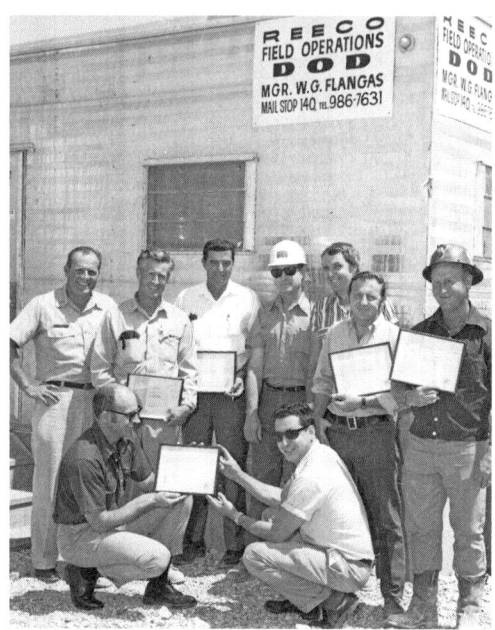

Reynolds Electrical and Engineering Company (REECo) field operations with Galen Adair, Bill Beam, and Bill Flangas, circa 1960s. The majority of Nevada Test Site (NTS) employees worked for private contractors that managed test preparations and operations, site maintenance, and industrial and radiological health and safety. Courtesy of Bill Beam Papers, UNLV Library Special Collections.

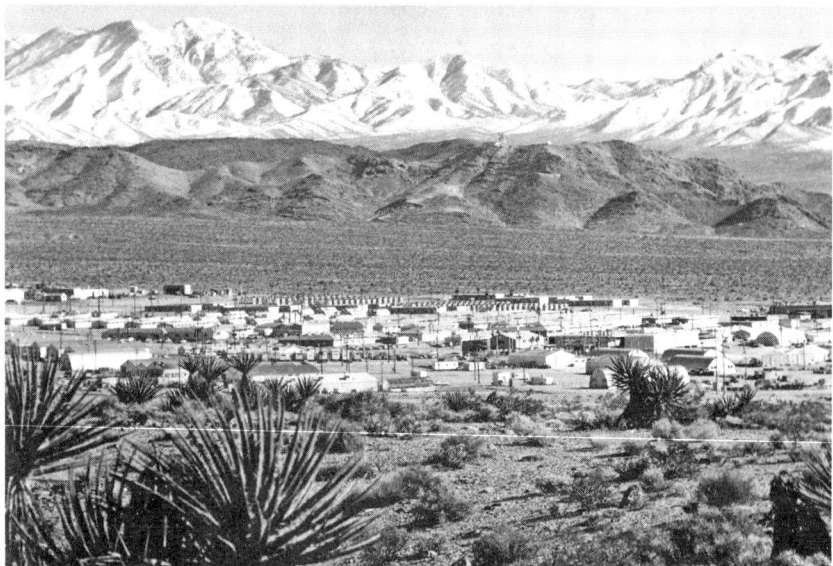

The Reynolds Electrical and Engineering Company (REECo) provided medical care for NTS workers, establishing medic stations throughout the site and a health, medicine, and safety building in Mercury, the main base camp pictured here, circa 1980s. Courtesy of U.S. Department of Energy Photograph Collection on the Nevada Test Site, UNLV Library Special Collections.

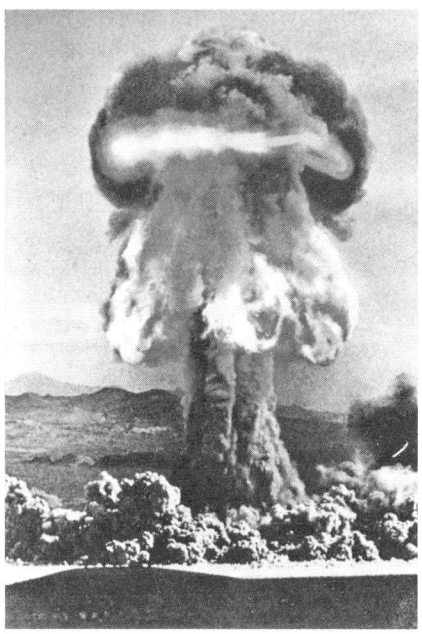

Shot Pricilla during Operation Plumbbob, June 24, 1957, the last atmospheric test series at the NTS. In Plumbbob, soldiers participated in tactical exercises monitored by rad-safe to ensure they did not exceed the permissible dose of radiation exposure. Courtesy of Central Nevada Historical Society Photograph Collection, UNLV Library Special Collections.

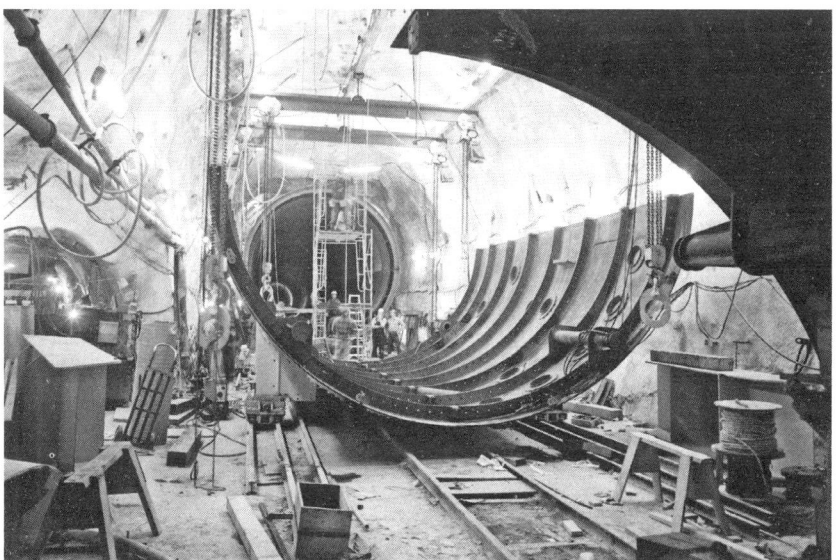

Line of sign pipes fabricated inside tunnels at Rainier Mesa, circa 1980s. Following the Limited Test Ban Treaty of 1963, nuclear testing shifted to underground tunnels at the NTS. The process limited fallout risk but presented new hazards associated with drilling and mining. Courtesy of U.S. Department of Energy Photograph Collection on the Nevada Test Site, UNLV Library Special Collections.

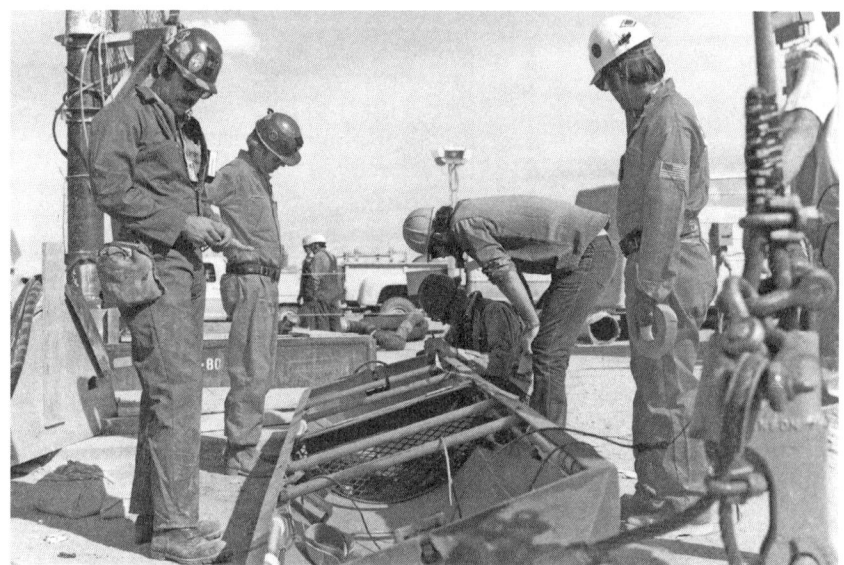

NTS workers setting up a mine rescue cage, circa 1980s. Courtesy of Bill Beam Papers, UNLV Library Special Collections.

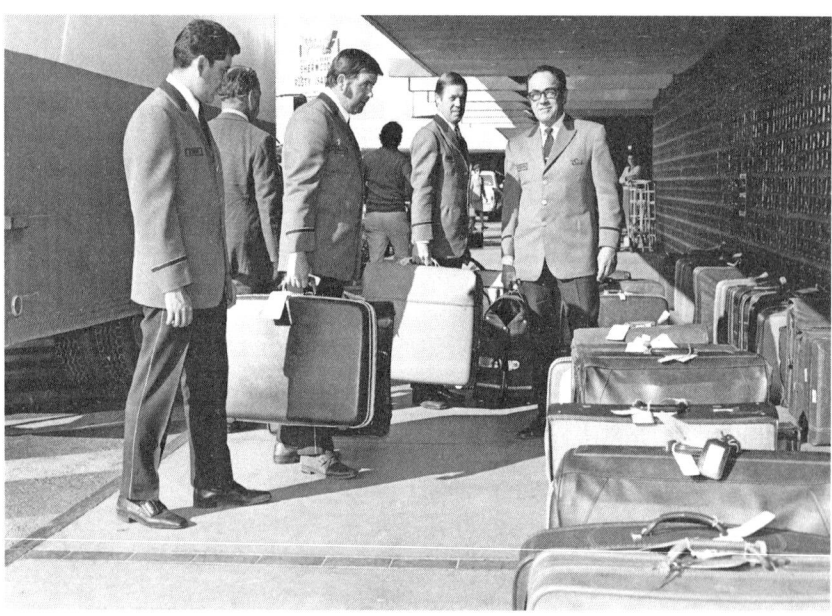

Bellmen at the Sands, circa late 1960s. The United States deindustrialized during the 1970s and 75 percent of Americans worked in postindustrial trades by the 2000s. The Las Vegas Strip exemplified the blurred occupational risks associated with service work. Courtesy of Sands Hotel Collection, UNLV Library Special Collections.

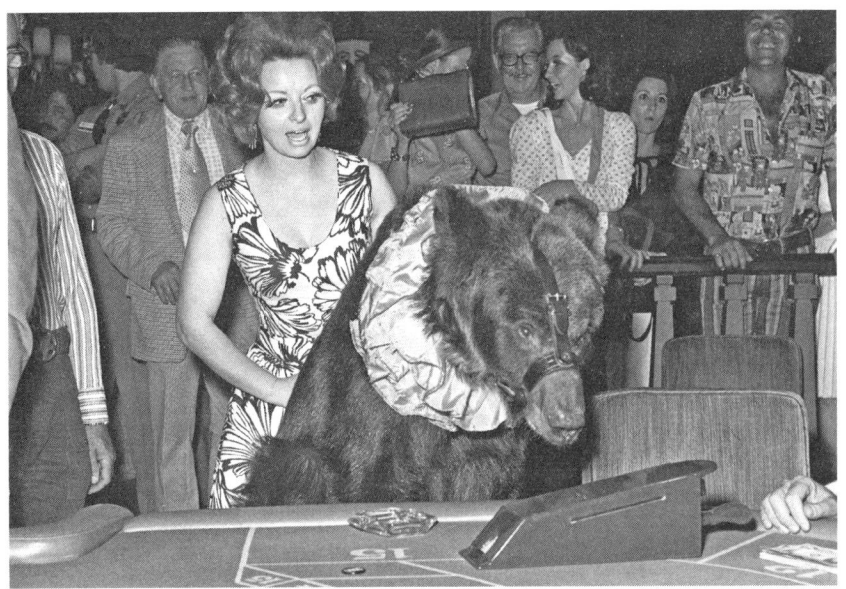

The Ruppert Bears appeared in Frederic Apcar's "Casino de Paris" at the Dunes during the 1970s. Between shows, a two-hundred-pound Scandinavian brown bear named Susie "played" the slots, baccarat, and craps on the casino floor. Courtesy of Dunes Hotel Collection, UNLV Library Special Collections.

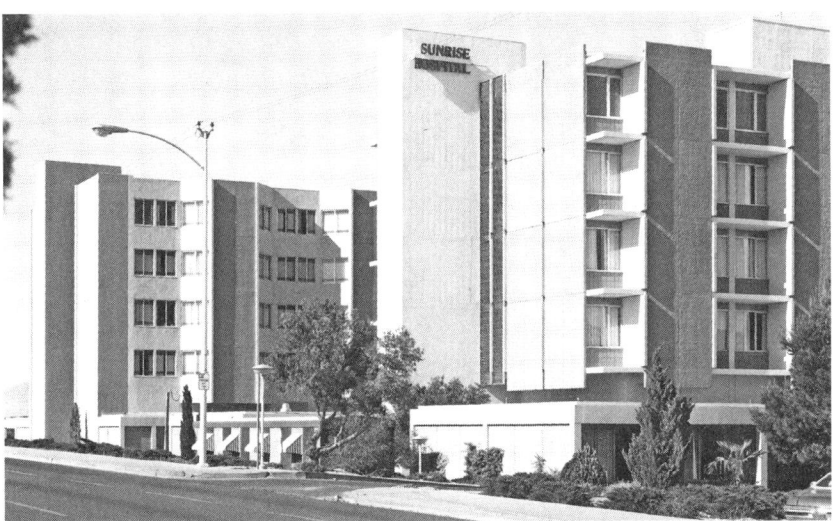

Opening in 1958 and funded by the Teamsters pension, Sunrise Hospital essentially functioned like a company hospital for the Strip until the 1970s. Courtesy of Single Item Accession Photograph Collection, UNLV Library Special Collections.

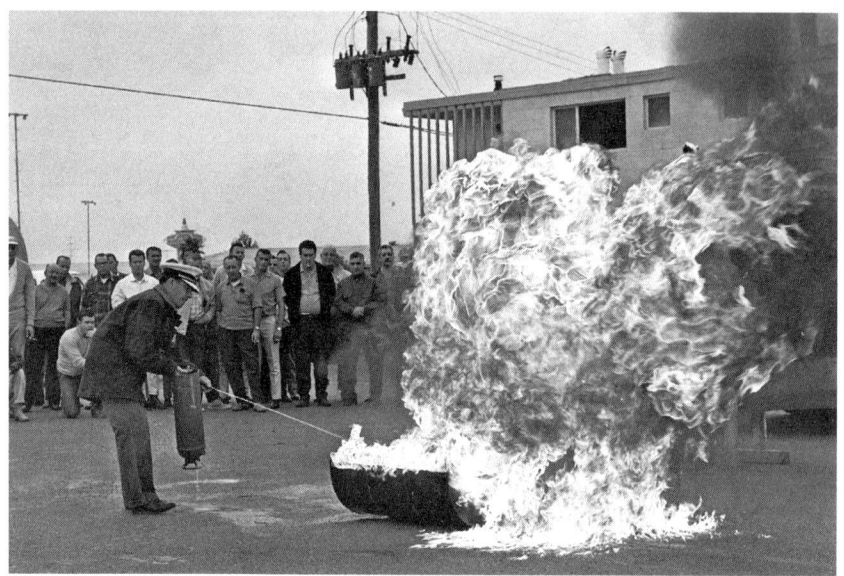

The Sands Hotel and Casino Fire Prevention Class, 1968. By the late 1960s corporate management streamlined health and safety awareness on the Strip, instituting new programs that stressed accident prevention. Courtesy of Sands Hotel Collection, UNLV Library Special Collections.

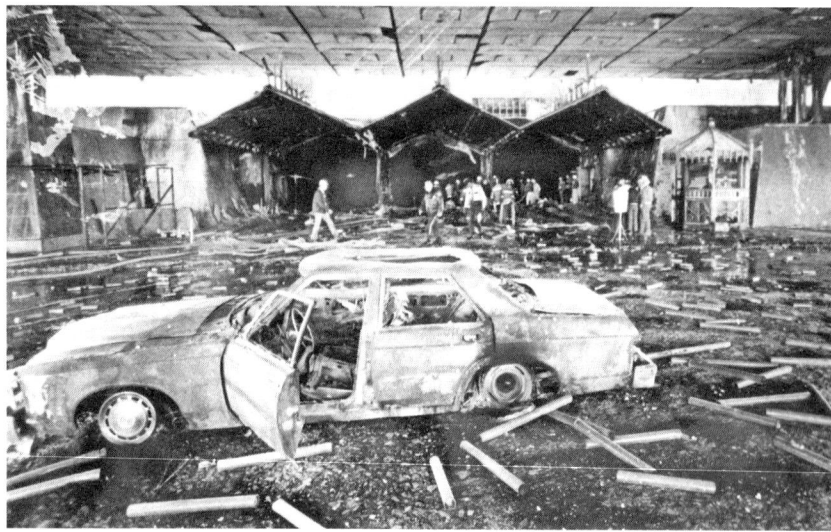

The charred entrance of the MGM Grand Hotel and Casino, November 23, 1980. Three days prior, eighty-five people died in a massive fire, most of them from smoke inhalation. The event, along with a subsequent loss-life fire at the Las Vegas Hilton, forced a global reevaluation of fire safety standards in the hospitality industry. Courtesy of *Las Vegas Sun* Archives.

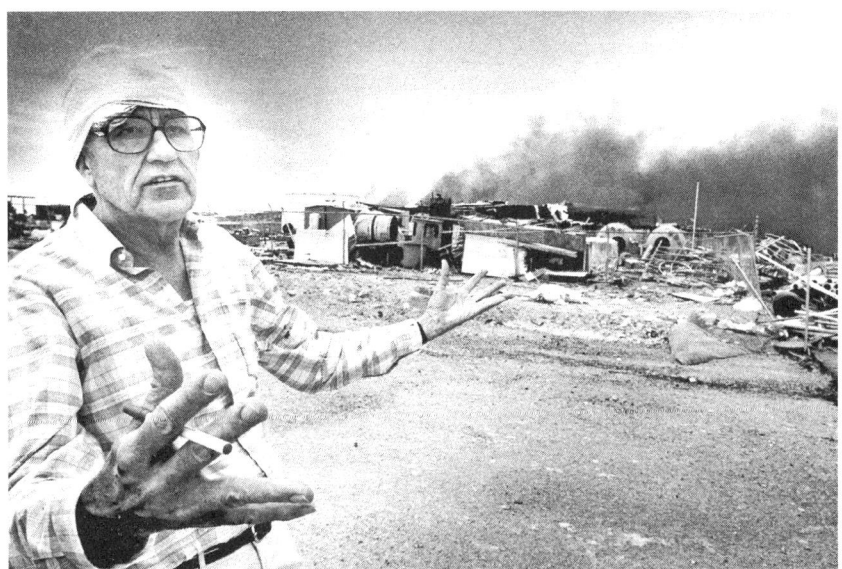

Fred Gibson Jr., president of Pacific Engineering and Production Company of Nevada (PEPCON), standing before the ruins of his rocket-fuel plant in Henderson, May 4, 1988. The PEPCON disaster produced the largest domestic, nonnuclear explosion in recorded history, killing two workers and injuring hundreds. Courtesy of *Las Vegas Sun* Archives.

# 4

# THE TEST SITE

AFTER WORLD WAR II there was an unspoken truce between labor and management with regard to health and safety in the workplace. The federal government dismantled most of its wartime programs, returning to the notion that regulation disrupted the work process. Still, the conversation did not disappear completely; the Labor Management Relations Act of 1947 provided employees with the provision to leave jobs that were deemed unusually dangerous. The act was ineffective, and President Harry Truman called the first Presidential Conference on Industrial Safety in 1948. When 119 coal miners died in a violent explosion in West Frankfort, Illinois on December 21, 1951, the discussion resurfaced. The tragedy garnered significant national attention, leading Congress to pass the Coal Mine Safety Act of 1952. For the first time, the federal government authorized the U.S. Bureau of Mines to conduct annual inspections of underground coal mines with more than fifteen employees, and granted the authority to close work sites in which employee lives were in imminent danger. While addressing only infrequent, large-scale disasters, it was progress nevertheless, and signaled a policy shift regarding federal responsibility to American labor.[1]

In the realm of health and safety, the scientific community rose to prominence as well. Industrial medicine specialists began rejecting so-called overdiagnosis by local doctors, arguing that laboratory science was the only method to discover the origin of a patient's condition. Toxicology became an independent specialty as well; toxicologists used the scientific method to diagnose workplace-related diseases, testing consumer products, pesticides, and chemicals in FDA and private sector laboratories.[2]

But while industry experienced relative autonomy during the postwar period, Americans began to question industry's methods in the 1950s, which marked the beginning of a second era of occupational health history. Postwar conditions prompted the shift, but the process took time. Until World War II the number of workplace-related deaths had steadily decreased, but after the war that trend reversed. From 1958 to 1968 the United States reported a rise in work-related deaths: in 1968 there were more than fourteen thousand fatalities annually, and 2.2 million injuries. Moreover, from 1961 to 1970 industrial accidents increased by 29 percent. It was during the 1960s that the crisis in workplace safety could no longer be ignored: the field of industrial health evolved, incorporating the link among workplaces, the community, and the environment. The field first transitioned to occupational health, including health and safety in all workplaces, and later became a part of environmental health. Certainly, industrial hazards threatened not only workers, but all Americans. During the postwar period the chemical industry dramatically increased the material production of polyesters, nylons, detergents, pesticides, plastics, lubricants, and herbicides in both consumer and industrial products. Prior to the war, synthetic, organic chemical production totaled less than 1 billion pounds a year; in 1976 alone production was 163 billion pounds. Most products were unregulated, departing factories untested for human health and environmental impact. The results were devastating, contaminating the air or water surrounding industrial plants, agricultural communities, and households across the nation.[3]

After World War II, one of the most visible threats to employees, the community, and the environment involved the nuclear industry, and there is no better example of the development of the notion of responsibility in the United States. The advent of nuclear testing introduced the threat of radiation to American labor. While research existed, very little was known about the effects of large doses of radiation to the human body. After the bombings of Hiroshima and Nagasaki, three teams of American scientists traveled to Japan to study the medical effects of the atomic bombs, working alongside a Japanese group led by Dr. Tsuzuki Maseo. Dr. Shields Warren headed the Navy team, while

Drs. Ashley "Scotty" Oughterson and Stafford Warren directed the Army and Manhattan District teams.[4]

As in Hiroshima, the bomb devastated Nagasaki, but the destruction appeared less pronounced because a local mountain range had shielded part of the city from the heat, shock waves, and fallout. Upon arriving, Shields Warren examined survivors sheltered in schools, barracks, and hospitals, and collected clinical and laboratory reports from autopsies that had been performed by Japanese doctors. It was immediately apparent to him that nuclear weapons would create "unprecedented problems in the field of medicine." Warren found the survivors' injuries "diverse and confusing"; most resulted from radiation-blast effects, gamma rays, and neutrons rather than from the explosion itself. In fact, the effects of radiation took hours, days, or weeks to appear. The importance of these injuries, according to Warren, was masked by the thousands killed by flash burns, fires, and wreckage. While his colleagues told Congress that radiation caused 5 to 7 percent of the deaths, Warren concluded that radiation caused the majority. Its lingering effects were the legacy of Hiroshima and Nagasaki.[5]

After his investigation, Warren reported to the American Association for Cancer Research on the latent effects of radiation exposure, revealing that more than fourteen thousand *hibakusha* suffered from hemorrhages, leukocyte destructions, bone marrow damages, anemia, and fertility disorders. He advised that it was "necessary to follow the populations of Hiroshima and Nagasaki for many years" and to use the Japanese cities as a laboratory to study the medical and biological effects of radiation. The doctor recommended creating a permanent commission beyond the control of the military, leading to the establishment of the Atomic Bomb Causality Commission (ABCC).[6]

In the spring of 1947 Warren returned to Japan to reexamine the survivors and their descendants, and found that most had recovered. He wrote in his diary, "People were more alert, many smiling, look fat, and well-fed. Striking change." The Japanese census of 1950 recorded that there were 283,000 survivors; most of these had received "only minimal" radiation exposures of "10 rads or less."[7]

Warren continued his research over the next thirty years. His role establishing the ABCC influenced the Atomic Energy Commission (AEC) to appoint him as its first director of the Division of Biology and Medicine (DBM). From 1947 to 1951 Warren directed all aspects of radiation safety for the AEC, emerging as one of the nation's most influential biomedical scientists. His most notable accomplishments were persuading the AEC to fund cancer and atomic energy research, prompting the funding of fellowships and grants in life sciences, and overseeing the construction of the Argonne Cancer Research Hospital at the University of Chicago and other medical facilities at the Oak Ridge Institute for Nuclear Studies and the Brookhaven National Laboratory. Under the wing of federal support, research in radiation flourished.[8]

But Warren was also a tragic figure in occupational health history, establishing policies at the DBM that affected the health of Americans for generations. Historian David Rothman has called 1945–1965 "the Gilded Age of research, the triumph of laissez-faire in the laboratory." The influx of federal funding and advances in medicine and science prompted a major shift in American medicine. Instead of saving a few lives, many doctors became biomedical scientists, aspiring to save the human race from cancer and other terminal diseases. In the name of science, human experimentation occurred in most medical fields. Warren opposed the practice when it was not good for the patient or if there was no other solution to the health problem. He also challenged using military personnel in Exercise Desert Rock from 1951 to 1957 at the NTS, although he expressed more concern for blast injuries and negative press than for fallout risks. He shut down the total body irradiation experiments as well, which sought to expose two hundred volunteers to whole-body radiation to learn the threshold a soldier could sustain in combat. But Warren continuously suppressed information to prevent lawsuits and protect the AEC's public image. While it horrified him that Manhattan Project scientists injected humans with plutonium, he prevented the news from going public.[9]

Moreover, Warren had a checkered history of protecting humans from radioactive fallout. In an interview with former secretary of

Interior Stewart Udall, who represented downwinders from Nevada and Arizona in a class action lawsuit, he admitted that as early as 1947 he knew that hazardous fission products contaminated the atmosphere during a nuclear explosion. He also suspected food chain dangers in Hiroshima and Nagasaki, a theory confirmed when scientists linked contaminated fish to the 1946 atmospheric tests in the Pacific. Initially he opposed continental nuclear testing, arguing that it posed a great threat to the American public. But the AEC eventually wore him down, reassuring him that the NTS would detonate only a few low-yield bombs.[10]

In 1952 fallout from high-yield bombs sprinkled the ranches and small towns of Nevada and Utah. One week after the twelve-kiloton Easy Test in 1952, Warren recommended that "we cannot risk any continental aboveground shots larger [than Easy]." His superiors ignored the appeal. But by the mid-1950s, Warren changed his mind. He had left his DBM position, but continued working as an AEC consultant. As concern mounted over nuclear testing and fallout, Warren aligned with prominent scientists like Ernest Lawrence and Edward Teller, publicly advocating the need for further nuclear tests to maintain superiority over the Soviet Union.[11] In 1956 he wrote to Lewis Strauss, chairman of the AEC, that "distinct or worldwide radioactive fallout is not a controlling factor in bomb testing. To permit us to fall behind Russians is disastrous; to wait for them to catch up to us is stupid."[12]

Warren supported the theory that low doses of ionizing radiation posed limited health risks, called the permissible dose. Damage occurred when radiation rose above a certain level. The nuclear testing debate faded after the 1958 Test Moratorium and the 1963 Limited Test Ban Treaty banned atmospheric testing. But low-level radiation remained controversial. Did a safe dosage exist for nuclear workers and the public? Beginning in 1956 studies linked radiation in pregnant women to childhood cancer, and the ingestion of radioactive fallout contributed to immune diseases. By the late 1960s, public debate had resurfaced about nuclear reactors and the threat of radioiodine. In 1971 Canadian physician Abram Petkau discovered that cell membranes suffered more damage with long-term, low-level radiation exposure than high level. Scientists in atomic research also spoke out about the dangers of low-level radiation, arguing that emissions from nuclear reactors posed a greater threat to human health than plant accidents. In 1978 President Jimmy Carter, himself a nuclear physicist, ordered the successor of AEC, the Department of Energy (DOE), to make its operational records public, leading to further government, journalistic, and scholarly investigations. Investigations included historian Barton Hacker's comprehensive study on radiation safety and nuclear testing, *Elements of Controversy*. Eventually, a two-year congressional hearing determined the unthinkable: "The greatest irony of our atmospheric nuclear testing program is that our only victims of United States arms since World War II have been our own people."[13]

A nuclear testing program developed out of Cold War tensions. In 1946 Congress established the AEC, a civilian agency that directed peacetime developments of atomic science and technology. On August 1, 1946, Truman signed the Atomic Energy Act, transferring most of the Manhattan Engineer District (MED)'s plants, laboratories, and offices in Oak Ridge, Tennessee; Hanford, Washington; and Los Alamos, New Mexico to the AEC.[14]

Seven-eighths of the forty-four thousand employees worked for private contractors, a model that continued under the AEC. As the Cold War escalated, the Los Alamos Scientific Laboratory (LASL), the research institution behind the Manhattan Project, eagerly waited to resume testing. Since the Trinity and Crossroads tests, theoretical developments revealed new techniques to create more-efficient bombs. However, the scientists needed further data to choose between the designs, and appealed to the AEC to sponsor large-scale tests. Los Alamos narrowed the location to the Enewetak Atoll in the Pacific Ocean, which became the Pacific Proving Grounds (PPG). Logistical problems of testing in the Pacific, including unpredictable weather, pollution that would result, and the expense of transporting men and materials, prompted the Department of Defense (DOD) to push for a continental proving ground. In 1948 the Armed Forces Special Weapons Project (AFSWP) sponsored Project Nutmeg to search for a new site. The survey evaluated atomic clouds and fallout patterns, and meteorology. It concluded that there was no site in the United States or North America that would not produce fallout on populated areas. However, the surveyors indicated that the less populated American West was more sound than the eastern coastal area. The report did not recommend a specific location. The AEC ultimately determined a continental test site was not an option due to domestic and international relations concerns, and decided to resume plans in the event of a national emergency.[15]

Following the detonation of the Soviet Union's first nuclear weapon in 1949 and the outbreak of the Korean War in 1950, the AEC renewed its search.[16] The location criterion required that population, economy, or industry could not exist within a 125-mile radius. Public opinion, logistics, and security were also considerations. Thanks to the influence of Senator Pat McCarran, the AEC determined the Las Vegas Bombing and Gunnery Range held the most promise. Located northwest of Las Vegas, the site consisted of dry lakebeds, Frenchman Flat and Yucca Flat, and other advantages, including natural barriers for improved security and a nearby government-owned airfield at Indian Springs. But Las Vegas was within a 125-mile radius, and the site was only 65 miles from downtown. A team of physicists conducted further studies, and determined that a tower-burst bomb with a yield of twenty-five kilotons could be detonated without exceeding the permissible dose. While meteorologists could predict the wind patterns and limit off-site exposure, there was still a risk. Physicists concluded that the human population would undoubtedly receive "perhaps a little more radiation than medical authorities say [was] absolutely safe."[17]

Despite the risk, the AEC accepted the recommendation and the U.S. Air Force permitted use of the site, but only on a temporary basis. Planning for Operation Greenhouse at the PPG also moved ahead. The operation was a giant feat, testing the first thermonuclear bomb. But scientists needed to conduct more experiments to determine the test design and safety criterion. With Greenhouse beginning in summer 1951, the AEC organized the first continental test series in southern Nevada, called Operation Ranger. The AEC established a safety criterion that minimized radiation exposure restricting the permissible dose to 3.0 roentgens cumulative for a thirteen-week period.[18] A Radiological Safety Section also issued the AEC, Los Alamos, and DOD personnel film badges to measure radiation doses and other protective equipment, and set up monitoring and decontamination equipment.[19]

Ranger's first shot detonated at 5:45 A.M. on January 27, 1951, and was codenamed Ranger Able. The explosion was relatively small; its blast yielded only one kiloton, the energy equivalent of a thousand tons of the conventional chemical explosive TNT. The following day Ranger Baker produced a more spectacular explosion, yielding eight kilotons. While both tests produced varying levels of radiation on site, radiation safety monitors found trace readings off site. But, like the Trinity test, Ranger actually blasted radioactive debris into high-altitude winds, contaminating the snowfall in the Midwestern and Northeastern United States. Radioactive fallout would contaminate most of the United States throughout the decade, and not only the Southwest. However, the tests produced no immediate accidents to personnel or significant radiation exposure. The seemingly successful operation prompted the AEC to greenlight forty years of nuclear testing in southern Nevada.[20]

After Ranger, the AEC turned the NTS into a permanent proving ground, hosting 928 tests and 1,021 detonations from 1951 to 1992.[21] To run the site, the AEC maintained private partnerships, contracting with construction, architectural, and engineering firms, and laboratories. Its structure can be somewhat confusing; the AEC did not actually run the site or conduct the tests. Instead, it owned the assets, established authority of security and labor expenses, and set guidelines on safety, employee relations, and working conditions. Despite some limitations, the AEC ensured that the NTS reflected "the best experience of American industry," aiming to achieve "stable, democratic labor-management relations." The real operators were the DOD, laboratories, and contractors. Los Alamos, the Lawrence Livermore National Laboratory, and Sandia National Laboratories designed the bombs and ran the tests.[22]

Los Alamos and Livermore were the principal organizations at the NTS, while Sandia operated the Tonopah Test Range. The laboratories functioned as friendly rivals; competition arose out of the need to win each government contract. When the DOD needed a nuclear weapon, it approached both laboratories to create and submit a design. In turn, it awarded the contract to its favorite. As the winning laboratory built the test sequence, the scientists enlisted construction and engineering firms to conduct the tests.[23]

The largest contingent of workers was therefore private contractors, providing labor, equipment, materials, and industrial safety and hygiene, radiation safety, sanitation, fire protection, and medical care programs. The various firms also managed maintenance and operation, communication and mapping, engineering, and security. Reynolds Electrical and Engineering Company (REECo) was the prime contractor, sharing the responsibly with Edgerton, Germeshausen, and Grier, Inc. (EG&G), Holmes and Narver (H&N), and Federal Services, Inc. (FSI). The contractors worked together, carrying out each test seamlessly. REECo supervised construction, maintenance, support operations, and health and safety, while EG&G handled timing, firing, measurements, and other scientific functions.[24] H&N provided engineer services and FSI outfitted security guard services at test site and affiliated facilities in Las Vegas. Wackenhut Services Inc. (Wackenhut) later assumed the security contract.

As the prime contractor, REECo maintained health and safety, outfitting the test site with an intricate network of programs designed to protect workers and the public. Founded in 1932 by Lou J. Reynolds, the contractor first participated in the Trinity test as a subcontractor, and had assumed a greater role by 1952. It developed the reputation of a "no problem" or "can do" contractor, getting the job done quickly for the DOD and laboratories.[25]

REECo handled the majority of testing support. It was a big job, an expansive 1,375-square-mile desert that needed power, communications, and water. REECo built and maintained the facilities, roads, fences, and utilities, and operated the motor pool and maintenance shops, and craft support. It also installed and fired the nuclear tests, and handled post-shot data collection and drilling. However, its most important job was establishing programs for occupational safety and health, sanitation, medical, and by 1955, radiation safety.[26]

The majority of test site employees worked for REECo. Total employment varied considerably, based on each series. In June 1961 the test site employed 2,300 workers. On November 8, 1961, the workforce totaled 5,800 to accommodate Operation Nougat, and at the height of testing in 1966, it was 6,500. Most contractors recruited local talent for each test. A 1959 survey of H&N employees reveals that most workers lived in Nevada for at least two years prior to employment. However, a common complaint was that the contractors imported men from out of state. Some contractors established qualifications for employment, like age limitations, but eventually terminated the practice. For example, Wackenhut based its employment decisions on a physician's recommendations that an applicant could perform specific duties, rather than on the applicant's age.[27]

REECo hired an array of job positions. Because of the unique hazards presented, its occupational health program alone recruited not only medical professionals, but also health physicists and safety engineers. Ken Case, known as the Atomic Cowboy, began working at the test site in 1954 and became one of REECo's first radiation safety monitors a year later. In 1957 he worked under Captain Scott L. Reynolds of the U.S. Army Veterinary Corps, a veterinary advisor for radiobiological aspects of test activities. Case drove cattle over ground zero to study the effects of radiation on wildlife. After watching the test on horseback, he was often the first one entering ground zero: "We would get over (ground zero, the epicenter of the blast at ground level) and bang, [the monitors were] off-scale. When we went back over, about thirty feet off the ground, the sand it would be melted just like glass. Those ground zeros in the spring, they bleed a big circle in the snow.... Rabbits would run across there and they would be on fire. It was something."[28]

The majority of workers other than health personnel were laborers—masons, electricians, ironworkers, painters, plumbers, and carpenters—as well as surveyors and architect-engineers. After underground testing began in 1957, REECo began employing miners and drillers. Numerous employees also held culinary, housekeeping, and office staff positions. Los Alamos and Livermore also retained scientists and laboratory technicians, and the Nye County sheriff patrolled the grounds, writing speeding tickets, responding to car accidents, and ejecting protestors. Security guards also managed the badge office, processing military and civilian clearances.[29]

During the 1950s the most visible employees worked for the DOD; these were the soldiers engaging in Exercise Desert Rock.[30] Instituted in 1951, the military exposed its troops to realistic atomic warfare training, hoping to learn how to tactically use nuclear weapons in combat. Scientists also studied the effects on military equipment and the soldiers, testing their psychological and physical reactions. During Desert Rock I, the troops watched a detonation seven miles from ground zero. One soldier described it "like someone had sneaked up on me and breathed heavily on my skin." After the test, the troops inspected the damage and took decontamination showers. The Human Resources Research Organization (HumRRO) then recorded their psychological responses. The soldiers filled out questionnaires inquiring about nuclear warfare, the Cold War, and radioactivity, asking, "Just how frightened would you say you were when the last test A-bomb went off?" Did you have physical reactions, such as "violent pounding of the heart" or "urinating in pants"? Most men answered no. One soldier remarked that he "wasn't even that nervous." The comments reveal the major problem with Exercise Desert Rock: a lack of reality. Despite the enormous health risk, the exercises continued throughout the 1950s.[31]

During the era of atmospheric tests, there were several housing options for the military and contractors. Camp Mercury began as a military camp during Operation Ranger, its name derived from its location in the Mercury Valley. Workers slept in bunks on platform units with canvas roofs. Robert "Doc" Campbell, a Navy hospital corpsman, said it was not "the Waldorf Astoria but being military, they never did promise a rose garden.... We survived." During the evenings, the workers met at the old Slop Shoot for beer and food, or drove to Las Vegas. After testing became permanent during the era of underground testing, the AEC invested $6.7 million in Mercury, constructing temporary housing, an office space, cafeteria, recreation facilities, laboratory facilities, and administrative offices. With the addition of the Nuclear Rocket Development System (NRDS) and the Plowshare Program in the 1960s, the AEC invested an additional $15 million to build permanent housing and dormitories, and administration buildings. Some workers resided there during the week, returning to Las Vegas on the weekend. Others commuted every day, leaving on buses from various points in Las Vegas. As Mercury expanded, it provided all the needs of a small town, including a chapel, bowling alley, swimming pool, and upscale steakhouse. But unlike the federally financed towns Boulder City and Henderson, the AEC restricted public access.[32]

Besides Mercury, Camp Desert Rock housed the majority of troops participating in Exercise Desert Rock. Private George Younkin described it as a typical field camp in which the soldiers slept on cots in tents and ate food out of mess gear. The bathrooms were open trenches, because there was no running water, and the men showered in canvas tents with suspended water pipes. The *Review-Journal* called the showers the encampment's most popular spot because of the overwhelming dust. After the completion of Exercise Desert Rock III, the DOD added substantial upgrades, installing water storage and sewerage systems, and electrical services. It also improved sanitation, constructing concrete bathrooms with flush toilets, showers, and sinks, and built a small hospital and mess hall with a five-hundred-person seating capacity.[33]

Given its isolation, the DOD also made recreation a priority at the camp. It established clubs, and arranged for various entertainment acts to visit the camp or it set up shows in Las Vegas. In 1953 the Jimmy Durante Show performed during Operation Upshot–Knothole. Two years later, Patti Page serenaded the troops before Operation Teapot's Doom Town APPLE-2 shot. Regardless, most soldiers disliked the post, for the most part due to concern over radiation exposure and extreme conditions. One soldier complained that he froze his "ass off" at night because his sleeping bag was poor quality. The wind was also an annoyance, forcing soldiers to salvage wooden boxes from trash areas to board their tents and use potbellied stoves to keep warm. In 1955 a windstorm flattened several barracks. During the Plumbbob series, summer temperatures reached nearly 120 degrees and a flash flood inundated part of the camp, resulting in numerous cases of heat exhaustion and food poisoning after refrigeration units failed.[34]

The biggest difference between the occupational health regimes discussed in previous chapters and the NTS was that the AEC, DOD, laboratories, and contractors always considered health and safety a primary concern, not an afterthought. It was well known that nuclear testing was a hazardous line of work. The occupational health regime therefore developed around three types of potential accidents. The AEC classified the first as "no way related to atomic energy," such as falls, electrocutions, and motor vehicle and construction accidents. The second covered "materials or the processes closely related to the program," or fires and explosions caused by noxious nonradiation-inducing materials. For example, when a Kiwi-B IA reactor produced a hydrogen explosion in a shed, it did not release radiation and was not considered a nuclear incident. The third classification involved radiation as a major factor caused from human error or faulty equipment. Workers entering hot test areas also produced injuries. Most instances fell between the second and third classifications.[35]

Other workers incurred damages because of safety oversight. In 1956 four workers in protective clothing entered a test area to recover samples without their rad-safe monitors, and received external exposures of 4 rads, 14 rads, 19 rads, and 28 rads, respectively. (Rad-safe, or radiological safety organizations in the nuclear program, is discussed below.) To put the exposure in perspective, the recommended permissible dose was a cumulative 3.9 rads over thirteen weeks for most nuclear tests. Other accidents involved radionuclides contaminating construction or laboratory areas, laboratory technicians handling radioactive material with torn gloves, or experiment-related explosions.[36]

Radiation exposures affected employees biologically, physically, and psychologically. REECo doctors diagnosed two categories. Most industrial, nuclear reactor, and medical accidents resulted from external exposure. Contamination also occurred internally by ingestion, inhalation, or absorption of radionuclides. The clinical name for external exposure was acute radiation syndrome (ARS); an illness caused by whole-body irradiation during a short period.[37] Classic examples of ARS were victims of Hiroshima and Nagasaki, and firefighters responding to the Chernobyl disaster. However, ARS in the workplace is extremely uncommon. According to international registries, only three hundred patients have developed ARS worldwide, excluding survivors of events in Hiroshima, Nagasaki, and Chernobyl.[38] Fatalities are also rare; affecting only 20 percent of all patients.[39]

ARS almost never occurred at the NTS because patients never received doses of more than 70 rads. Mild symptoms, however, occurred in workers as low as 30 rads. The AEC determined radiation doses according to curie, roentgen, rad, and rem units. The curie and roentgen evaluated radiation activity and exposure, while rad and rem determined the absorbed dose and dose equivalent that could cause biological damage to the human body. One rad equaled one rem.[40]

While the lethal dose for humans was uncertain, Dr. Shields Warren theorized in 1950 that it was 450 roentgens. Of course, the number was only an estimate and never tested experimentally, but scientists often referred to it as Dr. Warren's magic number. Besides a dose of 70 rads or higher, ARS patients received doses that penetrated the entire body, affecting all the organs. Most radiation-related injuries at the NTS involved exposure to the hands. Such localized exposure did not cause ARS. The dose also needed to be delivered in a short time period and at the same magnitude, usually in a matter of minutes.[41]

Throughout atmospheric testing, radiation accidents caused a very small percentage of injuries. From 1945 to 1964 99.8 percent of AEC, DOD, laboratory, and contractor employees received less than 5 rem annually. The majority of exposures more than 5 rem resulted from accidents. The AEC determined that out of 7,693 injuries, thirty-six were from radiation. Of the thirty-six, three died, eleven did not show evidence of radiation effects, and twenty-two showed clinical manifestations attributable to radiation. Of the latter group, two were put on permanent disability and two required amputation. All NTS employees received a fair amount of radiation exposure, but their tolerances varied. According to Dr. Leonard Kreisler, the medical director of REECo from 1973 to 1990, test site doctors did not treat workers based on a number system alone. Since the amount of radiation was not indicative of bodily damage, they theorized that the human body differed in dose tolerance and had a wide margin of safety. The types of ionizing radiation (alpha, beta, gamma, x-ray, neutron) were also factors, as well as distance and shielding. Kreisler provided an example:

A radiation monitor was giving a class on how to handle a radio-active source.... He came out and there is this lead-shielded box, [known as] a pig, and inside is radioactive material. The way you would normally take it out is you attach a cable to it, which is shielded, and this would pull out the radioactive material.... This guy opens up the container and pulls the thing out with his bare hand. With his bare hand! They reconstructed the time that he was exposed, the type of radiation, whether it was alpha which will not penetrate the skin, whether it was beta which really gets penetration, whether it is nasty stuff like gamma. They calcu-lated the dose and he had significant exposure to his hands from a physics point of view. We watched this guy for a month. We did blood tests. I looked at his daily for two weeks. He didn't even sunburn. He didn't even get redness! Nothing! He got no adverse medical findings. It just goes to show that there is a wide margin of safety, number one [and that] individuals differ. [42]

The key issue was therefore not exposure levels, but whether work-ers received damage. High doses of external radiation produced recog-nizable symptoms, but low-level exposures were problematic. During the 1950s scientists started using the term "low-level radiation" to refer to doses of whole-body radiation ranging from 25 to 100 rads. At that level, they believed there were no observable effects. All workers re-ceived low doses on a regular basis, sometimes so small that it defied detection. REECo doctors consequently treated low-level exposures statistically rather than clinically. It was easy to treat a worker blasted with high levels of radiation; ARS signs appeared immediately. But small doses on a regular basis could possibly induce cancer years later. The causal link also became blurred as the time between exposure and injury increased. The medical program therefore protected workers based on probability of injury. In January 1961 the AEC required that all contractors limit worker exposure to the permissible dose, which was 5 rem per year. [43]

While radiation posed a threat to workers, most doctors expressed more concern with traditional workplace hazards. Dr. Clinton S. Mau-pin, the radiological safety advisor to REECo, believed that the maximum permissible radiation exposure level was very low, and that it impeded the occupational health program. Maupin called it "unreasonable and unrealistic" to consider low-level exposures more serious industrial accidents, which he believed produced the most injuries and fatalities. From 1943 to 1964 the AEC reported 15,790 injuries, 7,364 of which happened during construction activities. The most common injuries involved dust inhalation, burns, cuts and lacerations, hernias, infections, strains from improper lifting, and fractures. Out of 251 fatalities, the majority occurred in construction and production. Most deaths occurred due to falls, electrocutions, and car accidents, which the AEC attributed to "lack of proper precautions, too much familiarity with the job, and failure to follow safety precautions." Motor vehicle casualties were also a menace. In fact, many workers identified "unsafe driving" as the biggest hazard at the NTS, not radiation. Cars flipped on site, killing drivers and passengers with burn and crush wounds, asphyxiation, or explosions. Accidents also occurred on the two-lane road connecting the test site and Las Vegas. Nicknamed "the Widowmaker," thousands of workers traveled it daily. The road had been poorly constructed, with innumerable dips preventing visibility. Most accidents resulted from fatigue, hurried driving, or binge drinking at saloons in Cactus Springs or Indian Springs, with workers crashing into oncoming traffic or sand embankments. The AEC and the state of Nevada recognized the problem, and expanded the road into a four-lane, divided highway. Still, the accidents continued. In 1964 the Widowmaker caused forty-five deaths.[44]

The occupational health regime that coalesced at the NTS loosely resembled the Boulder Canyon Project. As a remote, high-profile project, the AEC, DOD, laboratories, and contractors needed to prioritize health and safety to function correctly, and spare it from bad publicity. Similar to the Boulder Canyon Project, federal interests played a huge factor in the occupational health regime, but the AEC exercised broader influence over health and safety. As a self-regulating agency, it shielded the work site in the name of national security, barring state regulatory agencies and labor unions from exerting real influence. Still, knowing the considerable health risks, the AEC and its contractors took a more proactive approach than Reclamation and Six

Companies, and partnered with the PHS to manage off-site radiological safety activities and develop safety protocol to protect employees, the community, and the environment.[45]

Although the AEC felt a sense of responsibility to protect workers and the public, it was a different understanding from modern notions. Employers during the second period of occupational health history were not morally obligated to protect their employees from harm that could possibly develop years later. As a result, its program outlined basic health and safety standards that covered immediate, physical threats. The program had three categories: general safety, fire safety, and health protection. General safety set procedures for performing construction; handling explosives; mining and tunneling; operating motor vehicles, aircrafts, and firearms; and transporting radioactive materials. Fire protection mandated fire and building codes; and conducted inspections of appliances, equipment, materials, and nuclear safety involving AEC-owned reactor procedures. The final category, health protection, included occupational medicine, industrial hygiene, environmental sanitation, and radiological safety. On paper, the program appeared to protect workers and the public from radiation and other hazards. In reality, the test site was a giant laboratory, and the research was always more important than human life or ecological damage. With modern notions of employer responsibility still developing, the AEC, DOD, laboratories, and contractors lacked the moral and legal commitment to fully protect from perhaps the biggest threat, the cumulative effects of low-level radiation. In order to get the job done, they based their health and safety program on the vague scientific boundaries of a permissible dose, a policy they well knew could harm employees in the future.[46]

Still, the test site's occupational health regime had advanced from previous systems. With regard to the health and safety program, the AEC required the contractors to establish programs based on their individual work, and the DBM issued a guide of minimum standards.[47]

Doctors specializing in occupational medicine, industrial hygiene, and health physics were prominent members of the team, conducting regular inspections, recommending preventive and corrective measures, and supervising physical examinations. Three types of examinations were administered: preplacement, periodic, and sepa-ration. Like the LA&SL Company, Six Companies, and BMI before it, the AEC required preemployment examinations to record preexisting conditions, occupational history, and personal and family medical history. It insisted that the examinations helped in "suitable place-ment" in job positions. Periodic examinations were similar; doctors decided if an employees' health was "compatible" to their work and if their employment attributed to "ill health." In the event of employee terminations, doctors conducted separation examinations, especially in the event of radiation exposures or other injurious events. The doc-tors recorded skin lesions, cataracts, blood dyscrasias, internal radio-isotopes and other toxic materials. While the examinations helped maintain employee health, the files also documented a worker's time at the test site for potential liability suits. The AEC stressed that it was "highly desirable" for each contractor to maintain its own "accurate and complete" medical records, emphasizing to regularly record "data of exposures of hazardous physical (including radiation) and chemical agents."[48]

In the event of a workplace-related injury, the AEC expected con-tractors to furnish their own medical care. The program departed significantly from previous models of employee-funded care. Prior to 1950, employers offered medical benefits with company doctors and on-site hospitals in exchange for monthly salary deductions. As seen in previous chapters, the plans were hardly comprehensive, usually only covering workplace-related injuries. But after 1945, American medicine and health insurance coverage transformed significantly. During World War II, third-party health insurance companies like Blue Cross and Blue Shield increased market share significantly.[49]

A partial reason for their success was wartime wage restrictions; the War Labor Board declared that fringe benefits, like health insur-ance, did not count as wages. When employers had to increase benefits, they turned to third-party insurance companies. In 1960 70 percent of full-time employees received third-party benefits. As insurance companies competed to provide the most coverage, workers started viewing health insurance as a right, not a privilege. For the first time, any employed person could acquire quality medical care, regardless of personal wealth. Coupled with increased federal spending in medical research, the introduction of third-party insurance companies led to a huge expansion of the American hospital system, encouraging advances in medical technology, surgical procedures, and the quality of medical training.[50]

The test site merged the old and new system. REECo handled on-site medical care, providing on-site emergency diagnosis and treatment, physical examinations and immunizations, and health insurance with third-party carriers like Blue Cross. Employees benefited from the federal–state partnership, which provided worker's compensation for disability or death from radioactive material or industrial injuries.[51] If a worker received an injury on site, he sought treatment at the test site from REECo doctors. If a worker got a cold, he saw a primary care physician in Las Vegas, a visit covered by third-party benefits.[52]

The AEC made it clear that diagnosis and nonoccupational disorder treatment were "not the responsibilities of an occupational health program," but there were exceptions. REECo doctors regularly treated minor disorders, especially to prevent loss of life or limb. Caring for workers on a preventive basis, they also corrected ailments that could aggravate work. REECo established on-site medic stations throughout the site and a health, medicine, and safety building in Mercury, a hospital subsidized by federal funds. In the event of an emergency, REECo doctors stabilized critical workers, transporting them to Las Vegas or Los Angeles. While on-site health services changed throughout the test site's operation, the medical program was always directed by a physician trained in occupational medicine. The medical director dictated its development, interpretation, and implementation, managed units at the NTS, Groom Lake, the Tonopah Test Range, and Las Vegas, and handled all hiring. The number of staff ranged considerably based on funding and need. To be considered for employment, training in occupational medicine was desirable, but not mandatory.[53]

During atmospheric testing, medical personnel provided twenty-four-hour, seven-days-a-week physician coverage during each test series, which usually spanned two to five months. In the 1960s testing expanded to year-round underground series, and it became harder for REECo to convince doctors to stay nights and weekends. The contractor consequently limited coverage to only weekdays. The workers disliked the change and pushed for expanded care, but REECo could only hire "well-trained first aid men" to cover nights and weekends. Similar to the construction of Hoover Dam, medics were the most visible members of the medical staff. Positioned in remote stations to active work sites, they provided immediate medical assistance to injured workers. Doctors also provided consultations during critical emergencies with "around the clock [advice] via telephone or radio communication." REECo's medical program also offered education and counseling to the workers, educating on personal hygiene and health maintenance. The AEC considered health education to go hand in hand with safety education, and taught about cleanliness, weight control, nutrition, and mental health: "Experience has shown that health education is most effective when the employer demonstrates his sincere and continuing interest in the health of his employees."[54]

While industrial injuries caused the most injuries and fatalities, radiological safety remained the test site's primary focus. Nuclear testing posed unique problems for the AEC, potentially exposing employees and communities to deadly levels of ionizing radiation. Working alongside radiation was not a new concept. During the 1890s, the discovery of man-made radiation sources, the x-ray and radium, began exposing humans to high, dangerous levels.[55]

In the 1920s scientists discovered that radiation caused genetic mutations and radiologists experienced alarmingly high death rates, linking overexposure and mortality. In the 1930s scientists connected radon gas to high cancer rates among Central European miners. After Americans dropped bombs over Hiroshima and Nagasaki, there were numerous articles written on the effects of radiation. However, most of these articles provided qualitative not quantitative data.[56]

In the field of radiology, the concept of the permissible dose emerged in the late 1920s. Because x-ray apparatuses produced more-penetrating types of ionizing radiations, safety experts began setting exposure level guidelines. The working theory was that a safety threshold existed, a number at which radiation workers could work safely. Officials eventually applied this concept to nuclear testing, conducting dangerous experiments that could cause illness at a later date but not impose immediate harm. During the Manhattan Project, thousands of workers became vulnerable to unprecedented doses of radiation that scientists had haphazardly deemed safe.[57]

The development of radiation safety in America's nuclear program has been covered extensively by Barton Hacker in *Elements of Controversy*.[58] Two terms denoted the field of radiation protection. The first term, "health physics," emerged during the 1940s, and designated the physics section of the Manhattan Project Health Division. After the war, health physics symbolized how the medical profession would protect people and the environment from radiological hazards. The second term, "rad-safe," described radiological safety in the nuclear program. At the NTS, rad-safe was handled by a division devoted to radiological safety, which established safety standards, radiation detection, equipment monitoring, and decontamination plans in the event of radioactive fallout. It also issued safety equipment and film badges to workers.

Rad-safe evolved significantly from the early 1950s. During Operation Ranger, the AEC assembled the program in only two months, basing it on Operation Greenhouse's rad-safe at the PPG. Rad-safe management shifted considerably afterward. In subsequent test series, Los Alamos or the DOD handled operations. Both parties faced numerous challenges; it was difficult to develop firm standards due to urgent construction needs. The various contractors regularly instructed their construction crews to build testing support in close proximity to tests just conducted. Although management recognized the levels were probably unsafe, they needed to fulfill the testing requirements. In 1957 REECo assumed control of rad-safe, establishing a full-time division to accommodate Operation Plumbbob. It was an ambitious endeavor: Plumbbob consisted of twenty-four nuclear detonations or "shots," and six safety experiments, and involved eighteen thousand DOD personnel taking part in scientific and diagnostic experiments, observation exercises, and tactical maneuvers.[59]

While some DOD personnel assisted in Plumbbob's scientific experiments, most participated in tactical exercises organized by Exercise Desert Rock VII and VIII. At shot Hood, the Marine Corps partook in a helicopter airlift and tactical air support. At shot Smoky, the Army conducted an airlift assault; and at shot Galileo, it tested the psychological reaction to witnessing a nuclear explosion. Rad-safe limited exposure to 5 roentgens for each six-month period. Of this exposure, no more than 2 roentgens could be immediate radiation. The limit was much higher than the limits for REECo and other contract workers, which allowed 3 roentgens for a thirteen-week period, and 5 roentgens for one calendar year. The 50th Chemical Platoon supported Desert Rock's rad-safe section, providing materials, equipment, and rad-safe personnel. Before the shots, the soldiers attended safety orientations, and received film badges and protective equipment. During the tests, rad-safe performed surveys, limited access to contaminated areas, provided decontamination support, and removed hot material from personnel and equipment.[60]

At first, Plumbbob went according to plan. On June 24, 1957, the Priscilla shot involved large numbers of DOD personnel and an extensive military effects program. On July 5 Hood produced the largest atmospheric test explosion at the NTS, yielding 74 kilotons. Weather delays postponed Smoky until August 31. It performed differently than anticipated, producing significant fallout on ground zero. Shortly after, rad-safe entered the area to determine radiation levels and soldiers performed their exercises. The final test, Galileo, occurred a month later. Although Smoky did not expose troops to significant radiation levels, it contaminated the Galileo area with fallout. Most soldiers were also supposed to participate in Smoky, not Galileo, but scheduling issues and radiation concerns postponed their exercises. The DOD ultimately approved the exercises for Galileo. After watching the explosion, soldiers entered the trench area and performed an infiltration course test. By the end of Plumbbob, only 50 out of 14,880 soldiers had received greater than 5 rem exposure. The health and safety program appeared to successfully protect workers and the public, but it was far from it. The tests released 58,300 kilocuries of radioiodine into the atmosphere, exposing nearby communities to 120 million rads of thyroid tissue exposure, a level of exposure that statistically could cause up to two hundred thousand excess cases of thyroid cancer. A 1980 survey of the participating soldiers also reported higher rates of leukemia, ten cases instead of the expected four.[61]

Plumbbob marked the end of the Desert Rock Exercises and atmospheric testing. In the mid-1950s, public concern grew when radioactive fallout sprinkled ranches downwind of the NTS and the Japanese fishing boat *Daigo Fukuryū Maru* that was near the PPG. The first outside influence affecting the occupational health regime was an international campaign that called for a comprehensive ban on nuclear testing worldwide. In 1959 the United States, Great Britain, and the Soviet Union halted testing and began negotiating a treaty, but the Eisenhower administration cancelled negotiations at the end of the year when they stalled. The test site remained inactive until the de facto moratorium ended in 1961. After four years of negotiations, the three parties reached an agreement and the United States, Soviet Union, and Great Britain signed the Limited Test Ban Treaty in Moscow, outlawing all atmospheric, underwater, and outer space tests.

The treaty ended atmospheric testing, ushering in a new era of work at the NTS that altered the occupational health regime. The test site shifted to conduct testing underground, a method that limited the risk of fallout. However, the process presented new hazards for workers associated with drilling and mining. The AEC first discussed underground testing in 1946, selecting the island of Amchitka in the Pacific. It ultimately deemed the site unsuitable, but the topic resurfaced after testing commenced at the NTS. Dr. Shields Warren, then director of the DBM, objected to underground testing, arguing that it was not possible "to disregard a potential long-term inhalation hazard." Moreover, he cautioned that underground detonations could create "recurring problems of dust contaminated with material of long half-life being blown by the wind" and the "arid character" of the desert would "increase this hazard." Despite his reservations, the AEC authorized the testing of shallowly buried, underground devices, hoping to use atomic energy for excavation and demolition purposes. The site conducted its first underground test during Operation Buster-Jangle in November 1951.[62]

In 1955 Army engineers tested atomic demolition munitions (ADM) underground. The *Chicago Daily Tribune* described these tests as "the dirtiest of the series," producing radioactive dirt that contaminated the entire test site. With the help of both laboratories, Plumbbob hosted the first underground tests designed to be fully contained. Los Alamos conducted two tests, Pascal-A and Pascal-B, in unstemmed holes in Yucca Flat. Meanwhile, Livermore conducted a third test, Rainier, in the Rainier Mesa. Rainier was the first fully contained explosion at the NTS, with no fission particles vented into the atmosphere.[63]

Rainier served as a prototype for future underground detonations. But before the Limited Test Ban Treaty, tests were rarely contained. In 1958 the NTS conducted nine safety and four weapons underground tests during Operation Hardtack II. Only one of thirteen tests was fully contained. When year-round underground testing began, the numbers were equally grim, with only about half of 113 tests fully contained. After the introduction of tighter safety controls, 1964 statistics showed slight improvements, with 55 percent containment out of twenty-nine tests. Of course, venting was a huge safety concern, but it was also legally problematic. According to the Limited Test Ban Treaty, all radioactive debris from the underground tests needed to stay within the nation's territorial limits. The AEC subsequently revised its regulations, mandating deeper tests. At first, the changes did not fare well because a lower burial did not ensure containment. During Operation Niblick, the Pike shot created a fissure in the ground, venting a black cloud of radioactive dust that drifted toward the California–Arizona border. Besides obvious health concerns, the United States would have violated the treaty if the radioactivity had reached Mexico. Although a crisis was avoided, it forced the AEC to impose tighter regulations, mandating that firings occur only during optimal weather conditions.[64]

Pike demonstrated that deeply buried tunnels or shafts did not guarantee a fully contained test. It was not until the late 1960s that the NTS figured out a system that provided both treaty compliance and a safe work environment. Underground testing was an extensive endeavor. After merging with EG&G in 1967, REECo organized all drilling, mining, and tunneling. When a laboratory acquired federal funding for the test, it decided whether to conduct it in a vertical or horizontal tunnel. The laboratories conducted 90 percent of underground tests in vertical shafts, usually testing the development of new weapons systems. The vertical tests housed smaller-yields in Yucca Flat and larger-yields requiring deeper holes in the Pahute Mesa. Horizontal testing occurred in a testing complex located in the Rainier Mesa, hosting experiments that typically studied radiation and ground shock effects of military weaponry systems.[65]

In general, the methods followed the same steps. It took several months to a year to mine the test bed, field the experiments, execute the event, and reenter the location to collect the experiments. A common complaint among REECo miners was that the laboratories demanded impossible design scenarios. But according to superintendent John F. Campbell, the miners always delivered. The workers surveyed, staked, and core-drilled the site, and conducted geophysical, biological, and cultural inspections. After the preliminary steps, they mined or drilled the main experiment drift, instrument alcoves, and containment plugs. Each event required four thousand to five thousand feet of tunnel driving. Diesel locomotives pulled mine cars, hauling concrete underground and muck outside. REECo also handled engineering and construction, setting up structural steel and concrete to create extensive grounding systems, and installing utility power, instrumentation cables, diagnostic and radiation monitoring systems, and shock mounting. On experiment day, engineers transported an unassembled nuclear device in a lead-containment vessel known as a "pig."[66] When the device reached its destination, rad-safe and industrial hygiene technicians checked it for leaks and other safety requirements. Upon its approval, the laboratory took the device out of the pig and conducted a diagnostic assembly, reporting its findings to the Containment Panel. If the panel accepted the designs and preliminary tests, the device was ready for detonation. Security operations evacuated all nonevent workers prior to the test, and rad-safe activated its monitors and aircrafts to track potential venting activity. After a weather forecaster determined that the wind direction and fallout patterns would not threaten off-site populations, the test controller detonated the device remotely. Following the explosion, a reentry team containing miners, laboratory technicians, and rad-safe personnel checked for appropriate ventilation and opened the doors to enter the area. After safety was established, the workers continued their jobs according to event requirements. They recovered experiment instrumentation, reentered the drifts to permit visual examination of ground zero, and occasionally mined back to the detonation site.[67]

REECo drew from an eclectic workforce to support underground testing. After the laboratories had chosen a test location, they submitted work lists to local labor unions. Word quickly spread among the transient mining and construction community. The miners were a rough group, tramping from all over the world. They had a circuit, traveling from water projects and mines in Bakersfield, California, and Ely, Nevada, to the Coeur d'Alene District in Idaho, and Butte, Montana. At first snowfall, they headed to southern Arizona and New Mexico, and to other warm weather locations. John Campbell noted that most miners were single and did not have a real social life because of the mentality, "I don't know if I'm going to live tomorrow."[68] Many had been in the business for a long time, and several had worked in the tunnels at Hoover Dam. Their jobs were intense and time consuming. The men lived in a six hundred–bed camp established in Area 12 or commuted from Las Vegas.[69] Early conditions in Area 12 were rough. In 1962 Harry Adams described the discontent among miners in the encampment to Senator Howard Cannon. While the men were aware of the importance of their work, the conditions made it "difficult to be patriotic." Four adult men shared sleeping trailers with inadequate sanitary facilities, and the nearest entertainment area was in Las Vegas, leading to a dangerous commute when the men spent their free time drinking at bars. There were only two phones in the camp, which were usually out of order. The workers also regularly threatened food strikes because of high prices and quantity issues. REECo eventually resolved the problems as the testing program intensified. With the perceived threat of fallout diminishing throughout the 1960s, Area 12 eventually provided permanent living quarters with better amenities.[70]

Constructing the underground tests presented a host of new workplace hazards. However, most men considered the risk a natural part of their job and felt a patriotic duty to safeguard America from the threat of communism. Other than leaving work dirty, they never worried about the risk of their job. If workers started "dying at once en masse," commented Campbell, that would have "created panic." But with only sporadic reports of cancer or cardiovascular disease cases, they enthusiastically carried out their work. Most enjoyed the thrill of manufacturing an underground test. Campbell remembered his work fondly, especially when he handled big equipment and dynamite.[71] Still, the conditions were dangerous. During the summer, temperatures sometimes reached more than 120 degrees. The tunnels and shafts were also located two thousand feet under the water table, so they were threatened with water inflows. Since it was impossible to apply standard safety procedures with such limited space, they invented new communication equipment, and devices for filtering and cooling breathing air.[72]

Regardless, accidents were very common. Safety superintendent William Beam said the majority were "construction-type accidents... [with] lots of bumps and lots of back strains" that intensified as the workforce aged. The indoor drilling and mining equipment also created noise pollution. Ear protection was the hardest to enforce, as many miners refused to wear earplugs. This contributed to multiple cases of temporary or permanent hearing loss. However, drillers had the most dangerous job, experiencing numerous fatalities and accidents while attempting to maneuver the massive equipment underground. Miners were in close second, lacerating parts of their body with the drill rigs. The rigs also had the potential to overturn, causing falls from the derrick platforms or down the shaft.[73]

Environmental exposures were prevalent as well, but Campbell considered the conditions improved from the uranium, copper, and metal industry. The shafts and tunnels exposed workers to diesel and blasting smoke, chemicals (epoxies, silicone, exotic chemical hardeners), dust, asbestos, and radiation. Of course, the workers wore safety clothing, but they regularly breathed contaminated air. Concrete dust accumulated in their nostrils as they poured concrete and mined. Campbell remembered that one old miner, Marv Swena, used to say "it was so god-danged dusty in [the tunnels], you had to pick your nose with a nail." Working alongside radiation also posed a risk. External radiation exposure was certainly a threat, but radionuclides were concentrated underground. During pre- and post-shot drilling, workers regularly breathed tritium and radioiodine. In 1965 radioiodine escaped from an abandonment valve. During a post-shot drilling, two workers received an estimated thyroid exposure of 31 and 27 rads, and four others reported smaller varying doses. Despite these conditions, Dr. Leonard Kreisler believed the tunnels were safe. As medical director of REECo, he tracked the health of miners for eight years that recorded work-related illnesses, time lost from work over five days, and deaths. In comparison to the state of Nevada, Kreisler found no difference in the incidence of diseases, especially cancer and cardiovascular disease. In fact, he considered the tunnels "cleaner than most of the casinos downtown." Still, most workers expressed skepticism of the tunnel conditions in retrospect. While not directly killing anyone during employment, most accepted the cumulative dosage might have affected them in the long term.[74]

Since testing nuclear weapons underground was a new method, accidents were very common. Kreisler attributed most injuries to the workers not listening well. In 1964 the frequency rate of disabling injuries was 9.65 per million man-hours worked. Eventually, revised safety procedures produced a workplace that was more secure. By 1967 REECo had reduced the rate to 3.15, and to 1.63 in 1968. William Beam regarded 1967 to 1993 as "the best years of the test site" because "everybody worked hard" and "followed safety guidelines." Kreisler agreed, calling it "the safest place in the world," with an accident rate "probably lowest in the industry" thanks to the NTS's occupational health program. Besides radiation monitoring, industrial hygiene, and air and water sampling, REECo staffed industrial safety and safety training departments to handle mining, drilling, and construction safety. The departments advised, inspected, recommended, and investigated, and offered safety training classes. In the Area 12 camp cafeteria, Beam taught mine rescue and first aid training, and blaster certification for handling explosives. All courses were renewed periodically. Additionally, mining inspectors interfaced with rad-safe and industrial hygiene on the tunnel reentries.[75]

The medical department worked alongside the safety program. According to Dr. Savino W. Cavender, a REECo consultant and interim medical director from 1967 to 1973, the medical personnel worked very closely with the industrial hygienists and radiological science department. His motto on the job was to prevent injuries because it was "a lot easier and more profitable to prevent than to have to treat." Cavender worked as a miner in undergraduate school and knew the job well, calling the shafts "quite dusty," and exposing workers to "a number of potential agents." He recognized that some miners had worked in the industry for decades, being exposed to chemical solvents, hydrocarbons, and combustion residues over long periods. Even Cavender was reckless, often leaving his film badge in the lunchroom because he "didn't want to be taken off the job" if radiation levels exceeded the allowable dose. This was a common practice among all workers. In the 1970s REECo cracked down on it, collecting and processing all badges on time. As with most employers, the contractor also highly discouraged time-lost accidents, instructing the medical staff to return patients back to work quickly. If a patient was "laying in the hospital with his liver lacerated," Dr. Leonard Kreisler did not clear him. But if he "came in with a broken arm," the doctor regularly "put a cast on it [and] sent him back to work."[76] Kreisler himself subscribed to the philosophy of an employee's right to work. Workers' compensation was only a fraction of their salaries and it was unfair to "keep a man from doing his job."[77]

To diagnose and treat patients, REECo doctors developed creative plans. Since nuclear testing was a new line of work, associated diseases did not have a clear treatment plan. Testing underground complicated matters. In 1959 ten miners were exposed to tritium, an active isotope of hydrogen. Although it was a low-energy beta emitter and not dangerous externally, tritium was a hazard if inhaled, ingested, or absorbed in the skin. In the late 1950s tritium contaminated the test site's underlying soil and groundwater, and underground testing aggregated the problem. When thermonuclear devices detonated in confined spaces, gaseous and water-based tritium passed the permissible dose. The isotope did not pose a threat to the public; it usually flushed out within ten days. But breathing large quantities on a regular basis underground presented serious health risks. Atmospheric conditions bled tritium into the tunnel, exposing miners to very unhealthy doses. Since exposure was short term and at a high dose, REECo doctors theorized that the effects could be limited if they purged the isotopes from their bodies. After the rad-safe division discovered the exposure, they went to work, but immediately ran into a problem.[78]

Tritium was a new material and treatment was still undefined. During the 1950s Los Alamos conducted studies to understand how the body retained it, but it was still unclear how to swiftly remove it. REECo doctors enlisted the laboratories to search for a solution. In the meantime, the miners drank large amounts of water, tea, coffee, and cola. Nothing worked. Two days after the exposure, health physicists proposed another solution: drinking beer. The theory was based on alcohol increasing the rate of urine, flushing the tritium out of the body. Human beings also could drink more malt beer than any other liquid because it contains amylase, a digestive enzyme that converts starch into sugars. After learning the treatment plan, mining supervisor William Flangas told his coworkers the treatment. They figured he had lost it, but drank large amounts of beer in Area 12 for several days. Rad-safe took urinalysis samples every few hours, recording their levels. The treatment worked. Nine of the ten miners reached a tolerable dose within several days. One man refused to drink alcohol based on religious beliefs, and still recorded traces in his system months later. Beer continued to be the treatment of choice for tritium exposure until rad-safe invented a monitor recording air concentrations of the isotope during the 1960s. The new technique worked and limited tritium exposures henceforth.[79]

In the early 1970s the test site's occupational health regime seemed to have eliminated the threat of nuclear testing to human health. Of course, environmental concerns were never a consideration. To all appearances, moving the tests underground achieved both the goals of the Limited Test Ban Treaty and eliminated public concern over radioactive fallout hazards. From a public relations standpoint, the NTS conducted safe tests. In reality, most vented, posing serious risks to employees and the public. After the atmospheric ban, most people assumed underground testing was safe. But of the 475 underground tests conducted, sixty-two failures occurred. Of those, the AEC classified fifty-three as "leaks" and "seeps," or gradual escapes of radiation, and nine as "venting," defined as "a massive release of radiation."[80]

In 1970 a by-product of the seemingly safer conditions was an erosion of the occupational health regime. Since no major accidents had occurred since the atmospheric ban, health and safety became routine. Employees in the 1950s dealt with crises regularly, but employees in the 1970s never experienced a major disaster. To all appearances, the test site perfected underground testing; following basic requirements guaranteed a successful test.

Under these circumstances, the test site prepared for Operation Emery in 1970. As with other series, rad-safe limited workers to 3 rem per quarter, with a maximum of 5 rem a year. Livermore planned a number of tests, including the Baneberry shot. Geologist Richard D. McArthur selected the southwest corner of Area 8 for a shaft hole named U8d, predicting that the location was 2,200 feet northwest of the nearest fault line, first discovered during the Discus Thrower event in 1966.[81]

In October 1970 REECo began drilling under the engineering supervision of Fenix and Scisson Inc. On November 14 it finished an eighty-six-inch diameter hole that stretched 980 feet underground and began an extensive cementing program. Even from the beginning, problems surfaced. During excavation, workers used large quantities of water to remove displaced dirt and rock, and to clean its equipment, and drilled U8d on top of a fault line.[82] The water eroded the hole, causing fissures in the cement walls and depositing one hundred feet of saturated clay. Due to the water use and other issues, U8d's construction cost reached $586,564, five times its original budget.[83]

When REECo completed the shaft, Livermore scheduled the Baneberry shot for Friday, December 18. The NTS bustled with activity during the week prior, conducting three tests. During each other test, safety procedures mandated the evacuation of Area 12. However, Baneberry proceeded differently. Since the previous tests had run smoothly, rad-safe decided not to evacuate approximately nine hundred employees in the camp, situated only five miles from the detonation point. On the early morning of December 18, workers began reporting for duty in the tunnels or awaiting permission to enter their work sites. At the same time, Wackenhut security guards and rad-safe monitors manned stations seven miles from the test. Even though it was Livermore's test, its most experienced scientists were not there, and instead were supervising it remotely. Like previous tests, rad-safe positioned monitors and television cameras, and scheduled a helicopter to shoot aerial photographs and aircrafts for cloud sampling. Rad-safe also positioned remote camera stations at the trailer park sixty feet from ground zero. The Baneberry test detonated at 7:30 A.M. Wackenhut security guard Harley Roberts had just arrived for his shift, relieving Jack Cupples from the night shift. Both men felt the vibrations of Baneberry, and watched as a black cloud of dust swirled from the desert floor. At the same time, John Campbell was carpooling to work. At only five miles from ground zero, he looked up "just in time" to see Baneberry, describing it as "the desert floor just kind of bubbled up and then pshooo…things [were] flying through the air and it just kept going."[84]

The chaos began three minutes after the shot. Excess water created a clay formation in the shaft, and the device blasted through it and triggered the fault line. The detonation shifted the earth, spewing molten rock and ash through a 315-foot fissure. Radioactive gas burst eight thousand feet in the air and continued venting over the next twenty-four hours. Based on weather forecasts, rad-safe determined that radioactive fallout would occur in the south and southeast to Area 3, and the north and northeast to Area 51. But the wind unexpectedly shifted after the test, carrying low-level radiation from the base of the cloud toward Area 12. At 8:05 A.M., rad-safe determined that Area 12 fell dangerously within the fallout zone, and the test manager frantically issued evacuation orders.[85]

As security guards, Roberts and Cupples were instructed to evacuate Area 12. When they arrived, it was encased in a dark gray fog. Cupples walked into the first row of trailers, saw himself in the mirror, and did a double take. "My entire face was white," he recalled, and "[my] lips were all clogged up." With minimal rad-safe training, the guards entered the area without protective suits or masks. Although he had worked at the NTS for fifteen years, Cupples had never seen such a sight. His first instinct was, "My God…I'm breathing this stuff." He grabbed a towel and told everyone to "put something over their faces." The evacuation took about an hour. Roberts was then instructed to report to the Area 20 guard station. When he stopped by Area 17, a rad-safe monitor told him that he was "hot as hell" and to "get out of here." Despite the warning, Roberts followed his orders, continuing to Area 20. While driving a radioactive truck and wearing contaminated clothing, Roberts received exposures of 2 rads an hour. He continued working for another nine hours. At 5:00 P.M., a rad-safe monitor insisted on relieving him, reporting he had received 200 milli-roentgen an hour, 30 inches from his chest. He ordered Roberts to decontaminate.[86]

Meanwhile, Cupples and the other evacuees went to CP-2, a rad-safe building located at the control point. The condition of the facility symbolizes the neglected edges of the NTS's occupational health regime. Idle since atmospheric testing, health and safety had become routine, not a necessity. The hot water heater was broken, forcing the workers to take ice cold decontamination showers for thirty minutes to remove the radioactivity. After that, they were transported to the PHS's Radiological Health Building in Las Vegas for whole-body radiation and thyroid counts. Roberts arrived at CP-2 nine hours after exposure. After his frigid shower, rad-safe gave him a pair of gloves to cover his hands, which read 25 milli-roentgen. Roberts received the highest dose of whole-body radiation out of all the workers. Dr. Shields Warren calculated the number was at least 15 rads. He also never got whole-body or thyroid counts at the Radiological Health Building. In fact, the AEC did not treat him until he checked into Oak Ridge Hospital on August 16, 1973 after the onset of his preleukemia.[87]

Following the incident, the AEC immediately went on the defense. It issued a public statement claiming that no employees were affected by radiation sickness. This was a half-truth: while there were no cases of ARS, numerous workers received low-level radiation exposure. Out of nine hundred personnel in Area 12 and assisting in the evacuation, rad-safe detected eighty-six contaminations. Analytical Radiological Laboratory technician Robert Friedrichs participated in the monitoring and decontamination process, and called the experience a "key memory" of his career. "It was a once-in-a-lifetime event," he said. "We wanted to make darn sure that we got them decontaminated [and]... we got accurate information on the level of their exposure." Out of

475 vehicles, 413 were marked contaminated, and rad-safe impounded 33. Since the event was close to the holidays, technicians also confiscated Christmas presents stored in cars, and radioactive clothing from 106 workers, eighty-six of whom required showers. After monitoring, sixty-eight received additional decontamination and direct measurement of their thyroid radioactivity. Of those, rad-safe transferred eighteen to the Radiological Health Building for whole-body counts. The Southwestern Radiological Laboratory also studied off-site fallout under the auspices of the Environmental Protection Agency (EPA). An evaluation of external gamma radiation revealed higher-than-normal radiostrontium, plutonium, and tritium levels in snow samples, air filters, and milk. However, the highest estimated doses were well within permissible dose standards. Rad-safe considered conditions so safe that AEC chairman Glen Seaborg canceled additional field studies and protective actions, citing that the accident did not pose any threat to human health.[88]

Still, rad-safe continued to monitor the workers, evaluating their film badges, thyroid and whole-body counts, and urine samples. Technicians determined that no person received external or internal doses over the permissible dose: 3 rem per quarter and 5 rem per year limit. Moreover, their thyroid counts did not surpass 10 rem per quarter and 30 rem per year. According to AEC records, prompt action diverted a major crisis. But others saw it differently, including Dr. Shields Warren. After evaluating rad-safe's monitoring and radiation procedures, he affirmed, "I'm sorry to say, I would have to call it bad, judging by [Harley Robert's] detailed counts." Rad-safe monitors confronted numerous problems while conducting the evacuation. Warren noticed that their measuring devices and uniforms were not "where they were supposed to be." Additionally, "evacuation was not ordered adequately soon" and the monitors did "not agree with each other [about] readings." A veteran in radiology, Warren knew the difficulties of managing a crisis. But had he been in charge, the doctor "would have raised hell with whoever was responsible for this."[89]

After Baneberry, all testing ceased and the AEC closed Area 12. The botched shot exposed faulty procedures that developed during the underground testing program. After the atmospheric ban, the AEC allowed contractors to ease health and safety protocol, allowing the positioning of repair shops, field warehouses, and camp sites like Area 12 to be in close proximity to tests. During atmospheric testing, support facilities were strictly prohibited in forward areas, but underground testing supposedly improved the risk. Positioning workers close to testing was also beneficial to the AEC from a financial standpoint, saving time and money. Baneberry forced a reevaluation of all these policies. The rhetoric of occupational health also gained momentum on the national scale, culminating in the passage of the Occupational Safety and Health (OSH) Act on December 29, 1970 and the creation of OSHA and the National Institute of Occupational Safety and Health (NIOSH) the following year. For the first time, American employers were legally responsible for providing healthy and safe workplaces for employees. Since the OSH Act did not cover atomic energy workers, it will be discussed at greater length in the following chapter. However, the concept of employer accountability, coupled with the Baneberry disaster, certainly resonated at the test site, helping force the health and safety issue.

Prior to Baneberry, occupational health at the test site was a means to an end. While the AEC, laboratories, and contractors felt an obligation to protect workers and the public, their main goal was for the test site to function efficiently, to keep negative public opinion at bay, and to adhere to the Limited Test Ban Treaty. After Baneberry and the OSH Act, their responsibilities evolved, incorporating modern notions of employer moral and legal accountability. When testing resumed in June 1971, the test manager completely revised its procedures, mandating the evacuation of all areas north of the control point during shots. The AEC also founded the Containment Evaluation Panel, a team of experts that reviewed plans prior to approving the event. Robert Friedrichs described it as a "far more sophisticated level of review" than its predecessors. After determining the device yield, the panel chose a location that ensured the best overburden for containment. Overburden was the quantity of soil above ground zero, usually between seven hundred and one thousand feet.[90]

The panel then created a summary of worst case scenarios and determined its probability of containment. Baneberry transformed health and safety at the NTS, finally putting employee lives first. According to Friedrichs, a new motto emerged: "Economy of operations is subject to overriding consideration of safety." Afterward, the test site "never had a real serious leak again." Still, Baneberry left workers in disbelief. Friedrichs called it "a shocking way to find out that things were not as straightforward as people thought." But the revised standards worked; most underground tests were contained from then on. From 1961 to 1970, 122 nuclear tests vented radioactivity. After 1971, only three did not fully contain.[91]

As health and safety improved at the test site, the notion of responsibility began playing out in the public sphere. Baneberry sparked renewed interest in past rad-safe protocol, attracting intense criticism. Barton Hacker termed three general waves of testing concerns in the United States, all of which were important components of the occupational health regime. The first began in the late 1950s centering around radioactive fallout, but faded after the Limited Test Ban Treaty in 1963. Modern environmentalism developed at the same time, partly inspired by the publishing of Rachel Carson's *Silent Spring* in 1962, revealing the connection between the workplace, the community, and the environment. The American Medical Association (AMA) moved occupational health beyond the workplace as well, changing the name of its publication *Archives of Industrial Hygiene and Occupational Medicine* to *Archives of Environmental Health* to broaden readership. As shown by Allison Helper, once occupational health became connected to environmentalism, industry had two responses. Some employers developed a broad view, arguing that the positives of benefiting society outweighed the negatives of harming the environment. Others emphasized the only way to identify workplace hazards was laboratories rather than the court system. Consumers took another approach, which came to define the 1960s. Linking together the public sphere, big business, and employees, activism surged on behalf of environmental issues.[92]

But while underground testing temporarily silenced the testing debate, scientists continued to research the long-term effects of low-level radiation. Nuclear power expanded in the late 1960s, prompting a second wave of controversy over low-level radiation and radioiodine hazards. However, mainstream science still generally agreed that low-level effects posed limited health risks. The 1972 BEIR and UNSCEAR reports also endorsed this view.[93]

Meanwhile, the AEC split in 1975 to address a long-standing complaint about the agency, dividing regulation and safety from development and promotion. The Nuclear Regulatory Commission (NRC) focused on the former, while the Energy Research and Development Administration (ERDA) addressed the latter. Three years later, ERDA became the DOE.[94]

The third wave of controversy began in the mid-1970s. The scientific community did not collectively agree with the 1972 BEIR and UNSCEAR reports, prompting the issue of low-level effects to resurface, and inspiring scientific and historical studies on atmospheric testing from 1945 to 1962.[95]

By the mid-1970s, Drs. Samuel Milham, Thomas Mancuso, and Alice Stewart and statistician George Kneale began investigating the long-term health of workers at the Hanford facility. While working for the Washington State PHS, Milham produced the first study, arguing that excessive cancer fatalities occurred among the workforce because of repeated exposure to low-level radiation. When the AEC learned of his findings, it requested Mancuso, an epidemiologist and professor in the Department of Occupational Health at the University of Pittsburgh, to publicly refute them. Mancuso declined, and the AEC terminated his contract. The AEC had contracted with Mancuso since the mid-1960s to study low-level radiation effects on the nation's five hundred thousand atomic energy workers. Mancuso ultimately drew similar conclusions to Milham: Hanford workers receiving continued low-level exposures exhibited a 6 percent greater chance of developing cancer than the general public. In December 1977 Mancuso and his colleagues, Stewart and Kneale, published their findings in the journal *Health Physics*.[96]

The Mancuso study stunned the scientific community, but failed to arouse significant public concern. In 1975 the Veterans Hospital in Salt Lake City admitted Paul Cooper, a retired Army sergeant with acute myelogenous leukemia. Cooper had participated in the Exercise Desert Rock VII and VIII during Operation Plumbbob. After witnessing Galileo, he and 2,231 other soldiers completed the contaminated

Smoky exercise. The causal relationship between low-level radiation and cancer attracted the attention epidemiologist Dr. Thomas Cosgriff. Since leukemia was associated with radiation exposure, Cosgriff contacted Dr. Glyn Caldwell, chief of the Cancer and Birth Defects Division of Epidemiology at the CDC, to investigate a link. In May 1977 Caldwell identified three cases of leukemia among Smoky veterans, a higher rate than expected for a comparable group. When the Veterans Administration denied Cooper's claim that leukemia was a service-connected disability, he brought his story to the media. The media attention finally informed the public about the dangers of nuclear testing employment, and led to the publishing of numerous documents that vilified the AEC, charging that it willingly exposed workers to radiation levels detrimental to their health. It also prompted the CDC to conduct a detailed study on the fate of Plumbbob participants.[97]

Caldwell determined their various health statuses and risk of developing leukemia or other radiation-linked diseases. In 1980 he completed the study, reporting that participants contracted leukemia at a higher rate than expected. The cases, however, did not correlate with dosages or assigned units. Out of ten cases, only three participated in Smoky; the rest were involved in Exercise Desert Rock VII and VIII. An eleventh worked at the test site during Plumbbob. Caldwell also identified a higher-than-average incidence of a rare bone cancer among the participants. In the end, the findings were inconclusive, but scientists continued to dispute the dangers of low-level radiation. Moreover, the indecision did not end low-level radiation fears. The slightest possibility that it caused cancer was enough for workers to begin fighting for compensation.[98]

Since the Veterans Administration denied most radiation-related disability claims, atomic veterans first sought compensation in the courts. But they never won. In 1946 Congress passed the Federal Tort Claims Act, permitting lawsuits against the federal government. In 1950 the Supreme Court added the Feres Doctrine, or doctrine of sovereign immunity, granting the government immunity from injuries that members of the armed forces sustained while on active duty. Under these conditions, atomic veteran Stanley Jaffee sued for damages in 1979. In 1953 Jaffee participated in Desert Rock V during Operation

Upshot–Knothole; he developed terminal cancer decades later. *Jaffee v. the United States* was the first case that applied the Feres doctrine to veterans alleging radiation-connected injuries.[99]

The doctrine prevailed throughout the 1980s and was further solidified by the Warner amendment in 1985, disqualifying all suits against AEC contractors. It also barred civilians from alleging contractor negligence. In comparison to atomic veterans, civilians fared only slightly better; however, most lost due to a loophole in the Federal Tort Claims Act, which granted the government immunity from lawsuits regarding policy decisions. The federal courts continued to define nuclear testing as a policy decision. Ranchers in Iron County began suing the government in 1955, claiming that fallout from the Harry shot in 1953 killed forty-five hundred sheep. Although the ranchers lost *Bulloch v. the United States,* government investigators reopened it in 1980, eventually reversing the decision after uncovering massive fraud on the part of the AEC. Still, courts regularly rejected government liability for testing-related damages.[100]

The first civilian case alleging radiation-related injuries involved the Baneberry shot. Prior to the accident, Harley Roberts was a healthy fifty-year-old man. A test site employee since 1966, REECo doctors recorded in his physical examinations that he had an average health record based on his age and normal blood counts. But after Baneberry, Roberts felt exhausted. As his conditions worsened, he began suffering from frequent nosebleeds and skin bruising. In June 1972 a doctor at Loma Linda Hospital in California diagnosed him with blood abnormalities, with forty-five chromosomes instead of forty-six, lacking the C group chromosome. The treatment was unsuccessful, leading his doctors to transfer him to Oak Ridge Hospital in August 1973. At Oak Ridge doctors diagnosed him with pancytopenia, or too few blood cells, and indicated he was possibly in a preleukemic state. Still, they discharged him a month later. Over the following months, his health worsened. Shortly before his death on April 17, 1974, he was diagnosed with myeloblastic leukemia, cancer of the blood. The immediate cause of death was progressive interstitial pneumonia due to a fungal infection. The primary cause was leukemia. Over the next year, William Reed and William Nunamaker, REECo workers on site during

Baneberry, also died from leukemia. The three deaths exceeded the national leukemia mortality rate by twenty times.[101]

On their deathbeds, Roberts and Nunamaker insisted that low-level radiation emissions from Baneberry had caused their leukemia. Their widows, Dorothy Roberts and Louise Nunamaker, decided to fight for compensation. Represented by Alan and Larry Johns, they filed a $1.1 million wrongful death suit against the federal government.[102] The Johns brothers had represented Dorothy Roberts since 1974, along with twelve Wackenhut guards that swept Area 12 after Baneberry. But at first, low-level radiation was not central to the case. It charged REECo, ERDA, and Livermore with negligence and the suppression of information, and requested deleted information from the summary report, including the device yield, nearby fault line, worker medical records, and geological reports on the emplacement hole. The federal government's counsel responded that the information was classified in the interest of public defense. In 1976 Dorothy Roberts and Louise Nunamaker followed suit, charging gross incompetence in planning the event and willfully disregarding the safety of both workers. Their case focused on four categories: site selection, drilling and related activities, evacuation procedures and radiation protection, and decontamination. It also addressed the longstanding medical dispute on low-level radiation for the first time in the court of law, arguing that even small doses can stimulate biological damage in cell structures.[103]

The case rested on one question: Could low-level radiation cause leukemia? The Johns brothers enlisted several expert witnesses, including Dr. Shields Warren, radiation expert and former director of the DBM. His testimony provides an excellent example of how many medical professionals shifted their opinion of low-level effects, and employer and government responsibility during the 1970s. Drawing on thirty years of research, Warren derived a new conclusion. In contrast to his days working for the AEC, he cited that small amounts of radiation could have caused their leukemia. According to Warren, it was "highly probable" that a "smaller dose of radiation was adequate to induce leukemia" under special circumstances. Moreover, he questioned the validity of REECo's radiation records, which calculated that Roberts and Nunamaker received an exposure of only .4 rem and .1 rem. While rad-safe took seven separate readings, each varied considerably. The figures ranged from 200 milliradian per hour to 50 milliradian per hour, exhibiting a time-decay pattern. A reading at 4:00 P.M. recorded 1 rad per hour. Based on the latter figure, Warren determined that Area 12 camp received 11 rads per hour of fallout, and Roberts received a cumulative dose of 15 rads. The testimony provided the basis of the plaintiffs' argument; low-level radiation could have caused Roberts's leukemia because 1 rem and above could "produce a chromosomal change."[104]

Dr. John Gofman, medical doctor, professor emeritus of molecular and cell biology at the University of California, Berkeley, and a former associate director of Livermore Laboratory, reiterated Warren's conclusions. He supported the Linear No-Threshold (LNT) Model: radiation was always harmful and no permissible dose existed. In fact, the sum of small exposures could have the same effect as one large one. Gofman agreed with Warren that rad-safe took flawed readings. He found that the external dose was "100 times higher to the bone marrow" than the calculated amount.[105] Alice Stewart provided similar testimony. A coauthor of the Mancuso study, she added statistical calculations on the population involved in Baneberry. In 1978 Stewart conducted a follow-up study on the eighty-six workers requiring decontamination, observing the number of deaths. She determined that two deaths among eighty-six "in this rare form of disease [acute myeloid leukemia was] almost unheard of." Statistically, there should have been one. According to Stewart, the only possible reason for the statistical abnormality was radiation exposure. Roberts and Nunamaker were also more susceptible to the disease because of their advanced ages. Based on her research in Japan, she declared that it was common among Hiroshima and Nagasaki survivors to develop leukemia four years later.[106]

The testimonies concerned ERDA and the impact it might have on the testing program. Roberts's exposure was less than the permissible dose, calling into question the entire radiation safety program and putting exposure guides in doubt. Out-of-court or lost-in-court settlement was not an option. A settlement would disrupt operations, and significantly increase the cost of medical screenings and rad-safe procedures. It would also create a precedent for damage claims, raise public fears, and hurt public and press approval of operations. ERDA decided to fight the charges. To provide a counterargument, it enlisted health physicists and physicians to argue against a link between low-level radiation and myelocytic leukemia, and that the workers were within the maximum permissible dose. Roberts received less than 5 rads to his thyroid, not nearly enough to induce leukemia. Moreover, the diseases occurred too soon after Baneberry and therefore were co-incidental to the exposure, and not the cause.[107]

In January 1979 a three-month trial began. It was a nonjury case, with Judge Roger Foley presiding in the Federal District Court of Las Vegas. In June 1982 he rendered a partial decision. Foley found the AEC and contractors negligent in evacuation and decontamination procedures, and noted especially that they had failed to fully decontaminate the workers. However, he determined management did apply appropriate safety protocol in site selection, drilling activities, meteorological studies, and made the right decision to not evacuate Area 12 camp prior to the test because of its proximity to U8d. But Foley did not decide the issue of low-level radiation until seven months later. Based on the testimonies, he determined that the workers' maximum doses were .42 rem and .08 rem. At those doses, Foley believed that radiation exposure from the Baneberry accident did not cause their deaths. Moreover, he determined that that latency period following exposure was too short, calling Warren, Gofman, and Stewart's theories of causation "experimental, speculative, and lacking in credible empirical support" that had "little, if any, weight." Basing his opinion on "a reasonable degree of medical certainty," Foley ruled there was "no credible proof" that low-level radiation caused leukemia or chromosome abnormalities in Harley Roberts and William Nunamaker.[108]

The widows proved negligence but not causation. Still, they continued to fight. In May 1984 they filed a motion requesting a new trial or reopening the old one to introduce additional evidence. Foley denied the motion. In the late 1980s the widows decided to take their case to the Ninth Circuit of Appeals in San Francisco, arguing that the Federal

District Court in Las Vegas lacked jurisdiction. On October 27, 1989, Foley determined that his court indeed had jurisdiction under the Federal Tort Claims Act and reaffirmed his 1983 ruling.[109]

Although the widows lost their case, the new evidence helped another one. On the same day, Foley was set to decide *Prescott v. United States,* a consolidated radiation-related injury claim of 240 NTS workers. The government had sought a pretrial motion to drop the claim based on immunity in the Federal Tort Claims Act. Foley denied the motion because of two developments. First, Alan and Larry Johns revealed that the federal government and the NIC had contracted a secret agreement in 1956, allowing the AEC to replace the NIC in worker's compensation claims for radiation-related injuries. It also authorized REECo to bypass providing workmen's compensation insurance for such injuries, effectively barring workers from any benefits if they claimed to have radiation-related disabilities. Therefore, the only forum to seek damages was in the courts. Foley ruled the agreement illegal and void. The second development was a recent Supreme Court opinion. In 1988 it negated the clause in the Federal Tort Claims Act that protected nuclear testing as a policy decision, ruling that federal officials and contractors were not protected from negligence while carrying out the government programs. In *Prescott,* Foley determined that the government could be "held liable for breaching its duties to warn, train, and monitor, and provide medical treatment [at the NTS]." He recommended that a jury decide if the AEC failed to provide "objective standards of care for the protection of health and safety of human beings." The Ninth Circuit confirmed Foley's verdict in 1992, remanding the case for trial.[110]

Despite setbacks in the courts, government responsibility for radiation-related injuries emerged under the direction of Congress. After Dr. Glyn Caldwell's investigation, Congress began hearings on the Health Effects of Ionizing Radiation in 1978. The hearings inspired the formation of multiple advocacy organizations that demanded accountability and compensation from the federal government. Founded by Army sergeant Orville E. Kelly, the National Association of Atomic Veterans provided assistance to soldiers seeking damages for health abnormalities and genetic mutations. Benny Levy also established the

NTS Radiation Victims Association to support civilian workers. Both organizations had a difficult job, because the effects of low-level radiation continued to be contested throughout the 1980s. But Congress readily compensated high-level cases, providing ex gratia payments, or voluntary compensation admitting moral obligation but not legal responsibility. In 1964 it appropriated nearly $1 million to Japanese and Marshallese victims of the 1954 Bravo test during Operation Castle in the PPG. Since 1977 Congress also compensated thyroid cancer victims with $25,000 and provided up to $100,000 in death benefits. But the notion of responsibility to the test site's atomic veterans and civilian employees took longer to develop. In 1981 Congress approved the Veterans' Health Care, Training, and Small Business Loan Act, entitling veterans to medical care for service-related injuries. In 1984 it also passed the Veterans' Dioxin and Radiation Exposure Compensation Standards Act, outlining how to connect low-level radiation to military service. In practice, the act was ineffective because the doses were frequently too small to render compensation. In 1988 Congress eliminated the burden of proof. The Radiation-Exposed Veterans Compensation Act automatically awarded eligibility of thirteen types of cancer manifested within thirty to forty years after radiation-related service.[111]

Civilian employees benefited from congressional action as well, but the process took longer. In 2000 Congress outlined the struggles facing test site employees to receive workers' compensation. The standard policies of the DOE were to litigate occupational illness claims, a process that placed incredible financial burdens on injured workers and deterred most from filing claims. The DOE also encouraged and assisted contractors to oppose claims, essentially putting the private sector above the law. Moreover, nuclear testing involved unique hazards. Most third-party insurance carriers and state compensation programs did not have a uniform method to compensate aliments associated with the work. The Energy Employees Occupational Illness Compensation Program Act finally eliminated the burden of proof, linking illness to the job. It provided compensation and medical benefits to civilian employees who worked in nuclear testing and production over the past fifty years, and suffered from beryllium-related or radiation-related health conditions. On December 7, 2000, President Bill Clinton signed Executive Order 13179, which acknowledged that "too often these workers [in nuclear testing and production] were neither adequately protected from, nor informed of, occupational hazards to which they were exposed.... While the Nation can never fully repay these workers or their families, they deserve recognition and compensation for their sacrifices."[112] After a long process, test site workers received not only compensation but also the government accountability they deserved.

The growing recognition of the dangers of low-level radiation and chemical exposures during the 1970s marked a significant shift in American occupational health history. Deliberating workplace threats in various public forums convinced the public to place greater value in protecting its workers, communities, and environment. By the early 1980s, accidents were no longer considered a part of work, and employers and the government developed the moral and legal responsibility to protect not only workers, but also their surroundings. It also became commonsense that employees not only had the right to know about potential hazards at work but also could improve their conditions.[113]

Speaking in front of an OSHA fact-finding hearing in Washington, DC, on February 15, 1974, Dr. Thomas Mancuso outlined a dominant theme in occupational health history to Americans: "Invariably, whenever a new occupational cancer is discovered, it is played down for fear of alarming the workers and the general public.... In the first place, the worker doesn't even recognize an occupational disease when he sees one. In the second place, the general practitioner doesn't even recognize it. Consequently, it doesn't come to a compensation claim." Mancuso argued that OSHA and industry needed to change this historical pattern, acting to protect workers before the hazard materialized. With the institution of OSHA, it was now the federal agency's responsibility to "ensure that no harmful effects do occur as a result of exposures to various chemicals and the work processes involved."[114]

Although it refers to the regulation of vinyl chloride in the chemical industry, Mancusco's statement poses interesting questions when considering the history of occupational health at the NTS. What if an employer knew the risk and still exposed its employees? What if the employer was the federal government? In the case of the NTS, the size of the risk was an important consideration in developing health and safety policy, providing another example of gambling with lives in occupational health history.

When Congress established the Energy Employees Occupational Illness Compensation Program Act, it acknowledged that the American nuclear program had been recognized under federal law as extremely hazardous since World War II. Likewise, by the time the AEC founded the test site, the threat of radiation was very well documented. Hiroshima and Nagasaki demonstrated the immediate and long-term dangers, as with testing in New Mexico and the Pacific, and human experimentation determined the effects of radiation and radioactive contamination on the body. Most prior research was performed, funded, or supervised by the federal government. Still, the AEC authorized the contamination of civilian employees and atomic veterans, the surrounding community, and the environment with radioactive materials based on the scientific boundaries of the permissible dose.

While it can be somewhat understandable if employers exposed workers to untested chemicals later revealed to pose health risks, it is not fathomable that an employer approved known, harmful processes. It is even more alarming that a government body approved and promoted the practice. Yet this is a repeated scenario in occupational health history. Most scholarship is critical of AEC policies, especially with regards to health and safety. This criticism is merited. While occupational health guidelines protected from high-level radiation, it allowed repeated, low-level contact. The AEC, DOD, laboratories, and contractors knew the danger. As shown by historian Leisl Carr Childers, land use in the entire Great Basin region was based on "the size of the risk," an unfortunate decision that harmed the environment and people who lived there.[115]

When the NTS was founded, most scientists recognized that prolonged, small doses of radiation increased the possibility of dying from cancer and nonmalignant diseases. Studies also established a correlation between excess diseases and exposure to radiation. The AEC, DOD, laboratories, and contractors ignored the risk. If low-level radiation caused cancer in only a small portion of workers and the surrounding population, it was a chance they were willing to take.

Ninety-eight percent of radiation-induced cancers among the NTS's civilian employees and atomic veterans occurred at levels below the permissible dose. Scientific evidence also connected inhaling beryllium, a metal in nuclear weapons production, as dust particles, fumes, or vapor to developing incurable sensitivities that progressed into chronic beryllium disease (CBD). While the AEC, DOD, laboratories, and contractors established a health and safety program with capable medical, rad-safe, and industrial hygiene and safety personnel, it failed to completely protect the health of its workers. The program was advanced for the time, but was based on an uncertain safety threshold, and the employers involved lacked the moral and legal obligation to comprehend their own actions. An important lesson from the history of occupational health at the NTS is that it is virtually impossible for an industry to self-regulate. There needs to be a system of checks and balances. Until the 1970s, nuclear activities in the United States completely self-regulated with regard to health and safety. No other hazardous federal program has exercised such broad powers of self-regulation in American history. In doing so, the United States government put its citizens at risk without the proper education or consent, and contaminated thousands of sites with radioactive and toxic materials harmful to human and ecological health.[116] While the Comprehensive Nuclear-Test-Ban Treaty instituted a global ban on nuclear testing in 1996, the damaging effects of NTS operations will always remain, serving as a tragic chapter in America's occupational health history.

## NOTES

1. Barth, George, and Hill, *Environmental Health and Safety*, 4.

2. Markowitz and Rosner, *Deceit and Denial*, 156–57.

3. The petrochemical industry also accumulated nitrates, phosphates, toxic residues, smog, carcinogenic exhaust, and plastic waste in the workplace and environment. In later years, globalized production and the electronics revolution presented additional health and safety concerns. See Barth, George, and Hill, *Environmental Health and Safety*, 4.

4. For more on the Joint Commission for the Investigation of the Effects of the Atomic Bomb in Japan, see Ashley W. Oughterson and Shields Warren, *Medical Effects of the Atomic Bomb in Japan* (New York: McGraw-Hill, 1956); Barton C. Hacker, *The*

*Dragon's Tail: Radiation Safety in the Manhattan Project, 1942-1946* (Berkeley: University of California Press, 1987), 109-16; M. Susan Lindee, *Suffering Made Real: American Science and the Survivors at Hiroshima* (Chicago: University of Chicago Press, 1994), 17-38. Shields Warren and Stafford Warren were not related, but were often mistaken for one another. Stafford Warren was the chairman of the radiology department at the University of Rochester School of Medicine and Dentistry, and worked as a consultant to the Manhattan Engineering District.

5. Oughterson and Warren, *Medical Effects* (incl. "unprecedented problems," xi); Shields Warren and R. H. Draeger, "Patterns of Injuries Produced by the Atomic Bombs at Hiroshima and Nagasaki," *US Naval Medical Bulletin* (Sept. 1946) (incl. "diverse and confusing," 1350); Shields Warren, "The Pathologic Effects of an Instantaneous Dose of Radiation," *Cancer Research* 6 (1946): 449-53; Eileen Welsome, *The Plutonium Files: America's Secret Experiments in the Cold War* (New York: Dial Press, 1999), 115.

6. *Hibakusha* is the Japanese word that translates to "explosion-affected people" of Hiroshima and Nagasaki. See Warren, "Hiroshima and Nagasaki Thirty Years After," *Proceedings of the American Philosophical Society* 121, no. 2 (Apr. 29, 1977), 97; Paul Boyer, *Fallout: A Historian Reflects on America's Half Century Encounter with Nuclear Weapons* (Columbus: Ohio State University Press, 1998) (incl. "necessary to follow," 63); Lindee, *Suffering Made Real*, 32-34.

7. Warren, "Hiroshima and Nagasaki" (incl. "People were," "only minimal," and "10 rads or less," 98); Welsome, *Plutonium Files*, 197.

8. Boyer, *Fallout*, 69.

9. David J. Rothman, *Strangers at the Bedside: A History on How Law and Bioethics Transformed Medical Decision Making* (New York: Basic Books, 1991) (incl. "the Gilded Age," 51). The Human Radiation Experiments began during the Manhattan Project to determine the effects of radiation on the human body. The purpose was to develop a diagnostic tool to reveal how the human body reacted to plutonium and uranium. Officials believed the experiments were essential to protecting radiation workers; the idea was to figure out the point at which doses reached an unsafe level. The experiments continued until the 1960s, with researchers exposing children, pregnant women, inmates, mentally and terminally ill persons, and impoverished persons with radioactive iodine, calcium, and other radioisotopes. See William Moss and Roger Eckhardt, "The Human Plutonium Injection Experiments," *Los Alamos Science* 23 (1995); Jonathan D. Moreno, *Undue Risk: Secret State Experiments on Humans* (New York: Routledge, 2001), for a complete description of the experiments. See also Welsome, *Plutonium Files*, 264, 323-24.

10. Stewart L. Udall, *The Myths of August: A Personal Exploration of Our Tragic Cold War Affair with the Atom* (New York: Pantheon Books, 1994), 222-24.

11. Ibid. (incl. "we cannot risk," 224). For the most comprehensive scholarship on the controversies surrounding nuclear testing, see Barton C. Hacker, *Elements of Controversy: The Atomic Energy Commission and Radiation Safety in Nuclear Weapons Testing, 1947-1974* (Berkeley: University of California Press, 1994).

12. Welsome, *Plutonium Files* (incl. "distinct or worldwide," 260).

13. Hacker, *Elements of Controversy*, 276; Hacker, "Radiation Safety, the AEC, and Nuclear Testing," *Public Historian* 14, no. 1 (Winter 1992), 43; Welsome, *Plutonium Files*, 199, 260; Joseph J. Mangano, *Low-Level Radiation and Immune System Damage: An Atomic Era Legacy* (New York: Lewis, 1999), 4; John May, "How the United States

Turned the Bomb on Its Own People," *Sunday Age* (Melbourne, Australia), May 23, 1993 (incl. "The greatest irony").

14.  See Alice L. Buck, *A History of the Atomic Energy Commission* (Washington, DC: DOE, July 1983), 1, NV0410896, Atomic Testing Museum, Las Vegas (hereafter ATM). During World War II the MED spent more than $2.2 billion on production facilities, communities, and research laboratories in Oakridge, Hanford, and Los Alamos to build an atomic bomb. MED functioned like a large corporation, relying on public/ private partnerships. Oakridge and Hanford produced uranium and plutonium, the materials needed to build an atomic bomb. Private contractors built both the facilities and reactors in consultation with physicists at the University of California, Berkeley (Oak Ridge) and the University of Chicago (Hanford). Directed by physicist J. Robert Oppenheimer and in association with the University of California, Berkeley, the Los Alamos Scientific Laboratory (LASL) created the bomb design and diagnostic experiments. The site also hosted a proving ground, the Alamogordo Bombing Range. It exploded the first plutonium-based atomic weapon, codenamed Trinity. See G. B. Kistiakowsky to J. R. Oppenheimer, Oct. 12, 1944, NV0004059, ATM; Hacker, *Dragon's Tail*; "Project Trinity Fact Sheet," Defense Nuclear Agency (Washington, DC: Public Affairs Office, Dec. 15, 1982), NV0760126, ATM.

15.  Carroll L. Tyler to Dr. J. C. Bugher, memorandum, Aug. 20, 1953, NV0404908; Project Nutmeg, NV0411323; Review of Project Nutmeg, NV0404131 (incl. "more sound"); all at ATM. See also Sumner T. Pike to LeBaron, "Location of Proving Ground for Atomic Weapons," Mar. 8, 1949, as quoted in Hacker, *Elements of Controversy*, 40.

16.  See Hacker, *Elements of Controversy*, 36–49; Terrence R. Fehner and F. G. Gosling, *Origins of the Nevada Test Site*, History Division, Executive Secretariat, Management and Administration (Washington, DC: Department of Energy, Dec. 2000), 37–78, DOE-MA-0518, ATM, for a detailed discussion of establishing the test site in Nevada. See also J. P. Harahan and R. J. Bennett, *Creating the Defense Threat Reduction Agency* (Washington, DC: U.S. DOD, 2002).

17.  Mary Palevsky, "Establishing a Cold War Continental Test Site in Nevada," *Online Nevada Encyclopedia*, www.onlinenevada.org/; Hacker, *Elements of Controversy*, 41–42; Frederick Reines, "Discussion of Radiological Hazards with a Continental Test Site for Atomic Bombs, Based on Meeting Held at Los Alamos, Aug. 1, 1950," LAMS– 1173, Sept. 1, 1950, 5, 11–13, 21, 23–24; Fehner and Gosling, *Origins*, 43-46 (incl. "perhaps a little," 46).

18.  A roentgen is a unit of measurement to measure exposure to ionizing radiation. It was adopted in 1928, and was named after German physicist Wilhelm Roentgen.

19.  Fehner and Gosling, *Origins*, 50; Palevsky, "Establishing a Cold War"; Project Ranger Fact Sheet, Feb. 26, 1982, NV0760122, ATM.

20.  Atomic physicists referred to low-yield atomic bursts as "tickling the dragon's tail" rather than provoking a full-scale nuclear explosion. See "Nevada Atom Test Rocks Four States," *LA Times*, Jan. 28, 1951.

21.  The test site was first titled the Nevada Proving Grounds, but was changed to the Nevada Test Site (NTS) soon after. In August 2010 it was renamed the Nevada National Security Site to reflect its current goal of training troops rather than testing nuclear weapons. For continuity purposes, this chapter will refer to the site as the NTS. See Keith Rogers, "It's Official: Test Site Gets New Name," *Review-Journal*, Aug. 24, 2010. See also DOE, *United States Nuclear Tests, July 1945 through Sept. 1992*

(Washington, DC: DOE, Nevada Operations Office, Dec. 2000), xviii, DOE/NV-206-REV15, ATM.

22. AEC Employee Brochure, Howard W. Cannon Papers (hereafter HWC), 90th Cong., Box 16, Folder 260, UNLV SC (incl. all quotes). Los Alamos grew to fill the needs of the nuclear economy after 1945. The Z Division, which manufactured atomic weapons designed and tested by Los Alamos, moved outside Albuquerque to be closer to an airfield. In 1948 it became the Sandia Laboratory, a separate branch of Los Alamos. In the early 1950s physicists Ernest Lawrence and Edward Teller stressed the need for a second laboratory to enhance the efforts of Los Alamos, which led to the establishment in 1952 of the University of California Radiation Laboratory, renamed the Lawrence Livermore Laboratory, and a second Sandia Laboratory in 1956, in Livermore, California. Los Alamos, Sandia, and Livermore became national laboratories by 1979 legislation. See Sandia National Laboratories, "Sandia National Laboratories: A History of Exceptional Service in the National Interest," www.sandia.gov; "Nuclear Testing and Fallout Programs at the University of California Lawrence Radiation Laboratory," NV0402480, ATM; and J. L. Heilbron, Robert W. Seidel, and Bruce R. Wheaton, "Lawrence and His Laboratory: Nuclear Science at Berkeley," NV0724922, ATM.

23. The Tonopah Test Range in Area 52 was on the northern fringe of the Nellis Air Force Range. Like the NTS, the range conducted nuclear tests, including stockpiling research, and worked to develop fusing and firing systems. See "A Chronological History of Test Range Site Considerations Leading Up to the Selection of the Tonopah Test Range," ALSNLDE98056462, ATM; "An Analysis of the Role of Tonopah Test Range in Sandia Laboratories' Programs," ALSNLDE98040395, ATM; and Elmer Sowder interview, by Mary Palevsky, Apr. 29, 2004, NTS-OHP, UNLV.

24. *A Profile: Reynolds Electrical and Engineering Co. Inc: An EG&G Company* (Wellesley, MA: Corporate Communication and Information Department), NV0317251, ATM.

25. REECo hired subcontractors as well, including Robert E. McKee General Contractors, Inc., and J. S. Brown and E. F. Olds Plumbing and Heating Company in 1952, Eberline Instrument Company in 1955, and Lovelace Clinic in 1964. See Joe Ford, *REECo History*, NV0321540, ATM.

26. See *A Profile* for a summary of REECo's activities at the NTS. For a sample contract between REECo and the AEC, see *Reynolds Electrical & Engineering Co., Inc., Contractor At (29-2)-162*, NV0078994, ATM; "Application of Construction Conditions to Non-Construction Work," HWC, 86th Cong., Box 13, Folder 245, UNLV SC.

27. Deputy general manager of AEC to Howard W. Cannon, Aug. 31, 1959, HWC, 86th Cong., Box 13, Folder 245, UNLV SC. For letters regarding hiring complaints to Senator Howard W. Cannon, see HWC, 86th Cong., Box 13, Folder 245, UNLV SC; Background Information on Nevada Test Site, Nov. 13, 1961, HWC, 87th Cong., Box 12, Folder 159-61, UNLV SC; H. T. Herrick to Howard W. Cannon, Feb. 26, 1968, HWC, 90th Cong., Box 16, Folder 265, UNLV SC.

28. *NTS News* 7, no. 18, REECo Inc., Sept. 6, 1963; John May, "Expendable Americans," *The Independent* (Apr. 17, 1993) (incl. "We would get.")

29. There were many other job positions at the NTS. For a complete list, see REECo, EG&G, H&N, and Wackenhut contracts at the ATM. For example, *Reynolds Electrical & Engineering Co. Inc. Contract at (29-2)-162* outlines the company's general organization, and its departments and available positions in 1957. See also *NTS News*, Sept. 6, 1963; May, "Expendable Americans"; and James Merlino interview, by Suzanne Becker, Nov. 7, 2004, NTS-OHP, UNLV, for sheriffs' activities and issues with protestors.

30. See Hacker, *Elements of Controversy*, 7, 67–70, 74–77, 89, 92–99, 166–67, 187, 191–92, 267–68 for a discussion of Exercise Desert Rock. The topic garnered scholarly and journalistic attention during the 1980s after Plumbbob participant Paul Cooper claimed the test had given him leukemia. See Michael Uhl and Tod Ensign, *GI Guinea Pigs: How the Pentagon Exposed Our Troops to Dangers More Deadly Than War* (Chicago: Playboy Press, 1980); Howard Rosenberg, *Atomic Soldiers: American Victims of Nuclear Experiments* (Boston: Beacon Press, 1980); Thomas H. Saffer and Orville E. Kelly, *Countdown Zero* (New York: G. P. Putnam's Sons, 1982); Harvey Wasserman and Norman Solomon, with Robert Alvarez and Eleanor Walters, *Killing Our Own: The Disaster of America's Experience with Atomic Radiation* (New York: Delta Book, 1982). Other notable works include A. Costandina Titus, *Bombs in the Backyard: Atomic Testing and American Politics* (Reno: University of Nevada Press, 1986); and Welsome, *Plutonium Files*.

31. HUMMRO Psychological Tests, NV0750656, ATM (incl. quotes from questionnaire); "Armed Forces: Exercise Desert Rock," *Time* (Nov. 12, 1951) (incl. soldiers' quotes). See also Exercise Desert Rock I, NV0767719, ATM.

32. Robert "Doc" Campbell Jr. interview, by Suzanne Becker, Mar. 12, 2005, NTS-OHP, UNLV (incl. "the Waldorf Astoria," 28); William Flangas interview, Nov. 12, 2004, by Mary Palevsky, NTS-OHP, UNLV; "Mercury, Nevada, Fact Sheet," Nevada Site Office, DOE. The Plowshare Program sought to develop techniques to use nuclear explosions for peaceful construction purposes.

33. For a study on the archeological history of Camp Desert Rock, see Susan Edwards, "Atomic Age Training Camp: The Historical Archeology of Camp Desert Rock" (master's thesis, UNLV, 1997), 121, 126, 131, 139–42.

34. Robert Joseph Curran interview, by Suzanne Becker, July 18, 2005, NTS-OHP, UNLV (incl. "ass off"); Edwards, "Atomic Age," 122, 126–28.

35. See classifications in Daniel F. Hayes, "A Summary of Incidents Involving Radioactive Material in Atomic Energy Activities, Jan.–Dec. 1956," iii, NV0091411 (incl. all quotes); "Press Release Accidental Explosion," NV0143215, ATM.

36. "Press Release Accidental Explosion," 4.

37. Some authors use the word "illness" rather than "disease" or "sickness," but the terms are synonymous.

38. The Fukushima Daiichi Nuclear Power Station in Japan experienced equipment failures, nuclear meltdowns, and leaked radioactive gas after a devastating earthquake and tsunami on March 11, 2011, which claimed more than twenty thousand lives. Although it was the largest nuclear disaster since Chernobyl in 1986, the casualties at Fukushima were comparatively minor, with no immediate deaths due to ARS. See "Trauma, Not Radiation, Is Key Concern in Japan," Rebuilding Japan Series, NPR, Mar. 9, 2012.

39. CDC, "Acute Radiation Syndrome: A Fact Sheet for Physicians," https://emergency.cdc.gov/radiation/arsphysicianfactsheet.asp; Angelina K. Guskova, Alexander E. Baranov, and Igor A. Gusev, "Acute Radiation Sickness: Underlying Principles and Assessment," in *Medical Management of Radiation Accidents,* 2nd ed., ed. I. A. Gusev, Angelina K. Guskovo, and Fred A. Mettler (New York: CRC Press, 2001), 34.

40. These units are no longer the standards. The rad and rem equivalents are now Grey (Gy) and Sievert (Sv). But while Gy and Sv have superseded the rad and rem as industry standards, their use continues to be prevalent. See Barry N. Taylor and Ambler Thompson, eds., *The International System of Units (SI)* (Gaithersburg,

MD: National Institute of Standards and Technology, 2008), 37–38. For continuity purposes, this chapter will use the old units, because they were the standard for the majority of nuclear testing during the twentieth century.

41.  Dorothy Roberts et al. v. United States of America (1979), Deposition of Dr. Clarence C. Lushbaugh, 4045, Baneberry Collection, Box 4, Folder 4, UNLV SC; Guskova et al., "Acute Radiation Sickness," 33–51; CDC, "Acute Radiation Syndrome."

42.  AEC, *Operational Accidents and Radiation Exposure Experience, 1943–1964* (Washington, DC: U.S. GPO, 1965), 10–12, NV0015614, ATM; Leonard Kreisler interview, by Suzanne Becker, Apr. 20, 2005, NTS-OHP, UNLV, 19–20.

43.  J. Samuel Walker, "The Atomic Energy Commission and the Politics of Radiation Protection, 1967–71," *The History of Science Society* 85, no. 1 (Mar. 1994), 61. See also Hacker, *Elements of Controversy*, 272–76, for a discussion on radiation exposure versus radiation damage, and the low-level effects controversy.

44.  Clinton Maupin to J. E. Reeves, Nov. 15, 1961, NV0122450, ATM (incl. all quotes); "Test Site Worker Dies, June 17, 1958," Press Release, NV0034267, ATM; AEC, *Operational Accidents*, 6–7. For more on the Widowmaker, see Merlino interview; Kreisler interview, 46; R. Campbell interview, 29; "Widowmaker Records 44th and 45th Victims," *Review-Journal*, Oct. 17, 1964.

45.  Understanding between the AEC and PHS of the Department of Health, Education, and Welfare, memorandums, Jan. 25, 1954 and Feb. 1, 1954, SF–54–373, NV0004597, ATM.

46.  Hacker, *Elements of Controversy*. See also "AEC 0550 Codes for Standards for Health, Safety, and Fire Protection, 08/20/57" and "Operational Safety Standards, 11/08/68," *AEC Manual*, NV0092176, ATM. See also Mary Wammack, "Atomic Governance: Militarism, Secrecy, and Science in Post-War America, 1945–1958" (PhD diss., UNLV, 2010), for a discussion on how the hazards of the atomic program were not due to ignorance, but instead were based on the scientific boundaries of a so-called permissible dose.

47.  "NV Chapter 0528 Occupational Health Program: Vol. 0000 General Administration, Part 0500 Health and Safety, Approved May 2, 1962," *AEC Manual*, NV0058033, ATM; "NV Chapter 0528 Occupational Health Program, Vol. 0000 General Administration, Part 0500 Health and Safety, Approved Oct. 4, 1971," *AEC Manual*, NV0096021, ATM.

48.  "NV Chapter 0528 Occupational Health Program Approved May 2, 1962" (incl. all quotes); "$3,450 in Fees for AEC Doctor Told," *LA Times*, Mar. 13, 1952.

49.  For a history of Blue Cross and Blue Shield, see Robert M. Cunningham III and Robert M. Cunningham Jr., *The Blues: A History of the Blue Cross and Blue Shield System* (De Kalb: Northern Illinois Press, 1997).

50.  Engel, *Doctors and Reformers*, 316–17.

51.  For an example of the compensation for radiation workers, see Requirement Modification RE Workmen's Compensation for Radiation Workers, Feb. 10, 1967, NV0091818; W. B. McCool, Secretary, memorandum, Mar. 1, 1967, NV0908018; *Atomic Energy Commission Workmen's Compensation Record Keeping for Radiation Workers*, July 18, 1967, NV091817; F. T. Hobbs to Charles F. Eason, memorandum, Aug. 9, 1967, NV0091815; all at ATM.

52.  This practice changed by the 1970s. Leonard Kreisler established a system that treated not only occupational injuries or diseases, but also everyday ailments, to limit time-loss. See Kreisler interview, 20–21.

53. "NV Chapter 0528 Occupational Health Program, Approved May 2, 1962" (incl. "not the responsibilities"); Howard W. Cannon to Bob O'Neil, memorandum, Nov. 10, 1964, HWC, 88th Cong., Box 20, Folder 231, UNLV SC; Kreisler interview, 20.

54. Robert E. Miller to Howard W. Cannon, Oct. 23, 1970, HWC, 91st Cong., Box 28, Folder 348, UNLV SC (incl. "well-trained" and "around the clock"); "NV Chapter 0528 Occupational Health Program, Approved May 2, 1962" (incl. "Experience has shown").

55. Radiation is an energy released from unstable atoms, and is both natural and man-made. External radiation is emitted naturally in the environment from radium, thorium, and other materials. Radioisotopes also exist in water, food, and the air, but the levels are very low, producing little somatic effects. The discovery of radiation occurred in sequence in the last decade of the nineteenth century. German physicist Wilhelm Conrad Röntgen first discovered x-ray radiation in 1865 and French scientist Antoine Henri Becquerel discovered radioactivity in uranium salts the following year. In 1898 Pierre and Marie Curie discovered that polonium and radium emitted radiation. See J. Samuel Walker, *Permissible Dose: A History of Radiation Protection* (Berkeley: University of California Press, 2000), 1–28.

56. See Ruth R. Harris and Richard G. Hewlett, "The Evolution of Scientific Understanding of the Occupational Hazards of Ionizing Radiation," June 1983, 1–2, NV067984, ATM; Shields Warren, *The Pathology of Ionizing Radiation* (Springfield, IL: Charles C. Thomas, 1961), 3–5; Hermann J. Muller, "Artificial Transmutation of the Gene," *Science* 66, no. 1699 (July 22, 1929): 84–87.

57. The Manhattan Project anticipated the elevated hazards. In order to protect workers and the public, it instituted a comprehensive radiological safety program. But safety was never a priority; the scientists needed to help win the war and field-testing overshadowed it. At Los Alamos the risk of exposing the Southwest to fission particles seemed inconsequential to the potential result. When the Baker test in the Pacific Ocean blanketed the Bikini lagoon with radioactivity, it eventually became clear to the AEC, contractors, and laboratories that they needed to better prioritize safety. See Hacker, "Radiation Safety," 44–45.

58. Controversy mounted in the 1970s regarding nuclear testing, and in 1978 REECo hired a professional historian, Barton Hacker, to write a history of radiation safety in nuclear weapon testing. For the first time in American history, a historian gained access to classified memorandums, letters, studies, reports, and other documents outlining radiation protection and the AEC. The result is a comprehensive assessment of radiation protection in the United States. The first part of the manuscript became *The Dragon's Tail*, published in 1987, and the second became *Elements of Controversy*, published in 1994.

59. For a history of rad-safe operations from Ranger to Teapot, see Hacker, *Elements of Controversy*, 44–102, 164–69; and Seth R. Woodruff Jr. to Given H. Dugger, memorandum, Jan. 6, 1953, NV0404118; Rad Safe Control, NV0307267; Seth R. Woodruff Jr. to Given H. Dugger, memorandum, Jan. 6, 1953, NV0404118; H. E. Parsons to Los Alamos Scientific Laboratory, Jan. 10, 1955, NV0121275; Basic Guides for Radiation Protection, Feb. 26, 1954, NV092167; Procedures Governing Health and Safety Practices at Nevada Test Site, Dec. 8, 1952, NV030520; Plumbbob Series Fact Sheet, Sept. 15, 1981, RCC2.950425.007; all at ATM.

60. Plumbbob Series Fact Sheet.

61. Sowder interview, June 23, 2004, by Mary Palevsky, NTS-OHP, UNLV, 8; Plumbbob Series Fact Sheet; Exposure of Military Personnel from Nuclear Weapon Test at

Nevada Test Site, NV0705753; Analysis of Radiation Exposure for Task Force Warrior Shot Smoky, Exercise Desert Rock VII-VIII, Operation Plumbbob, May 31, 1979, DNA4747F; Advisory Committee Staff to Members of Advisory Committee on Human Radiation Experiments, memorandum, Apr. 4, 1995, ACH1.000013.046; Monitoring and Warning of Discharging Servicemen On The Long Term Health Effects Of Radiation Exposure, NV0755106; all at ATM. See also *Exposure of the American People to Iodine-131 from Nevada Nuclear Bomb Tests: Review of the National Cancer Institute Report and Public Health Implications* (Washington, DC: National Academy Press, 1999).

62. Welsome, *Plutonium Files* (incl. all quotes, 256–57).

63. "7th A Blast in Exploded Underground," *Chicago Daily Tribune*, Mar. 24, 1955 (incl. "the dirtiest"). Tests in unstemmed holes were conducted without protective features to prevent the flow to radioactive materials. Future underground tests were stemmed, a process that involved the positioning of plugs around in the encasement hole to prevent it from becoming a direct line for radiation leaks. Stemming also stopped gases from traveling up the emplacement hole, forcing radioactivity into the surrounding rock.

64. W. G. Flangas and L. E. Shaffer, "An Application of Nuclear Explosives to Block Caving Mining," June 2, 1960, Lawrence Radiation Laboratory, Contract No. W–7405-eng–38, UCRL5949, ATM; Bob Campbell, Ben Diven, John McDonald, Bill Ogle, and Tom Scolman, "Field Testing: The Physical Proof of Design Principles," *Los Alamos Science* (Winter/Spring, 1983), 177; Hacker, *Elements of Controversy*, 206–7, 231–35; Treaty Banning Nuclear Weapon Tests in the Atmosphere, in Outer Space and Underwater, signed Aug. 5, 1963, Art. I, Para. I.

65. DOE, National Nuclear Security Administration, "Underground Testing at the Nevada Test Site," Nevada Site Office, Office of Public Affairs, July 2005, doe/NV–1068, ATM.

66. Pigs are plastic shelled storage vessels with internal containers constructed of solid cast lead specifically made to contain radioactive material.

67. John F. Campbell interview, by Charlie Deitrich, Jan. 31, 2006, NTS-OHP, UNLV, 3–8; Kreisler interview, 23–24; *A Profile*, 4–9; Campbell et al., "Field Testing," 164–79.

68. John F. Campbell interview, Jan. 14, 2005, by Mary Palevsky, NTS-OHP, UNLV, 13, 58–59; ibid., 57; John F. Campbell interview, by Robert Nickel, July 23, 2004, NTS-OHP, UNLV, 14, 39.

69. The NTS was sectioned off into numbered Areas 1-30, dividing the site to create easily identifiable sections. However, not every numeral between 1-30 existed; omitted from the NTS map were 13, 21, 24, and 28.

70. Flangas interview, 42; William Beam interview, by Mary Palevsky, Jan. 20, 2005, 21–22, NTS-OHP, UNLV; Hacker, *Elements of Controversy*, 250; Harry Adams to Howard Cannon, Mar. 19, 1962 (incl. "difficult to"); Workmen Area 12 Nevada Test Site to Howard Cannon, telegram, Jan. 15, 1962; both in HWC, 87th Cong., Box 12, Folder 179, UNLV SC.

71. J. Campbell interview, July 23, 2004, 39 (incl. all quotes). See also J. Campbell interview, Jan. 14, 2005; J. Campbell interview, Jan. 31, 2006.

72. *A Profile*, 4–9.

73. Beam interview (incl. "construction-type," 24–25); "Worker Killed," Press Release, Nov. 14, 1968, NV0325062, ATM; "Operational Accidents and Radiation Exposure Experience Within the United States Atomic Energy Commission, 1943-1975," NV0001783, ATM; Kreisler interview, 35–36.

74. "A Summary of Industrial Accidents in USAEC Facilities," 1965–66, 17, NV0704455, ATM; J. Campbell interview, July 23, 2004, 19–20 (incl. "it was so," 19); Kreisler interview, 9–10 (incl. "cleaner than," 10).

75. *NTS News* 8, no. 12, REECo Inc. (June 19, 1964); Robert D. O'Neill to Howard Cannon, Mar. 3, 1969; both in HWC, 88th Cong., Box 20, Folder 231, UNLV SC; Kreisler interview, 35–36; Beam interview (incl. all quotes, 11–12); *NTS News* 12, no. 9, REECo Inc. (May 2, 1969), copy of document in HWC, 91st Cong., Box 28, Folder 338, UNLV SC.

76. Roberts et al. v. United States of America, Civil LV 76–259 RDF, Reporter's Transcript of Court Trial, 3867-27-3867-28, Baneberry Collection, Box 4, Folder 3, UNLV SC (incl. all quotes).

77. Kreisler interview (incl. "keep a," 36).

78. Flangas interview, 44–48; Human Studies Project Team Fact Sheet, Jan. 10, 1994, NV0701314, ATM.

79. Flangas interview, 44–48.

80. May, "How the United States" (incl. all quotes).

81. In 1966 the NTS embarked on a major exploratory program in Area 8, drilling thirteen holes. One of the holes housed the Discus Thrower test, which detonated on May 27, 1966. The device created a scarp northwest from ground zero about 1,200 feet long due to a fault line; it was later named the Discus Thrower fault. Although venting did not occur, an investigation revealed that the test had a high probability of venting. See Paul Duckworth, *Baneberry: A Nuclear Disaster* (Las Vegas: Harris Printers, 1976), 8.

82. Based on past experience, shots were routinely under the water table, even at 100 percent saturation of water content. Evidence also revealed that underwater shots in the Pacific contained nuclear particles. REECo and the laboratories therefore believed that water saturation was not important.

83. Summary Discussion of Test Series Applicable to Nevada Test Site and the Pacific, 3, NV0705726, ATM; *Baneberry: A Nuclear Disaster*, 7–10; Roberts et al. v. United States of America, 55–60, 75–78, Box 1, Folder 1.

84. J. Campbell interview, July 23, 2004, 34–35 (incl. all quotes); Duckworth, *Baneberry*, 3–4; Roberts et al. v. United States of America, Box 1, Folder 1, 60–70, 75.

85. Roberts et al. v. United States of America, Box 1, Folder 1, 95–97; Hacker, *Elements of Controversy*, 248–49.

86. Mary Manning, "Baneberry Decision Could Blast Legal Precedent," *Las Vegas Sun*, Jan. 31, 1982 (incl. all quotes); Duckworth, *Baneberry*, 4–6; Independent Guard Association of Nevada, Dorothy Roberts et al. v. Reynolds Electric and Engineering Company, Deposition of Dr. Shields Warren, June 9, 1975, NV0705909, ATM; Walter Pincus, "Rechecking 44 Exposed in '57 Urged," *Washington Post*, Aug. 11, 1977.

87. Manning, "Baneberry Decision"; Independent Guard Association of Nevada, Roberts et al. v. Reynolds Electric and Engineering Company, Deposition of Dr. Shields Warren; Pincus, "Rechecking 44 Exposed."

88. Robert Friedrichs interview, by Mary Palevsky, Feb. 25, 2005, NTS-OHP, UNLV (incl. "key memory," "It was a," and "We wanted," 11); Roberts et al. v. United States of America, Box 1, Folder 1, 95–97; J. Campbell interview, July 23, 2004, 35; Manning, "Baneberry Decision"; Friedrichs interview, 1–12; Summary Discussion of Test Series Applicable to Nevada Test Site and the Pacific, Topic A–5, 1–2; Hacker, *Elements of Controversy*, 248–49; Western Research Laboratory, Environmental Protection Agency, "Final Report of Off-Site Surveillance for the Baneberry Event," SWRHL-107r, ATM.

89. Summary Discussion of Test Series Applicable to Nevada Test Site and the Pacific, Topic A-5, 2; Hacker, *Elements of Controversy*, 249; Independent Guard Association of Nevada, Local 1 as a class, Dorothy Roberts et al. v. Reynolds Electric and Engineering Company; deposition of Dr. Shields Warren (incl. all quotes, 42–43).

90. "Overburden" is one of the many terms that miners used to describe their work. They invented many terms and phrases because there was no official name for what they did and how they did it. See J. Campbell interview, Jan. 31, 2006; and Friedrichs interview (incl. "far more," 8).

91. Friedrichs interview, 6–8 (incl. all quotes); Hacker, *Elements of Controversy*, 250–51.

92. Helper, *Women in Labor*, 111–12.

93. See the National Academy of Sciences–National Research Council Advisory Committee on the Biological Effects of Ionizing Radiation [BEIR], *The Effects on Populations of Exposure to Low Levels of Ionizing Radiation* (Washington, DC: GPO, 1972); United Nations Scientific Committee on the Effects of Atomic Radiation [UNSCEAR], *Ionizing Radiation Levels and Effects* (Geneva: United Nations, 1972).

94. Barton Hacker provides a complete discussion of the first two waves of concern over nuclear testing in *Elements of Controversy*. See Hacker's chapter "From Moratorium to Test Ban," esp. the sections on "Radiation Matters," "Testing Underground," and "The Issue of Low-Level Radiation," 211–26, 236–54.

95. For early publications questioning the effects of low-level radiation, see Harold A. Knapp, *Iodine-131 in Fresh Milk and Human Thyroids Following a Single Deposition of Nuclear Test Fallout*, Report TID-19266 (Washington, DC: AEC, 1963); Arthur R. Tamplin and John W. Gofman, *"Population Control" through Nuclear Pollution* (Chicago: Nelson-Hall, 1970); Ernest J. Sternglass, *Secret Fallout: Low Level Radiation from Hiroshima to Three Mile Island* (New York: McGraw-Hill, 1981). For a critique of Tamplin, Gofman, and Sternglass, see Robert W. Holcomb, "Radiation Risk: A Scientific Problem?" *Science 167* (Feb. 6, 1970): 853–55; Philip M. Boffey, "Ernest J. Sternglass: Controversial Prophet of Doom," *Science 166* (Oct. 10, 1969); and R. H. Romer, "Resource Letter ERPEE-1 on Energy: Resources, Production, and Environmental Effects," *American Journal of Physics 40* (1972), 805–29, esp. "The Low-Level Effects Controversy."

96. Walter Pincus, "Battle on Radiation Standards, Ever Bitter, Is Now Expanding," *Washington Post,* Jan. 16, 1978; Hacker, "Radiation Safety," 33–34; Hacker, *Elements of Controversy*, 276; Thomas A. Mancuso, Alice M. Stewart, and George W. Kneale, "Radiation Exposures of Hanford Workers Dying from Cancer and Other Causes," *Health Physics 33* (1977): 369–85.

97. See Uhl and Ensign, *GI Guinea Pigs*; Rosenberg, *Atomic Soldiers*; Corinne Brown and Robert Monroe, *Time Bomb: Understanding the Threat of Nuclear Power* (New York: William Morrow, 1981); Leslie J. Freeman, *Nuclear Witnesses: Insiders Speak Out* (New York: W. W. Norton, 1981); Saffer and Kelly, *Countdown Zero*; Wasserman et al., *Killing Our Own*; Titus, *Bombs in the Backyard*; Jim Lerager, *In the Shadows of the Cloud: Photographs and Histories of America's Atomic Veterans* (Golden, CO: Fulcrum, 1988).

98. Glyn G. Caldwell, Delle K. Kelley, and Clark W. Heath Jr., "Leukemia among Participants in Military Maneuvers at a Nuclear Bomb Test: A Preliminary Report," *Journal of the American Medical Association 244* (Oct. 3, 1980): 1575–78; Congressional Information of Operations, NV0755093; A History of the Nuclear Test Personnel Review Program, NV0051275; Military Participation in Atmospheric Nuclear Tests, NV705759; VA Assessment of Veterans with Military Service at Sites Temporarily

Augmented by Ionizing Radiation, NV0756892; Prepared Statement of Glenn H. Alcalay, NAAV Scientific and Medical Advisor to the House Committee on Veterans Affairs, May 24, 1981, NV0403135; all at ATM.

99.  Feres v. United States of America, 340 U.S. 135 (1950). See the succession of Jaffee cases: Jaffee v. United States of America, 592 F 2d 712 (1979); Jaffee v. United States, 468 F. Supp. 632—Dist. Court, D. New Jersey (1979); Jaffee v. United States, 663 F. 2d 1226 (1981).

100.  Bulloch v. United States (D.C. Utah 1955) 133 F. Supp. 885.

101.  At least one other worker at the Area 12 camp during the Baneberry accident developed lymphoma and died, but a REECo physician was of the opinion that the man's lymphoma existed prior to the event based on his physical examinations. See Roberts et al. v. Reynolds Electric and Engineering Company, Deposition of Dr. Shields Warren, 33–36; Roberts et al. v. United States of America, Deposition of Dr. Shields Warren, 1876–1888, Box 2, Folder 4; Manning, "Baneberry Decision"; "Summary Discussion of Test Series Applicable to Nevada Test Site and the Pacific," Topic A-5, 3.

102.  See Dorothy Roberts to President Jimmy Carter, May 9, 1977, letter, HWC, 95th Cong., Box 24, Folder 664, UNLV SC, for Mrs. Roberts's opinion on the Baneberry case and her husband's death.

103.  Roberts et al. v. United States of America, Deposition of Dr. Russell F. Miller, 2357–89, Box 3, Folder 1; "Widows Lose Baneberry Radiation," *Review-Journal*, Jan. 21, 1983; "NTS Hit with Second Suit," *Las Vegas Sun*, Dec. 28, 1976; Barbara Larson, "Government Hiding Information on Baneberry, Attorney Claims," *Las Vegas Sun*, Sept. 4, 1975; Duckworth, "Baneberry."

104.  Roberts et al. v. Reynolds Electric and Engineering Company, Deposition of Dr. Shields Warren, 38–39 (incl. all quotes); Buford L. Allen to Leon Silverstrom, Jan. 24, 1977, NV0705897, ATM.

105.  Roberts et al. v. United States of America, Deposition of Dr. John Gofman, Box 5, Folder 4 (incl. "100 times," 5242).

106.  Roberts et al. v. United States of America, Deposition of Dr. Alice Stewart, Box 1, Folder 1, 143–83 (incl. "in this rare," 157).

107.  See Bruce W. Church and Paul B. Dunaway to Roger Ray, letter, Jan. 7, 1977, NV0075899; Guy H. Cunningham III to James L. Liverman and Alfred D. Starbird, letter, Feb. 10, 1977, NV0705894; Leon Silverstrom to Guy H. Cunningham, letter, Jan. 24, 1977, NV0705896; all at ATM. See also Pincus, "Rechecking 44 Exposed" and appropriate testimonies in Roberts et al. v. United States of America.

108.  Roberts et al. v. United States of America, Conclusions of Law, Box 5, Folder 4, 104–18 (incl. "experimental," 114 and "a reasonable," 118).

109.  Dorothy Roberts et al. v. United States of America, 887 F. 2d 899 (1986). In the 1989 case, Foley ruled that the act was "actionable negligence" under the Federal Tort Claims Act, because no immunity existed when the government's choice was a "failure or refusal to follow safety standards." See Dorothy Roberts et al. v. United States of America, 724 F. Supp. 778 (1989) (incl. "actionable negligence" and "failure," 15). In 1996 Roberts's and Nunamaker's descendants attempted to reopen the case again, but the motion was denied.

110.  Keith Prescott v. United States of America and Reynolds Electrical and Engineering Company, Inc., 523 F. Supp. 918 (1981); Keith Prescott et al., v. United States of America, 724 F. Supp. 792, 798–99 (D. Nev. 1989) (incl. all quotes); Keith Schneider, "Nuclear Tests; Legacy of Anger: Workers See Betrayal on Peril," *New York Times*,

Dec. 14, 1989; Tim Dahlberg, "Attorneys Wage Marathon Battle for Nuclear Test Compensation," *Review-Journal*, Dec. 16, 1989; Keith Schneider, "Atom Tests' Legacy of Grief: Workers See Betrayal on Peril," *New York Times*, Dec. 14, 1989.

111.  Schneider, "Atom Tests' Legacy of Greif"; Titus, *Bombs in the Backyard*, 12; Howard Ball, *Justice Downwind: The Story of America's Atomic Testing Program at the Nevada Test Site* (London: Oxford University Press, 1986), 99–100; Wasserman et al., *Killing Our Own*, 118–20; "Veterans' Health Care, Training, and Small Business Loan Act of 1981," Pub. L. 97-72 (1981), Title I, "Veterans' Dioxin and Radiation Exposure Compensation Standards Act," Pub. L. 98-42 (1984); "Radiation-Exposed Veterans Compensation Act of 1988," Pub. L. 100-321 (1988); William J. Flor and Jerald L. Goetz, "DOD Experience with Dose Reconstructions for Atmospheric Test Veterans," in Proceedings of the HPS-ANS Symposium, "Environmental Radiation and Public Policy," Las Vegas 1990; Radiation Exposure Compensation Act, Pub. L. 101-426 (1990).

112.  "Energy Employees Occupational Illness Compensation Program Act of 2000," Pub. L. 106-398 (2000); William J. Clinton, Executive Order 13179 of December 7, 2000: Providing Compensation to America's Nuclear Weapons Workers, Federal Register (Dec. 11, 2000), v. 65 no. 238, 77487–77490 (incl. "too often these," 77487).

113.  Corn, *Response*, 1–2.

114.  Markowitz and Rosner, *Deceit and Denial* (incl. "Invariably," 197 and "ensure that," 358). See also Thomas F. Mancuso, "Cancer and Vinyl Chloride-Polymerization Implications, Problems and Needs (Feb. 1974), Vinyl Chloride Docket, H-036 Exhibit 3–11, DOL Docket Office; DOL, OSHA, *Informal Fact-Finding Hearings on Possible Hazards of Vinyl Chloride Manufacture and Use* (Feb. 15, 1974), 125–126; Manufacturing Chemists Association Papers, in Markowitz and Rosner, *Deceit and Denial*, 197, 358.

115.  Leisl Carr Childers, *The Size of the Risk: Histories of Multiple Use in the Great Basin* (Norman: University of Oklahoma Press, 2015) (incl. "the size," 64).

116.  "Energy Employees Occupational Illness Compensation Program."

# 5

# THE STRIP

BY THE LATE 1960S the United States could no longer ignore the crisis in occupational health. The numbers were staggering. From 1961 to 1970 the incidents of industrial accidents rose by 29 percent, with an estimated 2.2 million workers receiving injuries on the job over that period. Every year 14,500 employees died and 390,000 developed an occupational disease. The economic impact was huge. American workplace injuries and deaths resulted in $1.5 billion in lost wages annually and an estimated $8 billion loss to the GNP. With the growth of unregulated chemical and nuclear industrial activities, new technological processes were introduced faster than health experts could develop safety standards. In 1965 the PHS estimated that industries developed a new, potentially hazardous chemical every twenty minutes. Americans also embraced a social revolution, protesting the Vietnam War, demanding civil and women's rights, and bringing attention to ecological degradation and dangerous workplaces. Reports of asbestos-related diseases, coke oven emissions–related cancers, and black lung disease among miners infuriated the public. Although industry-specific regulations existed, inspections and enforcement occurred rarely.[1]

Organized labor was also left in the dark, unclear about health and safety statutes and what the law covered. For example, the Walsh–Healey Public Contacts Act of 1936 authorized regular inspections of workplaces under federal contract, but it covered few workers and was nearly impossible to enforce. Congress updated the act periodically, but the last major revision was in 1956. Most health and safety standards were consequently established by private interests via industry-affiliated organizations or voluntary agencies, not the federal government.[2]

Beginning in the early 1960s, the DOL started creating new guidelines for inspections, but without a coherent enforcement plan. At the same time, Congress deliberated proposals for revisions and laws, even considering tasking the AEC to establish health and safety standards, and monitor all workplaces. In 1965 the environmental movement inspired the PHS to act; without a clear mandate, its Division of Occupational Health did not have the authority to help workers. It published "Protecting the Health of Eighty Million Americans: A National Goal for Occupational Health," a study by the Division of Occupational Health revealing how modern technology changed the workplace. Besides reporting about new chemicals, the report revealed that older workplace problems in the United States had not been eliminated. The report concluded with a plea asking for a federal mandate and funding to build a national occupational health program with two goals: to eliminate "any factor" that threatened a worker's "health or life," and to promote the national economy through "the reduction of sick absence."[3]

Still, the movement stalled. Throughout the 1960s Congress introduced legislation but none advanced. In 1968 the rise of industrial accidents led to another bill but it was again defeated. Union leaders eventually prodded President Lyndon B. Johnson to take up the cause, which led to a task force drafting the first national health and safety bill. Johnson declared occupational health a national crisis, and proposed tasking the DOL with setting standards and inspection authority. His proposal never reached a vote.[4]

The war also escalated in Vietnam, forcing factories to institute speedups, and requiring long hours and overtime. Similar to World War II, the hurried pace increased the rate of accidents. The increasingly militant American workforce finally had enough, and organized strikes throughout the nation, stalling productivity. The strike action hurt production, encouraging industry to consider health and safety measures.[5]

On November 20, 1968, an explosion at the Consol Energy coal mine near Farmington, West Virginia, killed seventy-eight miners, and in early 1969, an oil spill in the Santa Barbara Channel off Santa Barbara, California, covered the coastline with crude oil, killing thousands of marine animals. The events further encouraged Americans to demand change. After the Farmington mine disaster coal miners marched on the West Virginia capital, inspiring the Coal Mine Health and Safety Act of 1969.[6]

In January 1969 Congressman James G. O'Hara (D-MI) introduced the OSH bill, Senator Harrison Williams (D-NJ) followed suit in the Senate in May, and the Nixon administration introduced a proposal in August. Although the bill originated among labor activists and Democrats, President Richard Nixon embraced it to lure blue-collar white Americans to the Republican party. However, his proposal called for minimal disruption of the work process, and recommended creating a nonregulatory agency, the NIOSH, to research and develop safety recommendations as part of the CDC and the Department of Health and Human Services (DHHS). Under the DOL, OSHA would handle enforcement, training, outreach, education, and compliance assistance. Nixon eventually conceded to the Democratic-DOL plan, but insisted on establishing separate agencies. After another year of revisions, he signed the OSH Act into law on December 29, 1970. It was a significant departure from previous legislation, creating OSHA and NIOSH, two federal agencies authorized to set standards "to the extent feasible," and protect employees from damages and regular exposure to hazards. Since its ratification, much debate has centered around the broad meaning of the word "feasible." Although OSHA has maintained that the word implied "capable of being done," conservative employer groups have adopted a more cost-benefit approach.[7]

Still, it was a significant step forward. For the first time in American history, a federal mandate protected employees in the private sector, safeguarding health and safety through inspection, regulation, and standard setting. It also authorized the imposition of fines and sometimes prison terms, ending the longstanding principle that workplaces were not under federal control; it also guaranteed employees access to information about harmful substances in their workplace. While controversial, the OSH Act underwent few modifications after its passing, with the exception of an amendment in 1990 increasing penalties sevenfold.[8]

As OSHA and NIOSH developed, and the growing recognition of risks involving low-level radiation and chemical exposures played out on the national stage, the American workplace evolved to embrace a new postindustrial economy. The various events marked the beginning of a third period in occupational health history in the United States. In 1970 the manufacturing sector held 17.8 million out of 71 million jobs in the United States. In 2012 only 11.9 million out of 133.7 million jobs represented manufacturing positions. The decline in industrial work occurred because of two factors: automation and imports. Multinational corporations also responded to environmentalism and OSHA by moving their factories to developing nations. The move terminated thousands of jobs, most of them among steel and automotive workers in the Midwest and Northeast. But as the economy deindustrialized, employment in services, research, information technology, health care, and finance grew. In 1973 sociologist David Bell wrote *The Coming of the Post-Industrial Society*, accurately predicting that service employees would surpass the number of industrial and agricultural workers, creating an economy based on the proceeding eras. Postindustrialism was therefore not an entirely new economic realm, but depended on manufactured products. Likewise, manufactured products generated services. In the 2000s 75 percent of Americans worked in postindustrial trades. Older jobs, such as jobs in health care, education, and engineering, developed new specialties. Scientific, technical, and finance occupations also grew, marked by the expansion of communications, information, and medical technologies, and computer software and pharmaceutical development.[9]

Employees with the strongest educational credentials fared the best in the postindustrial economy, obtaining the highest-paying jobs because of their ability to manage information and innovate. Those without college educations or special skillsets had fewer prospects, gravitating toward unskilled work. One of the largest sectors of the service industry that offered options for unskilled labor was hospitality. The Las Vegas Strip was the ultimate manifestation, combining gaming, lodging, food services, conferences, entertainment, and theme park attractions into one, over-the-top experience. Unlike an industrial workplace, it did not produce tangible goods, instead providing escape, pleasure, and self-indulgence to guests. The job was an often-difficult task. A factory could stop an assembly line to fix a defect, but Strip employees continuously produced experiences in a scripted environment but uncontrolled setting. With the experiences created and consumed at the same time, there was little margin for error. Success required high commitment from the entire staff.[10]

In the process, employees faced similar hazards to industrial workers, but the risks were harder to define and interpret. According to the Bureau of Labor Statistics, hotel workers reported higher rates and more-severe injuries than other hospitality employees. They were also 40 percent more likely to sustain injuries and require more days off, job transfers, and medically restricted work.[11] After the 1970s, the risk of postindustrial work increased in Las Vegas, simply because the new megaresorts provided more services and required a greater number of employees.

Nevada legalized gambling in 1931, but the industry did not generate huge profits until after World War II.[12] In 1941 hotelier Thomas Hull visited Las Vegas to expand his California El Rancho hotel chain to Las Vegas. In a surprise move, he decided against Fremont Street, picking land on Highway 91 outside the city and therefore not subject to municipal taxes. The El Rancho opened in 1941, emerging as a prototype for the roadside hotels that characterized the 1950s and 1960s.[13] The venture was marginally successful, but inspired the future of Las Vegas. As the first casino suburb, it revealed the profitability of combining casinos with resort hotels. Guy McAfee, a former vice policeman and entrepreneur, named the area the Las Vegas Strip because of its likeness to the Sunset Strip in Hollywood, California. He also helped solidify the location as a tax shelter, establishing the unincorporated township of Paradise in December 1950.[14] The Strip eventually became synonymous with gambling and entertainment in the United States. Over the following decades, it expanded from small hotels with enormous neon signs to a succession of massive, dense megaresorts. In the process, the Strip helped shift American perceptions of gambling. Although gambling was associated with criminals, the Strip provided gaming, a legitimate recreational activity.[15]

The Strip's occupational health regime varied considerably based on ownership, undergoing two general periods of history. Organized crime syndicates and the International Brotherhood of Teamsters dictated the first period, and corporate ownership defined the second.[16] In the mid-1950s most of the Strip was mob-owned because of the difficulty for casino owners to obtain large bank loans.[17] After 1958 the construction boom went into a lull after an economic downturn in Las Vegas and a federal investigation into Nevada gaming and its ties to organized crime.[18] The inquiry prompted the institution of stricter gaming regulations, establishing the Gaming Control Board in 1955, the Gaming Commission in 1959, and the Gaming Policy Committee in 1961.[19] It soon became apparent that illegitimate capital could no longer support the Strip. Blending legal and illegal practices, the Teamsters entered the business, investing in commercial development and the resorts. Instead of gangsters reaching for shoeboxes of money, the Teamsters offered loans from legitimate banking institutions, funding the construction of Caesars Palace, Aladdin, and the Landmark Hotel and Casino.[20] Opening in 1966 at the cost of $19 million, Caesars Palace inaugurated a new era on the Strip, outshining the first generation of resorts.[21]

The corporate era emerged after Howard Hughes purchased the Frontier, Sands, Castaways, Landmark, and Silver Slipper in 1967. The eccentric billionaire provided a symbol of change, legitimizing investment on the Strip.[22] In 1968 entrepreneur Kirk Kerkorian constructed the largest hotel in the world, the International, and simultaneously acquired the Flamingo. He was the first person to benefit from the 1969 Corporate Gaming Act, which allowed for corporate involvement in the gaming industry.[23] Historian Hal Rothman called the Act "the most important event in the history of modern Las Vegas," ushering in a new era of business.[24]

After completing the International, Kerkorian sold both resorts to the Hilton Hotels Corporation in 1970, marking the first time a publicly owned corporation owned a casino. The Las Vegas Hilton subsequently reported massive earnings, changing the hotel industry's perception of the Strip, and inspiring Sheraton and Holiday Inn to invest. In 1973 Kerkorian opened the MGM Grand, setting a new industry standard of size and luxury. Costing $120 million, it was the first megaresort on the Strip.[25] Despite its success, the MGM Grand was the only property constructed on the Strip until 1989. Various factors prevented new development; Kerkorian had elevated the amount of capital needed to construct a comparable property. The country also experienced a nationwide recession during the 1970s. Steve Wynn provided a solution during the 1980s, redefining corporate ownership on the Strip. With the help of financier Michael Milken, he constructed Las Vegas's second megaresort, the Mirage, in 1989. Costing $630 million, it doubled the MGM Grand in size. Wynn innovated the mega-resort design, making the resort the main source of entertainment. The result was an over-the-top, tropical-themed, volcano-fronted spectacular, with expensive décor, luxury rooms and villas, and a multitude of entertainment, gaming options, and wildlife habitats. His vision revitalized Las Vegas, inspiring corporations to invest billions in the Strip over the following decades. Most existing resorts were imploded or demolished, and dense megaresorts soon outlined the iconic cityscape. The corporate activity not only transformed the Strip, but also the community. When the Mirage opened, approximately eight hundred thousand people lived in Clark County. By 2010 the population had more than doubled.[26]

Given the scope of operations, the Strip required a large workforce. In 1955 six thousand of Clark County's thirty thousand wage earners worked there. In 1975 the hospitality industry was employing 40,000 of 150,000 wage earners in Las Vegas. The Desert Inn and Sahara retained twelve hundred each, and the MGM Grand had forty-five hundred. After 1990 service employment skyrocketed. In 2005 the Strip accounted for 109,689 employees, distributing a $4.2 million annual payroll. Nineteen of the largest resorts employed 34.5 percent of Nevada gaming employees and produced 47.4 percent of the statewide revenue.[27] Most required minimal educational requirements. As explained by historian Hal Rothman, Las Vegas solved a major problem associated with transitioning from industrialism to postindustrialism. It became the Last Detroit: with barely a high school education, employees could earn a middle-class income and could expect to work for the company the rest of their lives. One of the Strip's most coveted jobs—valet—achieved almost mythic status by the 2000s for its sup-posed earning potential. In 2006 the *Las Vegas Sun* investigated a popu-lar theory that valets could earn $100,000 or more—just for parking cars. Most did not earn that much, but the job paid well considering the educational requirements. As with many positions in the service industry, tipping was an integral augment to their income. A valet's base salary ranged from $9 to $15 an hour. A valet stand staffed around twenty employees at one time, handling between fifteen hundred to eighteen hundred vehicles a day. After each shift, tips were pooled and divided based on employment hierarchy. Supervisors and runners received the biggest cut, and ticket writers the smallest. Most valets collected between $150 to $500 a shift, a yearly tipping income of a maximum $60,000 at the highest-rated resorts. The *Las Vegas Sun* con-cluded that valets did not earn six figures, but the exaggerated income reveals a common perception of the Strip. As cities across the nation struggled to transition to postindustrialism, Las Vegas appeared to op-erate the perfect service economy with endless financial potential for employers and employees alike. As noted by Rothman, the city also developed higher employment rates, lower unemployment rates, and steadily rising per capita income.[28]

Management styles varied among the resorts, but each incorpo-rated new theories on organizing the postindustrial workplace. In 1960 psychologist Douglas McGregor theorized about two models of managerial motivation. Industrial jobs were mechanical, requiring little decision making on the part of the workers. Theory X was there-fore a standardized, segmented, and strictly supervised management style based on penalties. Postindustrial work required employees to think and make choices, encouraging a more discretionary approach to management. Theory Y was based on the theory that service work-ers were internally motivated, and needed to direct themselves. Man-agement also needed to be less paternalistic, necessitating supervisors to relate to employees on a personal level.[29]

Theory Y seemed optimal for most postindustrial work, but it was a risky model for the Strip. Individualism, lack of rules, and limited leadership could create an inconsistent experience for guests, and so hurt profits. The Strip therefore combined both models to achieve the most efficient production. In a workplace characterized by open-ended tasks, strong management–employee relationships, task structure, and authority figures became important constructs. The resorts structured operations like an industrial plant, with four categories of workers. The first were skilled professionals or semiprofessionals, such as executive chefs and orchestra leaders, and the second were white-collar workers like secretaries, clerks, and switchboard operators. The third encompassed blue-collar workers maintaining the gardens, slot machines, and security systems. The largest category were employees with guest contact, operating the gaming areas, restaurants, retail services, lounges and bars, and entertainment. Each resort maintained twenty-four-hour-a-day, seven-day-a-week operations, departmentalizing employees based on functionary lines: casino, rooms, food, beverage, management, entertainment, and retail. The departments interacted with one another on a regular basis, delivering one seamless experience to guests.[30]

Until the late 1960s, management ran the resorts like a family business with off-site investors that demanded quick returns.[31] Operations divided into two units: the casino and all other departments. Mob associates oversaw gaming while a separate management team ran the hotel. Both units generally managed their business well, running honest games and cultivating a harmonious working environment. Employees remembered having an almost familial relationship with management, being paid well, and with the opportunity to better their positions. The friendly relationship was also thanks to Culinary Union Local 226. Even though Nevada became a right-to-work state in 1953, which prohibited labor union–employer agreements that made union membership a condition of employment, Culinary maintained a strong presence in Las Vegas's hospitality industry, representing Strip and downtown employees in most job classifications. Negotiations between the two parties were generally easy since management was not concerned with the cost of operations. Mob associates were also familiar with establishing strong partnerships with unions; they were key institutions for immigrant neighborhoods in the East and Midwest. No one signed a contract or broke a deal. The system worked well, cultivating an atmosphere that allowed employees to design and construct their own work experiences without being micromanaged by management.[32]

Corporatization dramatically restructured this working environment. Elected officials began handling management, determining policy and profitability, not daily operations. When Hilton Hotels Corporation acquired the International, Barron Hilton explained that his company was not "involved in the day-to-day operations, [but monitored] the profit and loss statements of the hotel." Unlike the mob, he took a long-term outlook and was not interested in quick returns. The new model dramatically reorganized management divisions. In addition to the casino, hotel rooms, food and beverage, and housekeeping, the corporate model established marketing, accounting, auditing, and financial and legal departments. At the MGM Grand, Kirk Kerkorian's management was particularly intricate, with a board of seven corporate officers, nine senior directors, and fifty-seven lower-level managers and supervisors. Corporate provided each supervisor with clear job descriptions and authority, and communication between the various levels were well defined.[33]

The corporations also incorporated human resources management, a concept that gained popularity among employers during the 1960s.[34] Management theorists argued that achievement, recognition, challenge, growth, and job responsibility motivated employees.[35] Human recourses divisions merged management with modern psychology, reorganizing the workplace to maximize return on human capital investment and minimize financial risk. The programs focused on recruitment, hiring, and firing, but also developed strategies to inspire success and develop employer loyalty. One important component was expanding benefits, covering not only medical but also childcare, legal, and other assistance. After the MGM Grand opened in 1973, its human resources division administered a pamphlet signed by President Alvin Benedict outlining the resort's "objective and philosophy." The workplace relationship resembled a family, and employer and employee had similar objectives: "The secret to a successful organization is teamwork where people work together for common interests and goals." The pamphlet promised "positive personal recognition" and other benefits for exceptional performances.[36]

Most employees resented the corporate takeover and changes in management, which reflected national trends. *Work in America*, a 1973 report by Elliot Richardson, secretary of Health, Education, and Welfare, found that the work ethic had diminished as a whole among postindustrial employees, for the most part because of declining job satisfaction and fading opportunities to someday become a boss.[37] This was the sentiment among many Strip employees. When the mob conducted operations, employees easily gained promotions to higher-paid positions. If employees made money for the house, managers rewarded them. Dealers consequently easily rose to management level.[38]

Organized crime syndicates treated employees like extended family, offering jobs to their children and relatives. This practice ended after corporatization. Like the rest of the nation, employment became more stratified by the 1980s. Employees could enter management positions only with a business or hotel school degree. The change frustrated existing employees, for whom it was a major point of dissatisfaction. It also shifted employment patterns. Like industrial jobs in previous generations, Strip employment became a transitional step to white-collar status. The poor, uneducated, and immigrant populations took blue-collar jobs at the resorts, and sent their children to college. If their children wanted to work on the Strip, they returned later with management qualifications.[39]

To be considered for employment, the resorts required applicants to submit to physical examinations. El Rancho doctors determined whether applicants were "likely to be all hands and feet," examining dexterity, eyesight, and "ability to hear accurately and speak distinctly," and rejected those prone to "accidents, harming themselves or others, breaking or damaging furnishings and equipment." For a casino position, applicants took preemployment exams, testing for mathematical skills, dictation, and memory, and required certification from a gaming school.[40]

Once employed, management issued guidelines on appearance, ethical behavior, and conduct. The El Rancho required employees to appear "wholesome [and] clean, [which conveyed] good health" to their guests. The Stardust articulated that they represented their workplace, "regardless of position [and the importance of] neat dress, grooming, courteous behavior, and a smile and friendly word." Management also issued guidelines for appearance, requiring that females apply makeup in good taste and hairstyles that were business appropriate. All employees were expected to be polite, friendly, and dependable, and to engage briefly with guests because management believed that prolonged conversations resulted in employee errors. Considering the job's close proximity to vice, management also set strict conduct codes, stressing that employees needed to be vigilant and alert at all times. Drinking alcohol was strictly prohibited, and repeated tardiness or absenteeism resulted in immediate termination. Above all, management instructed employees to maintain a good image, because they were team members, even while off duty.[41]

The composition of the workforce varied, but the Strip had a historically checkered approach to employment equality. The state did not have laws requiring segregation and unequal treatment for minorities, but southern Nevada developed the dubious, and exaggerated, title of the Mississippi of the West after World War II. The resorts hired young, white males for the most visible jobs to appease white clientele, many of which were from California after migrating from the South. In 1960 Nevada had the most young, middle-aged white adults in the nation. A third of the population had lived in the state for only five years. Most employees had immigrated from California, Texas, east of the Mississippi River, and the Northern Plains. Since white men held positions with the highest paychecks and power, they had plenty of opportunity to better their position. Female employees faced discrimination patterns, a reflection of postwar conservatism. After the war, employers reasserted the traditional sexual division of labor, offering separate pay scales and job positions. One of the earliest critiques of the female postwar position was Betty Friedan's *The Feminine Mystique* in 1963, a book that reinforced the one-dimensional, conservative stereotype that postwar women were suppressed in a white, middle-class, domesticated suburban cage.[42]

Some women fit this stereotype, but most did not. Lower-class whites and minority women worked on the Strip, but were limited to housekeeping and cashier positions, or worked as entertainers, cocktail waitresses, keno runners, restaurant workers, and retailers.

Female sexuality also played an important role in Las Vegas as a whole. Instead of openly selling sex, the resorts sold the possibility. The sexual objectification of women by men became an accepted business model. Management retained a multitude of attractive white women to entertain guests in shows and topless revues. In the show "Casino de Paris," the Dunes had strict criteria for its perfect showgirl during the 1960s: 5 feet 10 inches, 134 pounds, and "harmonizes with the globe's curvature with 37-25-37 measurements." Most were twenty-three years old, with blue or hazel eyes. Only two had brown eyes. While the women were "imported from the world over," the majority originated from the United States; according to the show's Paris-born producer Frederic Apcar, "America [was] still in great shape." If a woman gained weight during her time of employment, the Dunes considered it a breach of contract and replaced her.[43]

While female objectification benefited some women, the work introduced a hard life to others. Many endured long hours, sometimes abusive bosses, and uninvited sexual advances from coworkers and guests. A pregnancy resulted in immediate termination. Unable to make ends meet, some turned to freelance work on the Strip, becoming strippers, escorts, or prostitutes. The Equal Pay Act of 1963 and the Civil Rights Act of 1964 eventually helped the situation, but the process took time.[44] Most resorts also refused to hire female dealers. The city of Las Vegas officially endorsed discrimination of women on November 5, 1958, passing a public ordinance recommending against the hiring of female dealers. The ban forced Sarann Knight, one of Las Vegas's only black female dealers, out of work, as well as her white coworkers. A year later, North Las Vegas banned the employment of female bartenders.[45]

In the 1970s Las Vegas finally ceased its citywide ban on female dealers. Under affirmative action pressure, the resorts also began employing women in jobs traditionally held by men. Yet most dealers remained male; out of 2,616 dealers, only 25 percent were women in 1976. The situation gradually improved by the 1980s. On January 13, 1981, the Equal Employment Opportunity Commission filed a complaint and at the end of the month, nineteen Strip resorts and four unions settled out of court, agreeing to end discrimination. Still, the marginalization of women continued in Nevada and the nation as a whole. A 2005 Census Bureau survey found that women earned $0.82 to every $1.00 earned by Nevada men. With 3.44 women who died from domestic violence per 1,000 residents, Nevada also reported the highest rate of any state in the nation.[46]

Las Vegas's history of minority discrimination has been well covered by historian Eugene Moehring and others.[47] After World War II the segregation policies enacted during the construction of Hoover Dam and BMI continued. Blacks lived in the Westside slums, and were prohibited from gambling, eating, drinking, and attending shows on the Strip. Of course, the resorts allowed the employment of blacks, but only in the lowest-paying jobs. Management famously ushered entertainers such as Sammy Davis Jr. and Lena Horne out the back door after headlining their showrooms. In 1953 the Hotel Last Frontier even drained the pool after Dorothy Dandridge intentionally dipped her foot in it. A civil rights movement also emerged in Las Vegas, led by the city's first black dentist, Dr. James McMillan, and physician Dr. Charles West, as well as a group of local ministers, teachers, businesspeople, and parts of the medical community. General surgeon Dr. Kirk V. Cammack Jr. delivered a speech in 1964 entitled "Shall They Not Protest" in Las Vegas and gatherings throughout the United States on his dedication to civil rights, highlighting his relationship with his anatomy cadaver, Evan Keesee, during medical school:

> Since that time, I have explored many human beings and one thing I can assure you—as soon as you cut through the skin you can't tell a black man's brain from a white man's brain. There is no such thing as a stomach that is black or a stomach that is white. There is no special chapter of negro physiology or negro biochemistry or negro neuroanatomy of the brain. They are the same as a white man's. What if Evan Keesee's skin had been white instead of black? Would he have died in a psychopathic hospital and ended up on a dissecting table? It is possible, but I think you will all agree with the completely illogical fact that his skin pigment affected Evan Keesee's life from the day he was born until his death.[48]

The growth of the resort industry during the 1960s encouraged the creation of more low-paying jobs, inspiring thousands of blacks to move to Las Vegas. The influx of new black residents assembled enough support to mobilize protests. Local rioting raised attention to the Strip's discrimination policies as well as a 1961 report by the Nevada Equal Rights Commission. After holding meetings in Reno and Las Vegas, this commission concluded that the casino industry was guilty of flagrant discrimination. The Strip had no black dealers, waitresses, waiters, bellmen, or office personnel on the payroll, and only a "scattering of Orientals." In response, executives insisted they did not have enough qualified, nonwhite applicants to fill the positions. Dunes owner Major Riddle reassured commission members that "things [were] changing…. Four or five years ago, there would have been considerable opposition to Negroes in some of the positions." He claimed that blacks made up 10 to 20 percent of the workforce at that time.[49]

Local activism and a nationwide civil rights movement helped improve conditions, but did not inspire immediate change. Throughout the decade, the Equal Employment Opportunity Commission and the Nevada Equal Rights Commission continued to prod the resorts, but failed to make progress until corporations assumed ownership of the Strip. In 1970 the Nevada Resorts Association offered a plan to promote minorities to higher-paying jobs. This was a positive step, but it did not end discrimination. Local NAACP attorney Charles Kellar, who had filed complaints with state courts and the gaming commission, took the issue to federal court, suing the Las Vegas gaming industry under Title VII of the Civil Rights Act. In June 1971 U.S. District Court judge Roger Foley forced the resorts and unions to enter meaningful negotiations, and required that blacks represent 12 percent of the workforce.[50] The state legislature also passed a fair housing act ending residential segregation. During the 1980s the work environment had significantly improved for blacks, whose efforts benefited a growing contingent of employees from Mexico and other Central and South American, and Asian countries. Still, minorities rarely held upper management positions. The Strip did not appoint its first black president until 2002, Lorenzo Creighton at the Flamingo.[51]

It might be difficult to visualize a connection between the health and safety concerns discussed in previous chapters—operating a railroad, constructing a dam, manufacturing chemicals, and testing nuclear weapons—and the risks associated with working on the Strip. Postindustrial trades appeared to be a safer alternative, a far cry from working around heavy machinery, explosives, chemicals, and the cumulative effects of low-level radiation. However, it is important to evaluate postindustrial work in occupational health history, especially since it dominated the American workforce by the turn of the century. Seventy-five percent of Americans held postindustrial jobs and the workplaces were not completely safe. A telling example of the threat of postindustrial work was the MGM Grand fire on the Strip, which resulted in the deaths of seventy-eight guests and seven employees, and over six hundred nonfatal injuries on November 21, 1980. As shown by historian Michelle Murphy, many postindustrial employees also developed health problems associated with time spent at their postindustrial jobs, but did not have specific diseases or chemical exposures to measure. Still, they suffered from various ailments— headaches, nausea, dizziness, dermatitis, couching, immune system disorders, muscle pain, and fatigue—which doctors referred to as sick building syndrome (SBS). A mixture of substances or sensitivities to low concentrations of contaminants appeared to cause the symptoms, often disappearing after an employee left the building. SBS was a controversial subject, and many experts disagreed about whether it was a syndrome or a psychologically related phenomenon.[52] With building-related illnesses and other postindustrial hazards entering the conversation, new problems emerged in the third period of occupational health that merited attention.

The Strip provides an example of the blurred risks associated with postindustrial work. Working in Las Vegas was glamourous and exciting, but it was also physically demanding. Most jobs required employees to work nights, weekends, and holidays, stand for long periods, and tolerate rude and insulting behavior from guests. A multitude of stressors also dotted the casino floor, such as spaces consumed with secondhand smoke and audiovisual and noise overload. As added pressure, most employees did not have a set income and depended on gratuities. Many reported chronic headaches, racing hearts, upset stomachs, and irritability during working hours.[53]

The Strip also operated around the clock, necessitating employees to work irregular hours. The shifts made it difficult for them to interact with people outside the industry, encouraging them to socialize with coworkers. During the 1960s registered nurse Barbara Ann Barnett worked as a cocktail waitress at the Hacienda and described her cohort as "a group…that mimicked the behavior of guests" and "only thought of the thrill of the moment." Personal relationships tended to change quickly and "it was not unusual to see one person being involved with two or three different people at the same time." Overall, Barnett remembered "a lot of drinking and a lot of partying," a lifestyle that inspired her to leave casino work.[54]

Being in close proximity to vice, many employees developed addictive behavior. Casino workers had a more increased risk of pathological gambling behavior than the general public. The threat was especially high among dealers, as the value of money tended to lessen among those constantly handling money. Cases of depression were also significantly higher among casino workers, as well as alcohol and cigarette dependency. While working at the Clark County Health Department, Dr. Otto Ravenholt found that there was a "freer atmosphere for indulgence of alcohol [among his patients].… The same historically was true as far as cigarettes go." In a random sampling of casino employees in 1999, two out of five casino workers smoked, 50 percent higher than the rate among the general population.[55] Employees with pathological gambling disorders, depression, and substance abuse reported higher rates of insomnia, intestinal problems, hypertension, and suicide, and an elevated chance of developing cancer, cardiac problems, or engaging in criminal behavior. The conditions also contributed to disability, morbidity, and even premature death.[56]

Of course, typical workplace accidents were also a part of the job. Most positions required employees to stand for eight hours, performing repetitive, awkward movements. Injuries usually occurred during mundane tasks, reflecting national averages. Based on OSHA's three hundred logs in 2003–2005, hotel workers experienced injury rates of 5.2 injuries per 100 worker-years. Trauma disorders, such as lacerations, fractures, and contusions, accounted for 52 percent of the injuries. Thirty-nine percent were musculoskeletal disorders or repeated trauma caused by repetitive strain, such as carpal tunnel syndrome, tendinitis, and back injuries. Females experienced higher injury rates, especially those working in housekeeping.[57] Housekeepers had especially poor health due to heavy workloads, stress, and work-related pain. In the 1980s the majority were non-English-speaking immigrants, with limited literacy and unfamiliarity with workplace rights. With little training in workplace safety, illnesses, and injuries, they rarely used protective equipment. Nearly all housekeepers reported job-related pain at some point in their career. At the El Rancho housekeepers tended to develop arthritis with age, so the resort "forbade [older women] to work any longer in damp atmospheres." The resort also found that janitors, window washers, and painters had a higher probability of developing blood pressure conditions, dizzy spells, and contracting lead poisoning.[58]

In comparison to the workplaces discussed in previous chapters, the Strip was relatively clean, because unsanitary conditions hurt business. However, some resorts cut corners to help the bottom line. In the early 1960s a number of restaurants imported second-hand appliances from Los Angeles that did not run correctly in the desert heat. The food spoiled, causing a string of food poisonings. The Clark County Health Department quickly intervened, prohibiting the use of second-hand restaurant equipment in Las Vegas. In 1964 the Flamingo tested the ban. An inspection by the Health Department revealed that one of their kitchens recently installed second-hand equipment, and had subpar sanitary conditions. When the Health Department threatened to shut the resort down, it immediately complied.[59]

The most common disorders connected with Strip employment were dermatitis and respiratory issues. Dermatitis, mild irritations of the skin, was very common among culinary workers. Although it was not fatal, the annoying condition took a long time to heal. Practicing in Las Vegas since the 1950s, dermatologist Dr. Harold Boyer "saw a lot of occupations with dermatitis among anyone who worked on the Strip." In most cases, employees handled "soap and water" and "fish and meat juice." Boyer treated two types of dermatological disorders: atopic and contact. Atopic conditions typically resulted from food allergies, biological factors, or the intake of allergens, while contact conditions resulted from touching irritating substances. Most cases on the Strip involved the latter. Management instructed employees handling food to sanitize their hands with ammonia-based solutions, an action that wreaked havoc on their skin. According to Boyer, dermatitis also afflicted doctors. He knew at least one that "had to give up surgery because he could not scrub [his hands]" anymore. Boyer typically prescribed cortisone to employees to heal their conditions, but usually received repeated visits after the irritation resurfaced.[60]

Respiratory issues resulted from poor indoor air quality and exposures to synthetic carpets, inks, adhesives, solvents, and other contaminants. Bakers, hairdressers, and animal handlers regularly handled chemicals, gases, fumes, and dust, and developed asthma. Combustion sources such as oil, gas, kerosene, coal, and wood contaminated the air, along with deteriorating building materials and furnishings, and asbestos-containing insulation. Microbial contaminants such as gases, fungi, and mold fostered adverse health conditions as well. However, the most hazardous indoor air pollutant in the resorts was secondhand smoke. As most of the rest of the nation banned indoor smoking, the Strip became a haven for smokers. It became a joke that Las Vegas was California's smoking section. But secondhand smoke was very dangerous, especially to employees exposed daily. According to the Surgeon General and the CDC, there was no risk-free level of exposure. Burning tobacco indoors released nicotine, particulates, carbon monoxide, tars, and chemicals to help regulate the burning rate. The compound attached to the air, was inhaled by employees and guests, and deposited onto surfaces as a film. The Strip did not designate nonsmoking areas for restaurants and gambling areas until the mid-2000s. Dr. Harold Boyer remembered during the 1950s "not being able to see across the casino because there was so much smoke-filled air." The women wore beautiful gowns, but when they came home they "smelled like a tobacco pot." But "that was the way it was [at that time], so you can imagine what it was like smoking and having it in our lungs." Another local doctor, Dr. Leonard Kreisler, had a similar impression, even determining that the NTS's tunnels had "better air quality" than local casinos.[61]

The resorts installed sophisticated ventilation technology, but it did not reduce the risk. The systems removed large particles, but small fragments and gases still remained in the air. The operation of heating, ventilating, and air conditioning systems also distributed secondhand smoke throughout the resort. Even a well-ventilated casino contained metabolized nicotine levels 300 to 600 percent higher than in other smoking workplaces. Secondhand smoke regularly affected employees' heart, blood, and vascular systems, and increased the prevalence of heart disease. Brief exposure contributed to respiratory symptoms as well, irritating and damaging airway linings and triggering asthma, cough, phlegm, wheezing, and breathlessness. Secondhand smoke was a human carcinogen as well, containing more than fifty chemicals that cause lung, breast, and other cancers. One study found that smoke-filled casinos contained fifty times more cancer-causing particles than highways and city streets congested with diesel traffic during rush hour.[62]

Dealers, waitresses, and security guards were most affected by secondhand smoke. Whereas guests had the option to smoke outside, employees could not leave their positions to breathe clean air or ask guests not to light up. The resorts facilitated the problem, selling tobacco products on the casino floor and gift shops, and providing free cigarettes and cigars to high rollers. Management also did not monitor employees for secondhand smoke complications because they were not liable; the law specifically allowed patrons to smoke freely indoors.

In 2005 a group of blackjack dealers from Bally's, Paris, and Caesars Palace contacted NIOSH to conduct a confidential study of secondhand smoke in their workplaces. Investigators conducted three on-site evaluations at each resort, conducting indoor air quality tests and biomarker assessments of more than a hundred nonsmoking dealers. The results were not surprising. NIOSH found numerous tobacco components in the air, including nicotine, 4-vinyl pyride, respirable dust, solanesol, benzene, toluene, p-dichloromethane, naphthalene, formaldehyde, and acetakdehyde. Although it determined that dealers were in the ninetieth percentile of exposure to secondhand smoke in comparison to the general population, it concluded that all employees were at risk. Dealers had a higher incidence of respiratory symptoms compared to administrative and engineering employees, but the difference was not statistically significant. Tobacco components above the EPA safety threshold were found in all areas of the resort. Since secondhand smoke traveled through air currents and air ducts, it even contaminated nonsmoking areas considered safe.[63]

Dramatic cases of indoor air pollution on the Strip were rare, but they did occur. The Landmark experienced a resort-wide failure involving carbon monoxide. On July 15, 1977, the resort hosted a national convention for the Disabled American Veterans, and had nine hundred guests and employees on property. At 4:10 A.M., a water pipe burst in the subbasement and short-circuited the main power panel, telephone system, air conditioning, and all but one elevator. The power surge also ruptured a refrigerator line in the butcher shop. When the emergency auxiliary generator turned on, carbon monoxide, phosgene, and Freon traveled through the ventilation ducts. Don Thompson, a guest staying at the resort, said the fumes smelled sweet, and he knew something was wrong. His friend Robert Schriever also became ill, and began sweating profusely. Thompson tried to call the telephone operator for medical assistance, but the line did not work. The elevators were out as well, so he took the stairs to the lobby to get help. On his way back up to his room, Thompson remembered having extreme shortness of breath. He knew something was wrong, and began knocking on room doors to alert other guests. Meanwhile, Schriever's wife Sue collapsed and had to be carried out with a wet cloth covering her face. At 7:00 A.M., hotel manager Robert Anthony ordered a resort-wide evacuation, instructing security guards to rouse sleeping guests and gamblers in the casino. Anthony recalled that the evacuees did not panic. Fifteen minutes later, an ambulance arrived for Schriever and the fire department sent an intensive care unit to inspect the situation.[64]

Five ambulances, three intensive care units, and the police and fire departments arrived, and Operation Disaster began. Outfitted in gas masks, firefighters entered the Landmark, evacuating hundreds of unconscious and semiconscious guests and employees, and providing oxygen bottles to those sickened by the fumes. Most evacuees sat on the resort's front steps and lawn, gasping for air, crying, and vomiting. Paramedics loaded the critically injured onto stretchers or wheelchairs, and transported them to local hospitals. Since so many patients had been sleeping, some were unconscious and incapacitated, and the hospitals admitted them as John Doe or Jane Doe. A spokesman for Sunrise Hospital reported that many patients had delayed responses to the exposure. One person went to another resort after evacuating and reported symptoms hours later. In the end, there were few serious complications. According to Southern Nevada Memorial Hospital's toxicology reports, 106 patients were treated with carbon dioxide levels varying from 10 to 20 percent. Most were middle aged and elderly individuals who had been attending the Disabled American Veterans convention. The event produced one fatality. Frank Gulla, an attendee of the convention, had a history of heart disease but no signs of recent activity. The county medical examiner determined that his cause of death was carbon monoxide poisoning.[65]

Indoor air pollution also tested entertainers' ability to perform on a daily basis. The poor air quality, coupled with the dry, desert climate, heavy air conditioning, and strenuous show schedules were especially troublesome for singers. Many developed laryngitis, a disorder that became known as Vegas throat. During or following a performance, their larynxes became inflamed, rendering them unable to talk or sing. The condition garnered considerable media attention during the 1970s. Headliners such as Dionne Warwick and Neil Sedaka complained about the risk. The only way Warwick could sing in Las Vegas was to speak as little as possible. Sedaka reportedly turned off his room's air conditioning unit and set up humidifiers. However, not all singers were afflicted. Wayne Newton called Vegas throat absurd, citing that he worked fourteen days straight and never developed it. He contended that most entertainers did not take care of themselves. They partied, drank heavily, did not get enough rest, and were not used to playing two shows a night, seven days a week. Bad behavior therefore strained their vocal chords, not the desert. Still, the resorts recognized that Vegas throat was a problem, and hired otolaryngologists to manage disorders of the ear, nose, and throat. Singers received treatment before their performances, at intermission, and after the show. During construction of the Colosseum in the early 2000s, Caesars Palace installed special technology, including a $2 million humidifier, to protect Celine Dion's voice.[66]

All entertaining jobs on the Strip involved an element of risk. Each show involved complex production with numerous moving parts. Musicians and dancers entertained large venues, lounges, and bars, and the stage crew unloaded and dismantled sets, and worked on elevated platforms, scaffold structures, ladders, and underground in the stage pit. Objects regularly fell from the elaborate sets, and ventilation issues were a common problem. Concert devices—lasers, pyrotechnics, fog and smoke machines—could also malfunction. Major productions required complex stunts and choreography on uneven platforms and stairs, aerial aerobatics requiring suspension on wires, swings launching performers into the air and water, and the use of roller blades, stilts, and cycles in confined spaces. The bigger the performance was, the more risk was involved. In 2012 alone, fifty-three performers in the Strip's Cirque du Soleil shows were injured, causing 918 missed workdays. During thirty years in the business, Cirque never experienced an onstage fatality until June 29, 2013 when, during the final scene of "KÀ" at the MGM Grand, veteran acrobatic performer Sarah Guyard-Guillot plummeted ninety-three feet to her death. It was the second time that a Cirque show had been halted due to safety concerns that week. During a preview performance of "Michael Jackson One," an aerialist slipped through a slack rope and suffered a mild concussion. Cirque was a reputable, safety-conscious company, and served as a reminder that Strip entertainment involved inherent hazards, even in productions considered safe.[67]

Onstage props like wild animals also put entertainers and guests at risk. Animal acts have been a longtime staple of entertainment on the Strip. The Stardust's long-running "Lido de Paris" paraded elephants on stage. During the 1970s, the Ruppert Bears appeared in Frederic Apcar's "Casino de Paris" at the Dunes; two-hundred-pound Scandinavian brown bears drove cars, rode bicycles, and walked on a tightrope. Between shows, a bear named Susie "played" the slots, baccarat, and craps on the casino floor alongside guests. Her trainer helped count her winnings.⁶⁸ During the 1980s, the Tropicana and Flamingo built a bird atrium outdoors and by 1989 the Mirage had put lions, dolphins, and other exotic animals on full display to complement their headliners Siegfried and Roy. During the mid-1990s, the MGM Grand put a lion habitat inside its casino; later, the Mandalay Bay constructed an impressive shark reef exhibit with fish and reptiles.

Elephants, bears, tigers, and sharks attracted business, but they were still wild animals. Any disturbance could provoke an attack. Besides flesh wounds, an animal bite or scratch could spread disease, increasing the risk of infections and infestations. The highest profile animal attack on the Strip involved a white Bengal tiger. For more than thirteen years, Roy Horn and Siegfried Fischbacher headlined at the Mirage. Their show "Siegfried and Roy" blended magical illusions with exotic animals, attracting international attention and acclaim. It was so popular that the duo signed a lifetime contract in 2001. Fischbacher worked as a traditional illusionist and Horn, a fearless animal trainer, handled the tigers. During a 7:30 P.M. show on October 3, 2013, a six-hundred-pound tiger named Montecore grabbed Horn's neck and dragged him backstage in front of a live audience. Horrified onlookers recalled him looking like a rag doll in the tiger's mouth and could hear his screams from behind the curtains. After the incident, Horn suffered substantial blood loss, had a massive stroke, and was partially paralyzed. At the UMC trauma center, doctors performed a decompressive craniotomy, removing part of his skull to relieve brain swelling, and transferred him to UCLA Medical Center in Los Angeles for long-term recovery and rehabilitation. The situation could have been much worse if the tiger had punctured a major artery. The incident demonstrated the risk of working with wild animals and the need for improved safety measures to protect audience members. No barriers existed between the tigers and guests, which could have provoked the attack. Steve Wynn believed the tiger became distracted by a woman with a large hairdo sitting in the front row. When she tried to touch the tiger, Horn jumped between them. Both Wynn and Fischbacher claimed that the tiger was trying to protect Horn, not kill him, dragging him offstage to safety like a cub. A year later, Horn claimed that the tiger sensed that he was suffering a stroke onstage. "I started feeling kind of weak...[and] Montecore saw that I was falling down. So he actually took me and brought me to the other exit where everybody could get me and help me." Audience members told a different story. Several remembered Horn hitting the tiger on the nose with a microphone to get his attention. The tiger got upset and dragged his trainer offstage like prey. Regardless of the tiger's motives, one thing was for sure: tigers are wild animals, even if they're well trained.[69]

Although working with animals involved risk, human beings were far more dangerous to employee and guest safety. According to the DOL, violence caused the most fatalities in the service industry. In fact, hospitality reported higher rates of occupational violence than the police department. Two types of violence occurred on the Strip: violence directed toward a specific person, or unintentional, implicit violence. Disgruntled employees, frustrated with coworkers, working conditions, or lack of upward mobility, were more likely to engage in threatening or violent behavior. Violence between coworkers was common, prompting the resorts such as Harrah's Entertainment to post rules forbidding "fighting or the use of physical force against another person."[70]

Casino heists were also a violent threat. When mob associates ran the Strip, robberies were rare. After corporations assumed ownership, takeover style robberies increased substantially. During the 1990s robbers were said to be more daring, and people more violent. Armed men approached the cashier cage, demanding cash payments. Some robberies involved minimal violence, with robbers collecting the money and retreating. Others involved bodily harm or ended in dramatic shootouts. From 1998 to 2000, a series of heists occurred at the Treasure Island, Bellagio, New York–New York, Mandalay Bay, Desert Inn, and MGM Grand. On October 30, 2000, a gunman at the Treasure Island jumped over a casino cage at 12:30 A.M., pistol-whipped the cashier, collected the money, and fired shots at security guards as he fled. After the incident, the Treasure Island installed bars to prevent entrance. A month later, a surprised robber saw the bars and fired shots into the cage. Frustrated, he shot a security guard in the back and left. Luckily, the victim survived.[71]

In many ways, violence became synonymous with the Strip's social environment. The site sold sin and excess, encouraging guests to gamble, drink, and dine. In return, Las Vegas promised, "What happens here, stays here." Patrons could party all day and night, engaging in sex and fantasy with no consequences for bad behavior. The setting naturally bred violence, fueled by intoxication, fatigue, loss of funds, aggression, sexual frustration, and other issues. Parking lot and hotel room muggings were common. Everyone was susceptible to unruly guests, even headliners. On February 18, 1973, four drunk men tried to jump onstage during Elvis Presley's midnight show at the Las Vegas Hilton. Bodyguards and hotel security immediately intercepted three of them, but one made it through. When Presley offered to shake the man's hand, he lunged at the singer. Presley dropkicked him and sent the man flying offstage, breaking a table. One witness said Presley was "so upset that it took all of his guys to hold him back once the fight got started." After the incident, he apologized to the audience: "All I can say to any of you is, if you want to shake my hand, fine. If you want to fight, I'll whup your ass." All four men were arrested on drunk charges, but later filed a $4 million suit against Presley and the Las Vegas Hilton charging battery. Other lawsuits followed; an audience member had suffered an eye injury while one of the men tried to climb onstage. Her suit alleged that the resort "negligently failed [to protect her] from riotous guests." The Las Vegas Hilton settled out of court.[72]

The Route 91 Harvest music festival shooting on October 1, 2017, one of the deadliest mass shootings in American history that killed fifty-eight people, was a grave reminder of the dangers associated with Las Vegas Boulevard, the main road connecting the Strip. Thousands of vulnerable, distracted, and mostly intoxicated tourists walked the street daily, watching street performers and the city lights, and documenting their experiences on social media, oblivious to oncoming traffic and endless threats around them. Las Vegas Boulevard and surrounding streets have always been prone to violence, but the violent crime rate increased during the megaresort era. Prior to the Route 91 shooting, the most infamous act of violence involved rapper Tupac Shakur in 1996: Shakur was at the Strip for the Mike Tyson versus

Bruce Seldon boxing match at the MGM Grand. After the fight, he had an altercation with a man near the resort's lobby, and headed to a nearby club in a BMW. While stopped at a red light at Flamingo Boulevard and Koval Lane, a shooter in a light-colored Cadillac fired twelve to thirteen rounds from a high-powered, semiautomatic handgun at his car. Four bullets struck Shakur in the pelvis, right hand, thigh, and lung. He died six days later. At a red light at Las Vegas and Flamingo Boulevards in 2013, Ammar Harris fired at least five rounds from his Range Rover at Kenneth Cherry Jr.'s neighboring Maserati. Cherry's car then crashed into a taxicab and exploded, killing driver Michael Boldon and his passenger, Sandra Sutton-Wasmund. In 2015 Lakeisha Holloway intentionally drove her vehicle into a crowd of pedestrians standing in front of Planet Hollywood north of Harmon Avenue. With her three-year-old child in the backseat, she plowed down the sidewalk until reaching Bally's, killing one person and injuring thirty-five.[73]

Given the risk associated with postindustrial work on the Strip, an occupational health regime developed to address the hazards and eventually the health requirements of the community. But the process took time. Until the late 1960s, the resorts did not emphasize health and safety, and only adopted basic industry standards. In comparison to other industries, hospitality appeared relatively safe, and the resorts were brand new. Management instituted safety guidelines outlining proper lifting and avoiding slips, trips, and falls, but provided little other instruction. Like the Boulder Canyon Project and BMI before it, the resorts also followed state mandate and supplied their employees with workers' compensation through the NIC. Eventually, high numbers of NIC claims and frequent labor turnover forced management to reevaluate their health and safety policy. The El Rancho moved disabled employees to new, safer positions, and distributed a booklet outlining workplace safety. The resort instructed their painters affected by lead poisoning or in advanced years to not stand on high scaffoldings due to the potential of dizzy spells. They also moved disabled employees to positions related to painting but without the hazards, such as wall washing or furniture polishing. The policies solved some of their compensation claims. The thinking was that longtime employees would have greater loyalty to the resort, limiting the number of hospitalizations and benefit payments. Management also offered new health and life insurance policies, as well as union benefits. For example, the American Guild of Variety Artists (AGVA), an entertainment union representing the showrooms and cabarets, provided welfare benefits to participating members. Its employment contract mandated a contribution from all the resorts, with the employees' duration of engagement days determining the amount.[74]

Corporate management streamlined health awareness and safety protocol. Although no department was completely devoted to safety, the new management hired inspectors to investigate conditions, outlined safety policies in the employee manual, and issued pamphlets and flyers that stressed accident prevention. They also established emergency procedures in the event of a fire, bomb threat, and civil disturbance. Howard Hughes's Summa Corporation told its Landmark employees that it was good business to prevent accidents, and safety was more important than expediency and taking shortcuts. Management instructed employees to report accidents to their department heads and security department, and file claims immediately with workers' compensation. The Summa Corporation strove to achieve a zero-accident workplace. Management at the Stardust applied a preventive approach to health and safety, instructing its employees to report hazards directly to their supervisors, regardless of how small. It offered safety classes as well, covering essentials such as heavy lifting. The Sands hosted a fire prevention class in its parking lot. Employee graduates received a certificate of completion.[75]

The Strip did not emphasize safety programs until the 1970s, but the resorts always supplied employees with medical care. Like industrial employment, management recognized that healthy employees ensured profitability, costing less than compensation payments. Management contracted to third-party health insurance carriers, or employees received union benefits. However, Las Vegas still needed more hospitals and medical talent. As in previous decades, the medical infrastructure struggled to accommodate the growing population. The Las Vegas Hospital operated throughout the postwar period, but failed to expand without the direction of Dr. Roy Martin. After the development of the Strip, hundreds of employees moved to Las Vegas, and the resorts needed to augment local medicine to treat them all. At first, its workforce sought care at Southern Nevada Memorial Hospital, later renamed UMC. The nonprofit, county hospital evolved significantly during the postwar period, thanks to federal funding during World War II and the Hill-Burton Act.[76] Hill-Burton loaned federal funds to improve America's hospital system to achieve a minimum of 4.5 beds for each one thousand people. The understaffed and overcrowded county hospital was a perfect candidate, desperately needing modernization. Hill-Burton ultimately invested more than $2 million in Southern Nevada Memorial, which eased the crisis somewhat. In the 1960s the hospital innovated trauma care, opening an innovative burn treatment unit. During that decade there were twenty-four burn units in the nation and the one in Las Vegas was the only one in a ten-thousand-square-mile radius, serving parts of Arizona, California, and Utah. Founding Drs. John Batdorf and Kirk V. Cammack Jr. hosted visiting doctors from UCLA and other top-tier hospitals who wanted to pattern their programs after it. Southern Nevada Memorial also expanded to accommodate 285 beds, an intensive care unit, and emergency and cardiac care equipment. It also finally had the capacity to host sophisticated surgeries, ending the need to transfer its most critical cases to Los Angeles. Thoracic surgeon Dr. Harold Feikes acquired a heart–lung machine as well, and performed the first open-heart surgery in Las Vegas. In the 1970s the hospital continued to grow, functioning as a major medical center in the West and teaching institution for physicians, nurses, and ancillary specialties associated with the University of Nevada School of Medicine.[77]

Eventually, the Strip also funded a for-profit, private, more luxurious facility for its employees and guests. As a county hospital, Southern Nevada Memorial required physicians to provide care to indigents. Many doctors resented the arrangement and desired to establish a private practice to expand their profits. The resorts agreed. Not only did they need a more cost-effective way to ensure the health of their employees, but management also wanted to send guests to a luxury facility located near the Strip, and not to a facility serving the poor. Local physicians therefore banded with several businessmen, including developer Irwin Molasky and casino executive Moe Dalitz, to create Sunrise Hospital. The group secured funding from First Western Savings and Loan Association and the Teamsters Union, and purchased a tract of land on Maryland Parkway. The location was carefully chosen; it was in close proximity to the Strip as well as to the Las Vegas Country Club, which could provide upscale housing and golfing to resident physicians. Since the Teamsters funded its initial construction and continued expansion, Sunrise became referred to by locals as the Teamsters Hospital. Opening in 1958, the hospital epitomized Strip luxury. It had sixty beds, a picturesque rose garden, water fountain, and mosaic tile finishes. To recruit medical talent, the hospital took another page from the Strip, offering significant perks to recruit top physicians from all over the nation. Besides considerable medical recourses, it offered free office space and cars, and the promise of getting rich. The promotion worked. Sunrise easily recruited young doctors from all over the nation, including Kirk V. Cammack Jr., who had just completed his surgical residency in Flint, Michigan. He became the second board-certified surgeon in the state of Nevada. Within a year, the hospital staffed fifty-eight physicians and surgeons.[78]

Sunrise was an immediate success, thanks to the Teamsters' funding as well as thousands of employees obliged to use the facilities. At first it functioned like a company hospital for the Strip. Jimmy Hoffa, the union's general president from 1958 to 1971, mandated that the International Brotherhood of Teamsters and Culinary Union Local 226's medical funds be paid for medical treatment only at Sunrise. Like most employee-funding health-care systems, the cost was deducted each month from the workers' paychecks. Besides caring for employees, the hospital had additional benefits. Sunrise allegedly helped the resorts in casino skimming operations and complementary medical services.[79]

Until the late 1960s, doctors regularly performed surgeries for the various crime syndicates in exchange for discretion and under-the-table cash. The practice was less frequent after the corporatization of hospitals. Kirk V. Cammack Jr. performed numerous comp surgeries at Sunrise, calling Las Vegas the "last Wild West of medicine." He once mended a gunshot wound to the abdomen for Perry "Gold-dollar" Rose, the 6-foot 6-inch bodyguard of Texas gambler Lester Ben "Benny" Binion. At a follow-up appointment, Rose overheard a family threatening Cammack with a malpractice suit over the death of their drug-addicted daughter. They dropped the suit several days later, asking him to tell "Mr. Perry Rose." When Cammack asked him about it, Rose said, "Doc, I don't know what you're talking about." Cammack called it "a malpractice suit avoided by Frontier Desert Justice, Texas Style."[80] The story is a telling example of Las Vegas medicine until the 1980s. There were seemingly no rules, and the profitability margin was huge. But the lifestyle also took a toll on the doctors' personal lives. Sin City changed them. Dr. Leonard Kreisler referred to it as becoming "Vegasized."[81]

Many doctors were family men, well trained in their specialties. But the Las Vegas lifestyle—money, sex, and glamour—consumed them. Cammack divorced his first wife after establishing his practice and went on to marry four more times. When Dr. Elias Ghanem, a thirty-three-year-old Palestinian immigrant and doctor at the Los Angeles County Hospital, arrived in 1971, he made $3,600 a month directing the emergency room at Sunrise. Within five years, he was earning $300,000 a year in private practice, got divorced, drove a $32,000 Stutz Bearcat gifted to him by Elvis Presley, wore expensive jewelry, and had a mirrored canopy over his bed. "Fast cars and beautiful women are my hobbies," he reportedly told *People* magazine in 1976.[82]

The Teamsters ultimately helped Sunrise become the largest proprietary hospital west of the Mississippi. The hospital underwent a five-story expansion in 1966, with 325 beds, and an intensive care and coronary unit. Following Hoffa's imprisonment in 1967, the era of the Teamsters abruptly ended, and Philadelphia-based American Medicorp (AMC) purchased the hospital in 1969. The acquisition marked a major change in local medicine, ushering in the expansion of corporately owned, for-profit hospitals to address the needs of the growing population. Similar to corporations taking over the Strip, the shift in management also introduced new forms of business administration. Without the Teamsters requiring its members to use the hospital, Sunrise's new management team reconfigured its marketing strategy, embarking on a very aggressive advertising campaign. One program offered a revolving charge courtesy card to entice patients on the weekend, providing a 5.25 percent rebate for Friday and Saturday admittance. Another scheme entered patients into a lottery that gave away a Mediterranean cruise if they scheduled surgeries on Monday but checked in on Saturday. Since managed care did not exist yet, there was very little oversight. Dr. Otto Ravenholt described Sunrise during the 1970s as, "[It was] like getting customers into your casino who had a credit card that you could charge everything to—and they did!" The programs were nevertheless controversial, garnering national attention for attracting patients. Eventually, advertising became a staple in American medicine, increasing in popularity during the 1980s and 1990s.[83]

Besides Sunrise, in-house and on-call physicians supported the occupational health regime, treating employees and guests on site. The concept of establishing in-house medical treatment on the Strip gained popularity during the 1960s, and became a staple during corporatization. Similar to industrial workplaces, the resorts hired company doctors trained in internal medicine as permanent members of the staff. The doctors maintained on-site offices, providing immediate medical treatment to workers and guests during daytime hours. A full-time, medical professional on site benefited the resorts twofold. The doctors could monitor and treat employee injuries immediately, ensuring a healthy workforce. As an added luxury, they also provided premier and immediate care to entertainers and guests. Dr. Thomas Newman, the Las Vegas Hilton company doctor, earned the nickname "Flash" because he seemingly appeared instantly to supply headliners with drugs. Dr. Joseph L. Fink, the Caesars Palace company doctor, treated employees and guests in a medical suite built exclusively for him. When Fink, an internist and diagnostician, noticed that most of his house calls were on the Strip, he moved his entire practice on property in 1972. He practiced there for more than three decades.[84]

The resorts retained on-call doctors as well, a service reserved for guests and entertainers. On call at nine resorts, Elias Ghanem famously treated headliners Elvis Presley, Robert Goulet, Liberace, Tom Jones, and Johnny Cash. When asked about his practice on the Strip, he said, "A lot of people come here and they gamble two or three days straight. They want something to make them sleep. They have heart attacks, sometimes while they are at a show. And there is hysteria. One girl at Elvis' show was so hysterical we had to hold her down.... I think it is the personal touch that [the headliners] like [from on-call treatment]. They call at 2 o'clock in the morning and I go."[85]

Besides on-call services, Ghanem augmented the occupational health regime by innovating a Preferred Provider Organization (PPO)–style of medical services, establishing the first of many outpatient clinics, Las Vegas Medical Centers, in 1977. After the opening of the MGM Grand, more employees moved to Las Vegas and, once again, local hospitals could not accommodate the influx of patients. Ghanem provided a solution, opening a clinic behind the Hilton that contracted with the resorts to provide health care to guests and employees. His style of quick, clinic-style care became a staple in Las Vegas medicine, expanding throughout the valley during the 1990s. From 1991 to 1998, Ghanem's clinics offered complimentary medical care to 550 Frontier employees on strike, delivering more than one hundred babies for free. During his fourteen-year tenure with the Nevada Athletic Commission, he also protected the health and safety of the Strip's prize-fighters, instituting important safety measures; mandating HIV, Hepatitis B, and Hepatitis C testing; and enhancing protection in the boxing rings. When reports surfaced that Evander Holyfield had a hole in his heart, Ghanem refused to let him fight until further testing. "I have to wear hats because I am on the commission and we generally want fights," he explained, but "I am also a doctor."[86]

With corporations assuming ownership of the resorts and the continued expansion of occupational health regimes, the Strip appeared to be a safe, postindustrial workplace. The institution of OSHA and NIOSH also extended protection to all private sector employees, researching and implementing improved methods for health and safety. After the passage of the federal OSH Act, states followed suit. Before 1970, every state had passed an assortment of workers' compensation and health and safety laws, but most lacked an administrative agency completely devoted to occupational health. Nevada passed its first Nevada OSH Act in 1955, but it was largely ineffective. In 1973 it redrafted its Act and became one of twenty-seven states approving a statewide agency, the Nevada OSHA. Operating under the NIC, its federal counterpart

OSHA provided up to 50 percent of its operating costs. After becoming operational, Nevada OSHA tried to establish a presence in Nevada industries, outlining a program to eliminate known hazards that could cause serious injury or death. It distributed handbooks on accident prevention, began conducting inspections, and published a pamphlet, "Occupational Safety and Health Standards." On the Strip, it set new requirements for management to hire an employee or department entirely devoted to health and safety, and establish programs based on four components: employee education, self-inspection, accident investigation, and recordkeeping.[87]

The resorts were initially resistant to the suggestions. In comparison to industrial workplaces marred by mechanical and chemical dangers, the newly built Strip seemed like a refuge from occupational diseases and hazards. Moreover, the financial cost of establishing departments devoted to safety seemed excessive and unneeded. Nevada OSHA eventually rescinded its costlier requests, compromising with the resorts to enhance existing programs, and devoted increased energy to education about the importance of workplace safety.[88]

OSHA and NIOSH concentrated their efforts on curtailing the risk of radiation, chemicals, lead, vinyl chloride, and industrial hazards throughout the 1970s, but tragedies continued across the nation, including the Love Canal neighborhood pollution disaster and partial nuclear meltdown at the Three Mile Island Nuclear Generating Station. A new risk also loomed in the postindustrial realm. Prior to the 1970s, resorts on the Strip resembled beachfront hotels, built low and sprawling. As the structures increased in size, so did the hazards, increasing the rate of construction-related injuries. Taylor Construction Company was the most prominent construction contractor in Las Vegas, building Caesars Palace, Riviera, International, and MGM Grand. The latter two were the largest megaresorts in the world, with 1,512 rooms at the thirty-story International and twenty-two hundred rooms at the twenty-six-story MGM Grand. During construction, construction workers faced similar hazards to past jobs, but on a grander scale. Electrocutions and falls were common, as well as injuries from heavy equipment and inhalation of dust or other toxic particles. Kerkorian also put immense pressure on the crew to finish both resorts in record time. Coupled with inadequate risk perception, accidents increased tenfold.[89]

The size of the megaresort increased construction hazards, but the real threat involved building code deficiencies, a problem horribly evident during the MGM Grand and Las Vegas Hilton (formally the International) fires in 1980 and 1981. Fires regularly occurred on the Strip, but were usually small and quickly contained. The first major fire occurred at the El Rancho on June 16, 1960; a kitchen fire ignited the resort's trademark fifty-foot windmill, engulfing it in flames. After the roof collapsed, the windmill dramatically crashed into the casino. Structural damage closed the resort permanently, but there was only one reported injury, a fireman with a cut hand. The sprawling, low de-sign of the resort helped minimize damages, allowing employees and guests to easily locate exits. Most guests were also sleeping in cottages 150 feet away, and not affected by the smoke and flames. In another incident in the early 1960s, a welder accidently lit the Sahara's roof-top on fire during an air-conditioning install, resulting in $1 million in damages. Similar to the El Rancho, the hotel portion of the resort was not connected to the casino. The *Las Vegas Sun* reported that "life went on as usual at the swimming pool [as] swimmers splashed and floated on their backs while firemen scampered along the roof fight-ing the flames." Several people were adversely affected by the smoke, including hotel executive Herb McDonald, an employee, and a few firemen, but there were no casualties. Small fires continued to occur throughout the decade. In 1969 a blaze at the Stardust injured seven-teen people. One died during the incident from a heart attack. Several years later, a Holiday Inn manager died from smoke inhalation after falling asleep while smoking in a bed at the resort.[90]

Since the resorts were built horizontally, fatalities were few. Verti-cal construction changed everything. The MGM Grand fire and deadly outcome was directly related to deficiencies overlooked in the new megaresort design. During its construction from 1970 to 1973, Taylor Construction Company followed the Uniform Building Code (UBC) Standard, 1970 edition. But the resort met only minimum code re-quirements that were intended for much smaller structures. There was also little oversight evaluating its construction, because OSHA was just established and Nevada OSHA did not yet exist. The job rested on Clark County fire marshal Carl Lowe, who inspected the construction site but did not have the authority to enforce safety precautions. Lowe suggested installing a comprehensive sprinkler system throughout the property, but the resort put sprinklers only in the basement, showrooms, and a twenty-sixth-floor high roller casino converted into meeting rooms. He also recommended following the UBC Standard that all materials be made of fire resistant or noncombustible materials. The resort ignored the suggestion, and installed highly flammable cellulose acoustical ceiling tiles and adhesives throughout the resort. In the early 1970s there was ample evidence that adhesives were a fire-spread substance; the state of Connecticut had already banned their use. In terms of décor, the resort also approved use of carpets and slot machines containing harmful plastics. During the fire, the materials fueled the flames, creating a deadly combination of toxins. Moreover, the new construction design turned the stairwells and HVAC system into chimneys, spreading smoke throughout the casino and upper floors. The fire system amplifier failed, delaying notification to employees and guests, the exits were unclearly marked, and emergency doors and exit routes locked. The resort had not installed a paging system or automatic smoke detection system, and did not have a fire control room. The gigantic resort also had failed to outline evacuation instructions.[91]

In the early morning of November 21, 1980, an electrical fire in the MGM Grand ignited a pie display case in the Deli restaurant and smoldered for several hours. An employee discovered the fire and opened the door, after which the flames quickly spread to the ceiling. The flammable ceiling tiles, carpet plastics, wallpaper, PVC piping, and adhesives fed the fire, forming a massive fireball multiplying nineteen feet per second that burst through the front entrance, engulfing valet attendants, guests, and parked cars with flames. As the casino turned into an inferno, oblivious players continued to gamble. Firefighters removed most of them without sustaining significant injuries, but guests sleeping in the tower were not as lucky. The smoke raced up the stairwells and elevator shafts, cultivating lethal conditions from the eighteenth floor up. Faulty smoke dampers also circulated the fumes throughout the HVAC system, accelerating the toxicity. No alarm sounded, leaving the guests completely unaware of the advancing fire. A National Fire Protection Association study later revealed guests did not exhibit panic behavior, and rationally attempted to save their lives. After smelling the smoke, most guests banded together, knocking on doors, offering refuge, putting towels around the doors, and opening balcony doors or breaking windows to disseminate the smoke. Several groups attempted to escape, one of the most tragic stories of the MGM Grand fire. Reminiscent of the 1911 Triangle Shirtwaist Company fire in New York, the doors locked behind them after they entered the stairways. Trapped, the majority succumbed to carbon monoxide poisoning. Others fought the conditions and reached the roof. The most fatalities occurred on the twentieth and twenty-third floors, with fourteen deaths each.[92]

At 8:00 A.M., Dr. Otto Ravenholt, director of the Clark County Emergency Medical Services (EMS) system and coroner, heard the Strip had an all-alarm fire. He arrived to a shocking and "chaotic sight.... One didn't need details to know that this was a major disaster in progress.... Dark plumes of smoke" rose from the resort as firefighters and victims scrambled around equipment pieces. Since five thousand guests and employees occupied the resort, Clark County firefighters enlisted the help of Nellis Air Force Base helicopters to contain the blaze and rescue victims. Two-thirds had been evacuated when Ravenholt arrived. Most guests wore pajamas and no shoes. All of them were in a state of shock.[93]

At 9:00 A.M., Ravenholt entered the resort to help the evacuation effort. The first thing that surprised him was that supposedly noncombustible materials fueled the fire. He remembered seeing sculptures not considered flammable burning because the temperatures were so high. According to Ravenholt, the rescue mission was physically demanding. The twenty-six-story resort had no working elevators, and rescuers climbed the stairs looking for survivors. Worried about the media coverage, Ravenholt instructed firefighters to move the deceased to a side room instead of to the front of the hotel. Physically moving the dead also competed with saving victims that were still alive. Ravenholt described the evacuation process as a "very dramatic business." Firemen extended ladders to rescue victims on the first ten floors, and helicopters evacuated floors 11 to 26. Employees and guests leaned "out of the windows with black soot coming from their nostrils or towels over their faces" while the firefighters tied ropes around them and pulled them to safety. The rescuers evacuated more than seven hundred people. Still, there were many casualties. Ravenholt found a bell captain looking out an open window in a tipped-back chair. He was "sitting on the chair with his toes sticking up, dead," which "was the case with ten to twenty people." They died "completely unsuspecting in their rooms" or while waiting for the emergency to pass. Even survivors were "essentially walking wounded"; while not brought out on stretchers, they were exposed to high levels of poisonous gas and lacked oxygen.[94]

Ravenholt eventually retreated for the temporary fire department headquarters at the Barbary Coast, tasked with the job of determining the number of deceased. The figure started at twenty. At 10:30 A.M., he raised it to seventy. The number was difficult to determine. Ravenholt explained: "Only the bodies in the casino had been burned. A half dozen were severely charred, having been near the registration area when the fire swept across the top of the casino. There had [also] been several earlier Air Force helicopter transports of bodies from the roof to the morgue." Ravenholt initially determined eighty-three people died. Two days later, a female employee was found in a service elevator on the twenty-sixth floor. An eighty-fifth victim died several weeks later. Fatalities in the tower were attributed to asphyxiation secondary to carbon monoxide poisoning, with levels ranging from 25 to 66 percent saturation. The rest succumbed to smoke, burns, and myocarditis.[95] One woman died of a massive skull fracture after she jumped from the tower. More than six hundred people suffered major fire-related injuries, most of them due to smoke inhalation.[96]

The fire was devastating for the Strip, calling into question major concerns about the safety of the megaresort design. Governor Robert List appointed a panel chaired by Kenny Guinn and Thalia Dondero to recommend reforms to prevent it from happening again. But the effort stalled; at the urging of several state senators and resort management, the panel recommended against installing and retrofitting the hotels with room sprinklers due to cost concerns. It took another tragedy, the Las Vegas Hilton fire, to force change. After the MGM Grand fire, tensions ran high on the Strip. Two arson attempts occurred at the Royal American and Dunes. In both cases, an arsonist ignited drapes and bedspreads, but employees were able to extinguish the flames. On February 10, 1981, Philip Bruce Cline, a busboy at the Las Vegas Hilton, claimed he dropped a cigarette while engaging in sex. It torched nearby drapes, burst out the window, and dramatically climbed up the side of the thirty-story resort. Small fires also started in a storage room and service elevator on the second and third floors, and somebody stuffed a hose with combustible material on the ninth floor. The smaller fires discredited Cline's story, clearly pointing to arson. Like MGM Grand, the Las Vegas Hilton had no sprinklers, smoke detectors, or public warning systems. It had a manual pull alarm, but it malfunctioned. Unlike the previous fire, mass panic ensued. Many guests broke their windows, scaling the tower on ropes of sheets, or rushed stairwells to escape the suffocating smoke. There were 242 reported injuries. Eight people died. One person jumped or fell to his death onto the tennis courts, and the others succumbed to smoke inhalation.[97]

During the months following the fires, there was panic on the Strip. Another arson attempt occurred at Caesars Palace, but employees confined the flames to one hotel room. During Cline's trial, copycat arsonists set dozens of small fires to buildings on and adjacent to the Strip. In one weekend, the fire department reported sixteen separate fires at two resorts and an apartment building. Acts of violence also threatened other postindustrial sites, including the bombing at Harvey's Wagon Wheel at Lake Tahoe in August 1980. The event put the resorts on high alert after receiving several threats. In 1984 management refused to expand employee health insurance coverage, prompting a violent strike involving seventeen thousand workers. "It was an interesting time, but a difficult one," remembered Senator Richard Bryan. "It was protracted, and it was ugly. Las Vegas received a lot of negative publicity." On April 12, 1984, an explosive detonated in the MGM Grand swimming pool, causing minor damage and no injuries. When police investigated bomb threats at the other resorts, they discovered a small bomb between two slot machines at the Tropicana.[98]

As the resorts increased security, the occupational health regimes united to make the Strip safe again. The MGM Grand and Las Vegas Hilton fires revealed that the new megaresort design required a massive reevaluation of safety protocol. The UBC Standard, used at both resorts, contained codes dating back to the 1940s. Most importantly, it did not deal with the dangers of high-rise buildings. The megaresort was a different kind of postindustrial space, with high-rise towers, shopping malls, atriums, and the widespread use of harmful plastic materials. Moreover, the MGM Grand and Las Vegas Hilton were not the only resorts needing fire protection; the entire Strip was at risk. A Clark County manager report named eleven resorts that lacked comprehensive sprinkler systems. Five months after the MGM Grand fire, the Nevada state legislature passed the strictest fire protection standards in the nation, mandating comprehensive sprinkler systems in buildings more than fifty-five feet high. Even before the new standards, the MGM Grand voluntarily installed a $5 million fire and safety system. Although it had been a "long trying time," President Bernard Rothkopf promised employees that their workplace would bounce back as the "most luxurious" and "one of the safest hotels in the world." It marked the first time management emphasized safety to their employees, rhetoric that became a key feature of employment on the Strip thereafter.[99]

The MGM Grand and Las Vegas Hilton fires also inspired an unprecedented industrywide response to raise fire protection standards across the nation. Both resorts were newly built and code compliant, debunking the misconception that fires were only a concern in old buildings and postindustrial workplaces were completely safe. In 1981 the National Fire Protection Association published a detailed overview of the MGM Grand fire, exposing the widespread threat throughout the hospitality industry, and issuing a set of code compliance and safety requirements. Slowly, hotels and motels across the nation began to install or retrofit existing sprinkler systems. In 1980 only one out of nine hotel and motel fires in the United States had sprinkler systems. Detectors existed in one-fourth. In 1997 two-thirds of high-rise buildings had installed sprinkler systems and three-fourths had fire detectors. The new level of protection helped dramatically lower the number of hospitality fires as well as fire-related deaths. After 1983 there have been only two hotel fires in the United States that killed ten people or more. The influence of Nevada's strict fire standards spread globally as well. Hilton and other multinational corporations voluntarily retrofitted sprinklers in their international hotels as well, and other countries began mandating the use of sprinkler systems in high-rise buildings.[100]

Besides inspiring fire protection standards, the MGM Grand fire had profound legal ramifications, helping further prioritize health and safety in postindustrial spaces, and establishing important legal precedent for mass disaster litigation and retroactive insurance policies. The restitution trial, In re MGM Grand, had two thousand plaintiffs and more than one hundred defendants, including the resort and its construction contractors, architects, engineers, and suppliers. The claims consolidated into 1,327 lawsuits against 118 companies. Special Master Michael A. Cherry supervised the scheduling and handling of more than 4 million documents and fourteen hundred depositions, with Judge Louis C. Bechtle of the U.S. District Court for the Eastern District of Pennsylvania presiding. MGM Grand executives knew that their existing $30 million insurance policy would not cover the claims, so they acquired a retroactive insurance policy for an additional $170 million. Backdated to November 1, 1980, this type of supplementary insurance was unprecedented; it involved approximately thirty insurance carriers in four different insurance layers. The companies authorized the deal based on the assumption that it would be a long settlement process. In the meantime, money could be made in other investments. However, Kerkorian had other plans. He wanted to settle the lawsuit quickly, because it was bad for business. In 1983 he took matters into his own hands, directly settling all wrongful death, personal injury, property damage, and business-lost claims. The global settlement included most of the defendants, totaling $134 million. The MGM Grand alone settled its claims for $30 million, agreeing on $75 million for the remainder. Not one defendant admitted negligence.[101]

After the settlement, the retroactive insurance carriers refused to reimburse Kerkorian, so he assembled his corporate counsel and hired attorney Bill Shernoff, a specialist in insurance bad faith litigation.

Headed by Patricia Glaser, Kerkorian's counsel sought full reimburse-ment and punitive damages. But with so many insurance companies involved in the case, no courtroom existed in Las Vegas to accommo-date them all. Nevada District Court Judge Paul Goldman ordered a novel solution, requiring the companies to hire local counsel and pay $5,000 each, totaling $150,000, to build an eleven-thousand-square-foot courtroom next to the Thomas and Mack basketball arena at the University of Nevada, Las Vegas. Due to the sheer number of lawyers and parties involved, it was to be the largest trial in history. To keep order, Judge Goldman ran a strict courtroom, fining attorneys thou-sands of dollars for frivolous motions, and for not properly marking and identifying documents. According to Shernoff, "It was [Judge Goldman's] strict handling of the matter that created the climate for settlement." Beginning in the spring of 1985, the case was expected to last eight to ten months, costing approximately $345,000 a day. How-ever, after jury selection the parties approved an $87.5 million out-of-court settlement in less than a month. It was reportedly a festive affair. Shernoff recalled that "the settlement itself was quite an occa-sion. There was a big signing ceremony, after which [Judge Goldman] brought in a band for a celebration." "Champagne, rock music, and laughter filled the special courtroom," and the judge received a gift, a shirt inscribed in Latin from the lawyers that said, "You can never have too much insurance."[102]

The restitution trial and retroactive insurance suit were both land-mark cases in American legal history. *In re MGM Grand* established legal precedent in mass tort litigation, cases in which hundreds of plaintiffs sue multiple defendants for negligence. Michael Cherry, who later became a chief justice for the Nevada Supreme Court, observed that "the things we learned from [MGM Grand] paved the way for how we conduct today's massive consumer trials." Over the following decades, mass tort litigation involving toxic substances, catastrophic events, or faulty pharmaceutical products and medical devices—radioactive fall-out, chemical plant pollution or explosions, breast implants, tobacco products, and airplane crashes—all cited *In re MGM Grand*. The retro-active insurance case was also the first and last of its kind. Accord-ing to Shernoff, retroactive insurance was bad policy because it made insurers insensitive to quick settlements." Insurance carriers never sold retroactive insurance again. Fortunately for Kerkorian, he also had interruption insurance, which helped him renovate the resort and reopen it in August 1981.[103]

After the MGM Grand and Las Vegas Hilton fires, health and safety emerged as a top priority on the Strip, fostering a dramatically safer, postindustrial workplace. There were close calls, but no major disasters. Small fires, originating from electrical malfunctions, kitchen grease, cigarettes, and arson continued in isolated cases. In 1986 a jury convicted Thomas Edward Little Owl of several cases of arson, including one at the Sands. During the 1990s the under-construction Stratosphere caught fire and another Las Vegas Hilton blaze forced the evacuation of six floors and reported $1 million in damages. In 2003 a lit cigarette ignited a laundry chute, with six people treated for smoke inhalation. In 2008 the roof of the Monte Carlo, another Kerkorian-owned hotel, caught fire. As the most significant event on the Strip since the MGM Grand and Las Vegas Hilton fires, it revealed the improvements made in fire safety since 1981. While constructing a bridge on the roof, welders accidently ignited a fire that spread to the architectural façade. Since there were no detectors on the roof, the fire alarm did not sound. When president of the Monte Carlo Anton Nikodemus noticed the fire, he manually triggered the alert system and ordered an evacuation. The resort evacuated five thousand guests and nine-hundred and fifty employees. Security guards and engineers entered more than three thousand rooms to ensure every guest evacuated. The fire itself was brief, burning for only seventy-four minutes thanks to the quick response of the Clark County Fire Department. Following the incident, Fire Chief Steven Smith remarked that the MGM Fire dramatically changed fire protection and protocol on the Strip: "We have the best fire safety in the world in the resort corridor of Las Vegas." The Monte Carlo fire ultimately produced no life-threatening injuries, with only five guests and eight employees treated for smoke inhalation. Still, the hotel remained closed for several weeks due to water damage sustained from the sprinkler system on all thirty-two floors.[104]

Besides improved fire protection, the Strip's occupational health regime continued to adjust and evolve throughout the 1980s in respect to workers' compensation and employee-funded health-care options. Beginning in the 1970s, critics scrutinized the effectiveness of the NIC's state-funded workers' compensation. Both employees and employers alike voiced frustration. Employees complained of incompetence regarding the evaluation of injuries, hearing delays, and approval of surgical procedures. Frustrated with skyrocketing costs and bureaucratic hurdles, employers urged the state to allow businesses to purchase three-way coverage: the state fund, self-insurance, and private insurance. In the early 1980s reform measures began to address both parties' grievances.[105] The legislature voted to allow qualified employers to purchase self-insurance, abolishing the NIC and replacing it with the State Industrial Insurance System (SIIS), a public corporation providing workers' compensation and safety and rehabilitation services. However, the new system had disappointing results, and failed to address core issues. Medical and indemnity benefits costs continued to increase. The average SIIS premiums, per $100 of payroll, rose from $2.47 in 1988 to $3.31 in 1991. In 1999 legislatures authorized the privatization of SIIS, renaming it the Employers Insurance Company of Nevada (EICON), and allowed private companies to enter the market. With privatization, Nevada adopted a two-way workers' compensation model composed of private carriers and self-insured employers, ending the state monopoly of injury compensation that began in 1913. But while deregulation of the workers' compensation market seemed to stabilize rates and benefits, employees continued to cite problems, including poor communication, frequent changes in claim adjusters and coverage, and delays in reimbursements.[106]

The Strip's employee-funded health insurance also received a major overhaul, reflecting national trends. In the beginning, the resorts purchased fully insured plans for employees, essentially hiring insurance carriers to assume the financial risk. The plans reduced liability, but were very expensive. In the 1970s the American health-care system reached a crisis point. With no mechanisms to control prices, medical inflation increased the cost of care, hospital construction, physician salaries, pharmaceuticals, and thus, fully insured plans. President Richard Nixon attempted to fix the problem in 1973, approving the Health Maintenance Organization Act to institutionalize health maintenance organizations (HMOS). The organizations departed from their predecessors, requiring businesses with more than twenty-five employees to offer federally backed, managed care plans. Modeled after the Kaiser Permanente Medical Care Program and similar plans, HMOS established guidelines for doctors and limited the treatment available. In the 1980s costs continued to rise, prompting the Reagan administration to encourage HMOS to engage in private capital sources, and Reagan to sign the Preferred Provider Healthcare Act in 1985, which eased restrictions for PPOS. PPOS enlisted providers to agree to offer services at a discounted rate and pay a higher percentage of the costs when subscribers used in-network providers. However, unlike HMOS, PPOS also allowed subscribers to seek health care outside the plan at a higher rate.[107]

In the 1980s the Strip felt the financial burden of providing employees with fully insured benefits. Tensions reached a boiling point in 1984 after management refused to negotiate improved health insurance coverage and wages. A subsequent strike turned violent, prompting hundreds of arrests, bomb threats, and assaults. The violence had serious economic repercussions for the resorts, prompting them to reach a compromise several months later. Employees received most of their demands, resulting in an expansion of the Culinary Health Fund, a multi-employer, Taft-Hartley labor management trust fund. Members of Culinary Union Workers Union 226 received coverage for themselves, their spouse, and children, paying nothing out of their paychecks. The union also sponsored a program in which employees could purchase supplemental life, disability, and critical illness insurance.[108]

The Las Vegas medical community was initially resistant to the idea of managed care because it threatened their incomes. But as the number of organizations increased, the doctors became active participants for the guaranteed pay. Dr. Elias Ghanem in particular suggested a solution for the Strip's health insurance woes, founding his own PPO-style organization, Prime Health. In 1984 Ghanem and his associates proposed to Circus Circus Enterprises to enroll employees in a self-insured plan, a plan in which employers assumed the financial risk. The self-insured market had grown substantially since the Employee Retirement Income Security Act of 1974, reorganizing the plans and exempting them from most state-mandated benefits. Circus Circus management accepted and the program was a success, reportedly saving the resort $1 million in its first year. A year later, the Culinary Union entered a multimillion-dollar contract with Ghanem to provide health care to more than thirty thousand union members and their families. In the 1990s managed care programs like Prime Health steadily increased in popularity, but it was not a permanent solution. The plans initially helped decrease costs, but the cost of health-care premiums increased 98 percent from 2000 to 2007. In 2010 President Barak Obama signed into law the Patient Protection and Affordable Care Act (ACA), intending to reduce the number of Americans without health insurance. But rates continued to increase 20 percent in most states; Nevada had an average premium increase of more than 80 percent during the Act's first year. The insurance companies blamed the increase on the fact that new customers were more ill than they had expected.[109]

As health-care costs soared, the Strip began integrating employee wellness programs into the occupational health regime to promote healthy living, and thereby decreasing the probability of illnesses or injuries. The employee wellness program at MGM Resorts International sought to create a culture of health, articulating that Chairman Jim Murren was personally dedicated to a healthy lifestyle for himself, his employees, and their families. Management stressed its commitment ran deeper than typical employers, outlining a Healthy Living Wellness Program that fostered employee emotional and physical well-being through financial incentives. Each property provided Jim's Plate in the employee dining room, healthy options for employees to eat a balanced meal, and developed a mobile app, Healthy Eating Healthy You, on iTunes for employees to cook recipes at home. It also built a wellness center with a fun room of treadmills and computers, and contracted with Life Time Fitness to provide full-scale fitness amenities and health coaching. Employees had access to an on-call nurse that offered medical advice, and assisted in finding a physician and triage. Health professionals also provided free health screenings, such as monograms, dental care, and blood pressure checks, and a confidential Employee Assistance Program covered substance abuse, gambling addiction, grief, and weight and stress management.[110]

Harrah's Entertainment (later Caesars Entertainment) also took a proactive approach to increase employee wellness. Management developed a two-pronged plan, offering employees better health services that also cut costs for the employer. The result was Harrah's Health and Wellness Center (later Caesars Entertainment Health & Wellness Center), a $2.5 million venture operated by Whole Health Management, Inc. Opening in 2007, the nineteen-thousand-square-foot health center had a fitness complex and medical clinic. Clinical staff diagnosed and treated chronic conditions, provided vaccinations, filled prescriptions, and offered nutrition education, counseling, and physical therapy. Employees also had access to treadmills, weightlifting equipment, and yoga classes. According to Chairman Gary Loveman, the corporation wanted to provide an accessible and affordable health and wellness service directly to employees. Likewise, Boyd Gaming established a wellness program; its Healthy Rewards plan offered financial incentives to employees who lowered their blood pressure and cholesterol, and who lost weight if they had been overweight. Bob Berglund, Boyd's vice president of benefits, said management wanted to facilitate not only a culture of health, but also a culture of healthy behavior. Its main purpose was reducing health-care costs, but the culture of health had an added benefit. Along with advances in medicine, it helped increase life expectancy. In Nevada life expectancy rose from seventy-one years to almost seventy-nine years from 1980 to 2010. In 2013 the average for Clark County women was eighty-one years and eight months, and for Clark County men, seventy-six years and four months. The only problem was the longer people lived, the more health costs continued to expand.[111]

By the mid-2000s the Strip had successfully altered its regime, reinventing itself in size and amenities, as well as prioritizing health and safety in a postindustrial space. Occupational health in southern Nevada had evolved significantly from early-twentieth-century regimes. Employees no longer risked their lives for a paycheck; most perceived that the danger of working in a hazardous environment outweighed the threat of not working at all. They also held the notion that accidents were not a part of a job, and their employer was obligated to inform and protect them from harm. However, there were also similarities between the regimes that existed throughout the century. After receiving bad publicity and statistical analysis concerning hazards, productivity, and profits, employers began to embrace health and safety during the early twentieth century. Employers and employees realized it was a mutually beneficial cause, combining their interests to respond to the risks. This concept continued in subsequent regimes. Moreover, late-twentieth-century employers repurposed the idea of integrating employee wellness programs to promote healthy living, thereby decreasing the probability of illnesses or injuries. The programs were reminiscent of Los Angeles and Salt Lake Railroad (LA&SL) models, a mixture of on-site medical care and health screenings, and recreational activities to support healthy bodies and minds. The railroad expected it to help facilitate an efficient workforce, and to reduce workmen's compensation and medical costs. The Strip's goals were parallel, employing the same techniques, only expanded.

But similar to the early twentieth century as well, old problems resurfaced in a neglected part of the regime. The new set of megaresorts rose during the 2000s at the expense of the workers who built them. Twelve fatalities occurred in eighteen months during the construction of the CityCenter, Cosmopolitan, Trump, Fontainebleau, Palazzo, and Echelon, revealing serious gaps in the occupational health regime. The congested, frenzied, twenty-four-hour construction sites led to the deaths, but the contractors were not the only ones that failed workers. For an occupational health regime to function correctly, multiple groups need to reinforce health and safety. Nevada unions did not demand change. A leader of the Ironworkers Union Local 433 told the *Las Vegas Sun* that the contractors performed "in workmanship-like manner," and the deaths were "just the sheer number of man-hours" and the unfortunate results of human error.[112]

The union local also did not attend informal conferences between Nevada OSHA and the contractors to discuss each incident, missing an important opening to better conditions. Moreover, OSHA and Nevada

OSHA disappointed the workers, a reflection of both agencies' ongoing struggle to protect every workplace in the United States. Federal and state OSHA plans had only 1,938 inspectors in 2013—873 federal and 1,065 state—to inspect more than 8 million workplaces. With one inspector per 66,776 workers, it would take approximately 131 years to inspect every work site in the United States. When the Strip construction deaths occurred, twenty-five budgeted inspector positions existed in Las Vegas. Five were unfilled. The number of positions also did not increase from 2001 to 2007, even though all occupations increased from 200,000 to 927,000 workers.[113]

Still, the megaresort construction boom kept inspectors busy. Behind Oregon, Nevada OSHA performed the second-most statewide inspections in the nation. From 2006 to 2007 Pernini Building Company, a division of one of largest general contractors in the United States, Tutor Pernini Corporation, received twenty-five inspections on its largest Strip projects, with the state agency issuing it thirty-eight violations. But in each case, Nevada OSHA reduced or withdrew the fines, a trend occurring throughout the nation. OSHA civil and criminal penalties simply did not deter employer violations. Congress had not increased civil penalties in decades, and the Inflation Adjustment Act exempted the OSH Act. Criminal misdemeanors were rarely prosecuted as well.[114]

After Harold Billingsley's death, Nevada OSHA concluded that Pernini subcontractor SME Steel Contractors violated several safety laws, and issued three citations totaling $13,500. Later, SME met with the state agency in a private, informal conference with no family members and withdrew the citation. This scenario occurred repeatedly, essentially determining the worker was at fault. OSHA also weakened safety requirements that could have prevented the deaths altogether. After 1971 the federal agency issued compliance directives that taught field officers how to implement the laws. But OSHA's construction standards division started applying broader understandings in the 2000s, instructing employers in new ways to avoid violations. The modified use of directives dramatically changed construction safety protocol. It also could have prevented Billingsley's death. In 2002 OSHA eliminated the requirement to install temporary decking or netting if other safety measures failed. The federal agency determined that workers did not need decking if they wore safety harnesses. Of course, Billingsley's harness was not fastened. After establishing the new directive, the International Association of Ironworkers reported that fatalities tripled among its members, from approximately five to fifteen deaths every year. In 2008 there were eleven fatalities in the first four months alone.[115]

In response to the Strip construction deaths, the Nevada legislature passed two measures to strengthen workplace safety, requiring educational standards for construction workers and providing support to family members after fatal construction accidents. The state law expected regular and supervisory workers to complete courses in construction safety, and hazard identification and prevention, entitled OSHA-10 and OSHA-30. Attendees needed a completion card to gain employment. In the end, the history of occupational health on the Strip revealed several important lessons. First, the OSH Act had not eliminated the risk of working in the United States, but it certainly bettered conditions, saving approximately 472,000 lives over forty years. Employee deaths, injuries, and illnesses also decreased in a workforce that doubled in size. Still, improvement was needed.[116]

Another important lesson was that workplaces were constantly evolving, and new dangers could emerge. Building dense megaresorts on the Strip significantly changed the nature of construction work. Although environmental and public health laws underwent considerable amendments since the 1960s, the OSH Act remained unchanged for the most part. Megaresort construction created unforeseen complexities that were unimaginable in 1970, necessitating a reevaluation of the Act. The Strip construction deaths also demonstrated that even with the lessons learned over the past century, the nation needed to revive its dedication to occupational health.[117]

## NOTES

1. Barth, George, and Hill, *Environmental Health and Safety*, 6.

2. Markowitz and Rosner, *Deceit and Denial*, 159.

3. Division of Occupational Health, "Protecting the Health of Eighty Million Americans: A National Goal for Occupation Health," Special Report to the Surgeon General of the United States PHS, Washington, DC, 1965 (incl. all quotes); Benjamin W.

Mintz, *OSHA: History, Law, and Policy* (Washington, DC: Bureau of National Affairs, 1984); Frederic B. Siskind, "Twenty Years of OSHA Federal Enforcement Data: A Review and Explanation of the Major Trends," DOL/Office of the Assistant Secretary for Policy, Washington, DC (Jan. 1993); Corn, *Response*, 18–23, 42–46. See also HWC, 91st Cong., Box 30, Folder 376, UNLV SC.

4. Barth, George, and Hill, *Environmental Health and Safety*, 6.

5. Markowitz and Rosner, *Deceit and Denial*, 156–57.

6. Barth, George, and Hill, *Environmental Health and Safety*, 6.

7. For example, the word "feasible" has been controversial with regard to workplace noise. Adopted two years after the passage of the Act, the standard required employers to use "feasible administrative or engineering controls" to limit noise. By the early 1980s, OSHA allowed the use of personal protective equipment (PPE), such as earplugs and earmuffs, if the cost was less than administrative and engineering controls. In 2010 OSHA petitioned to reinterpret the standard, citing that the definition of "feasible" was "capable of being done." This meant that employers had to apply engineering and administrative controls before using PPE. The petition received a considerable amount of backlash and OSHA withdrew it a few months later. The agency cited that it was sensitive to the "possible costs." See OSHA, "Interpretation of OSHA's Provision for Feasible Administrative or Engineering Controls of Occupational Noise," Standard Number 1910 and 1926 (Oct. 19, 2010) (incl. "capable of being done" and "feasible administrative"); OSHA Trade News Release, "U.S. Department of Labor's OSHA withdraws proposed interpretation on occupational noise: Agency examines other approaches to prevent work-related hearing loss," DOL, OSHA, Office of Communications (Jan. 19, 2011) (incl. "possible costs"); Corn, *Response*, 18–21, 43.

8. The OSH Act covered all private sector employees working in manufacturing, construction, longshoring, agriculture, law, medicine, charity, and disaster relief, and religious groups with secular workers. It did not include the self-employed, immediate members of farm families, mine workers, certain transportation workers, and atomic energy employees covered by other federal agencies, and public employees in state and local governments. Markowitz and Rosner, *Deceit and Denial*, 164.

9. David Bell, *The Coming of the Post-Industrial Society: A Venture in Social Forecasting* (New York: Basic Books, 1973). See DOL, *Report on the American Workforce* (Washington, DC: DOL, 2001); Robert J. Samuelson, "Myths of Post-Industrial America," *Washington Post*, Apr. 7, 2013; Nina Brown, "Postindustrial Workforce," in *Work in America: An Encyclopedia of History, Policy, and Society*, ed. Carl E. Van Horn and Herbert A. Schaffner (Santa Barbara, CA: ABC-CLIO, 2003). For more on the transition to postindustrial society, see Bell, *Coming of the Post-Industrial Society*; Barry Bluestone and Bennett Harrison, *The Deindustrialization of America: Plant Closings, Community Abandonment, and the Dismantling of Basic Industry* (New York: Basic Books, 1982); Katherine S. Newman, *Falling from Grace: Downward Mobility in the Age of Affluence* (Berkeley: University of California Press, 1999); Robert K. Reich, *The Work of Nations: Preparing Ourselves for Twenty-First Century Capitalism* (New York: Alfred A. Knopf, 1991); Jeremy Rifkin, *The End of Work: The Decline of the Global Labor Force and the Dawn of the Post-Market Era* (New York: G. P. Putnam's Sons, 1995).

10. See Clayton W. Burrows and Robert H. Bosselman, *Hospitality Management Education* (Binghamton, NY: Haworth Hospitality Press, 1999), 21–28, for further description of the hospitality industry.

11. Bureau of Labor Statistics, "Survey of Occupational Injuries and Illnesses," 2002, 2005, and 2007, DOL.

12. Gaming had been common among the state's mining camps during the nineteenth century, and in 1868 the state legalized it and provided for its regulation. At the turn of the century, anti-vice movements gained momentum across the nation, prompting the legislature to pass a bill prohibiting all forms of gambling in 1909. By 1915 public protest prompted the state to add an amendment allowing card games and slot machines. But the law was unevenly enforced, leading to a rise in illegal gambling establishments. By the 1930s unemployment crippled Nevada, and the legislature began entertaining a controversial option to generate revenue. Passing in March 1931, the legalization of gaming allowed the state to capitalize on tax and economic benefits, and promote tourism. See Shannon Bybee, "History, Development, and Legislation of Las Vegas Casino Gambling," in *Legalized Casino Gaming in the United States: The Economic and Social Impact,* ed. Cathy H. C. Hsu, 3–22 (Binghamton, NY: Haworth Hospitality Press, 1999), for the development of gaming in Nevada. For a history of gambling, see David G. Schwartz, *Roll the Bones: The History of Gambling* (New York: Gotham Books, 2006).

13. The El Rancho was an Old West–themed hotel that offered gaming, a restaurant, swimming pool, and entertainment. Thanks to wartime business from defense workers, the resort prospered at first. But management issues led to labor turnover, prompting Hull to sell the resort in 1942. Over the following decades, it changed ownership several times and closed for good in 1960. See Moehring, *Resort City,* 45–46.

14. Eventually, the unincorporated township of Paradise split into two. Paradise A was founded in April 1951, followed by Paradise B in January 1952. In 1953 Paradise A became Winchester and Paradise B became Paradise. The resorts on the Strip were in both Winchester and Paradise. By the time of the 2000 census, Paradise was the largest unincorporated community in the United States. See Rothman, *Nevada,* 106–18; Moehring, *Resort City,* 43–45, 47, 49, 50, 55, 65, 108, 112, 116–17, 124; Moehring and Green, *Las Vegas,* 111–12; Bybee, "History, Development," 7–10.

15. For further discussion on American perceptions of the gambling industry and its emergence as the gaming industry, a legitimate form of recreation tourism, see Hal K. Rothman, *Devil's Bargains: Tourism in the Twentieth-Century American West* (Lawrence: University Press of Kansas, 1998), 287–337; Rothman, *Nevada,* 101–24; Hal K. Rothman, *Neon Metropolis: How Las Vegas Started the Twenty-First Century* (New York: Routledge, 2003).

16. The mob era on the Strip is covered extensively by popular literature. See esp. Ed Reid and Ovid Demaris, *The Green Felt Jungle* (New York: Pocket Books, 1964); Sally Denton and Roger Moore, *The Money and the Power: The Making of Las Vegas and Its Hold on America* (New York: Vintage Books, 2001).

17. During the postwar period, the economy boomed because banks and bond issues provided loans to support the nation's growth. But most financial institutions did not fund the vice industry. Only in rare cases did regional banks fund casinos because the stigma was far too great. Consequently, capital was the biggest obstacle that faced creating the Strip.

18. See "Las Vegas Hedges Its Bets," *Business Week* (Aug. 11, 1956), 157–58, for an overview of Las Vegas's economic downturn during the mid-1950s.

19. For the difficult job of regulating gaming in Nevada, see *U.S. Senate, Hearings Before the Permanent Subcommittee on Investigations, Gambling and Organized Crime, Part 1 and 2* (Washington, DC: GPO, 1961).

20. See Jack Sheehan, *Quiet Kingmaker: E. Perry Thomas* (Las Vegas: Stephens Press, 2009) for details on the Bank of Las Vegas's (Valley Bank) relationship with Jimmy Hoffa, and the building of the Strip resorts during the 1950s and 1960s.

21. Rothman, *Nevada*, 115–18, 127, 131, 133, 136, 137, 149; Moehring, *Resort City*, 86–87, 117, 119, 243; Steven Brill, *The Teamsters* (New York: Pocket Books, 1978), 213–19; Reid and Demaris, *Green Felt Jungle*, 85–88.

22. See "News of Reality: Las Vegas Sale," *New York Times*, Aug. 15, 1967; "Hughes Sinks Another $55 million in Vegas," *LA Times*, Aug. 27, 1969.

23. From 1955 to 1969 the Gaming Commission performed background investigations of each casino stockholder, a practice that discouraged corporate ownership. However, Kerkorian found a solution to the problem. Unlike a traditional corporation, he was the sole stockholder of the International Leisure Corporation. As the lone stockholder, he was the only person required to pass the gaming inspection. After the Flamingo flourished under his legitimate management, the Securities and Exchange Commission permitted the sale of 17 percent of his stock to the public. Offered at $5 a share, the stock jumped 600 percent in three days. See "Kerkorian Unit's Stock Jumps 600% in 3 Days," *LA Times*, Feb. 18, 1969.

24. See Rothman, *Nevada*, 125–46; Rothman, *Devil's Bargains*, 287–88 (incl. "the most," 287); John Wilen, "LV Historians Compile Top Gambling Event," *Las Vegas Sun*, June 10, 1999; Moehring, *Resort City*, 118–22. See also "Las Vegas Is Getting a Huge Hotel," *New York Times*, Oct. 27, 1968; "Largest Resort Hotel Under Construction," *LA Times*, Feb. 18, 1968; "Las Vegas Rivalry Escalates," *LA Times*, June 30, 1969.

25. A megaresort is the ultimate manifestation of the hospitality industry. It is a huge hotel that offers rooms, gambling, entertainment, shopping, fine dining, and other amenities on one property. Megaresorts also typically adopt fantastic or mythical themes.

26. U.S. Census Bureau, "Population Change and Distribution, 1990 to 2000," Census 2000 Brief, Issued Apr. 2001, CZKBR/01-2. The 2010 population estimate of the Las Vegas metropolitan area was 1,951,269. See Brian Haynes, "The Face of Nevada," *Review-Journal*, Feb. 25, 2011.

27. See James P. Kraft, *Vegas at Odds: Labor Conflict in a Leisure Economy, 1960–1985* (Baltimore: Johns Hopkins Press, 2010), 34; *Las Vegas Report, 1965, A Compendium of Statistical Commercial and Social Facets of Las Vegas for Year 1964, Complete Though Dec. 31, 1964* (Las Vegas: Research & Statistical Bureau, Las Vegas Chamber of Commerce, 1965); David G. Schwartz, *Las Vegas Strip Casino Employment: Productivity, Revenues, and Payrolls, A Statistical Study, 1990–2009* (Las Vegas: Center for Gaming Research, University Libraries, UNLV, 2010), 3; Hsu, *Legalized Casino Gaming*, 17.

28. Rothman, *Devil's Bargains*, 314–16; Marshall Allen, "It's a Myth, Now Park It," *Las Vegas Sun*, Aug. 27, 2006.

29. Douglas McGregor, *The Human Side of Enterprise* (New York: McGraw Hill, 1960).

30. Kraft, *Vegas at Odds*, 34–35. For information on the various jobs and departments at the resorts, see documents in UNLV SC, esp. the Department Series, Boxes 21 and 23, and Miscellaneous Series, Box 155; Stardust Collection; Employee Records, Box 27, Folders 3–20, Box 28, Folders 3–17, Box 29, Folder 7, Sands Collection; Series 2, Employees, Box 4, Dunes Collection.

31. The pattern of financing, ownership, and management became institutionalized at the Desert Inn in 1950. Wilbur Clark, part owner of the El Rancho, bought land on the Strip in 1945. Envisioning a luxury resort that rivaled the Flamingo, he ran out

of money during construction and turned to a group of Cleveland businessmen. Led by Morris "Moe" Dalitz, they invested $1 million in the Desert Inn in return for 74 percent ownership. Clark became the front man of the Desert Inn, a locally respected businessman and owner of the resort. But in reality, he had limited control.

32. Kraft, *Vegas at Odds*, 16–17; Michael Green, "Las Vegas Mob," *Nevada Online Encyclopedia*, www.onlinenevada.org.

33. Kraft, *Vegas at Odds*, 16–17, 29–31 (incl. "involved in," 29).

34. Although the term "human resources management" did not garner widespread use until the 1960s, personnel management had existed since the late nineteenth century. During the 1950s the term designated the expansion of personnel management to include modern psychology. Behaviorists determined that employees could not be regarded as replaceable; they needed job security, self-expression, communication, and recognition. Nurturing an employee's psyche thus would create a more stable and productive workforce. See Rudiger Pieper, *Human Resource Management: An International Comparison* (Berlin: Walter de Gruyter, 1990), 42–43.

35. See Frederick Herzberg, Bernard Mausner, and Barbara Bloch Snyderman, *The Motivation to Work* (New York: John Wiley and Sons, 1959).

36. For the resorts' human resource management programs, see Jill Heintz to All Department Heads, memorandum, Nov. 5, 1991; Definitions of Hiring Standards and Interviewing Manual; Jim Hippler to Distribution, memorandum, Mar. 2, 1992; Jim Hippler to Employees Covered Under The Boyd Group Employee Benefit Plan (PERCS), memorandum, Oct. 5, 1992; all in Box 21, Stardust Collection, UNLV SC. See also Housekeeping Retreat Material, Box 23; Emergency Procedures to All Departments, May 5, 1988; Emergency Recall Roster to All Departments, Mar. 23, 1987; both in Miscellaneous Series, Box 155, Stardust Collection, UNLV SC; Kraft, *Vegas at Odds*, 31 (incl. "Objective and philosophy, "the secret," and "positive personal").

37. See Tom Luz, *Do Nothing: A History of Loafers, Loungers, Slackers, and Bums in America* (New York: Farrar, Straus, and Giroux, 2006), 272–74; U.S. Department of Health, Education, and Welfare, *Work in America: Report of a Special Task Force to the U.S. Department of Health, Education, and Welfare* (Cambridge, MA: MIT Press, 1973); Daniel Yankelovich and John Immerwahr, "Putting the Work Ethic Back to Work: A Public Agenda Report on Restoring America's Competitive Vitality" (New York: Public Agenda Foundation, 1983).

38. See Alan Balboni, *Beyond the Mafia: Italian Americans and the Development of Las Vegas* (Reno: University of Nevada Press, 2006) for a good source on networking in the casinos.

39. Rothman, *Devil's Bargains*, 314–16.

40. "Chapter V: Selection of Employees," *Housekeepers' Guide to Selecting and Training Employees*, 50–55, El Rancho Collection, NSMA (incl. "likely to," 50; "ability to," 53; "accidents, harming," 50–51).

41. "Chapter V: Selection of Employees" (incl. "wholesome"); Employee Orientation Program (incl. "regardless of position"); Stardust Collection, Box 155, UNLV SC; *General Procedures: All Employees and You and Your Job*, Harrah's Entertainment Collection, UNLV SC.

42. Betty Friedan, *The Feminine Mystique* (New York: W. W. Norton, 1963). See also Joanne L. Goodwin, *Changing the Game: Women and Work in Las Vegas, 1940–1990* (Reno: University of Nevada Press, 2014) for oral histories on the female postwar employment experience in Las Vegas.

43. "Vital Showgirl Statistics Stagger Vegas Showgoers," Box 9, Folder 16, Information for Publicity Releases, Box 9, Folder 8, Dunes Collection, UNLV SC (incl. "harmonizes with," "imported," and "America"). For sample showgirl contracts, see Folders 2, 4, and 5 in the Virginia James Collection, UNLV SC. See also Joanne L. Goodwin, *Changing the Game: Women and Work in Las Vegas, 1940–1990* (Reno: University of Nevada Press, 2014) for oral histories on the female postwar employment experience in Las Vegas.

44. The 1964 Civil Rights Act prohibited discrimination on the basis of race, sex, and national origin in employment. The Act created the Equal Employment Opportunity Commission and assigned enforcement to the U.S. Justice Department. See Nancy MacLean, *Freedom Is Not Enough: The Opening of the American Workplace* (Cambridge, MA: Harvard University Press, 2006) for a discussion on the changes in the American workplace because of racial and sexual equality.

45. Kraft, *Vegas at Odds*, 34–36; Moehring and Green, *Las Vegas*, 201; Natasha Zaretsky, "Feminists in the 1960s and 1970s," in *Women's Rights: People and Perspectives*, ed. Crista DeLuzio and Peter C. Mancall (Santa Barbara, CA: ABC-CLIO, 2010), 192; Moehring, *Resort City*, 201–2. For the debate surrounding Las Vegas's decision to ban women dealers, see City Commission, Minutes, XI, Nov. 5, 1958; and Roske, *Las Vegas, NV*, 122. The complaint, filed on Jan. 13, 1981, is entitled "U.S. Equal Employment Opportunity Commission v. Nevada Resorts Association et al.—Case No. CV-LV–81–12 RDF."

46. Filed on Jan. 13, 1981, the Equal Employment Opportunity Commission complaint is entitled "U.S. Equal Employment Opportunity Commission v. Nevada Resorts Association et al.—Case No. CV-LV–81–12 RDF." For corporate records on appointing women to traditionally male-held positions, see Roger Wagner to Al Guzman, June 6, 1976, Box 27, Folder 11; Al Guzman to Forrest Duke, Press Release to *Review-Journal*, Oct. 1, 1975; both in Box 28, Folder 3, Sands Collection, UNLV SC. See also Michael W. Bowers, *Sagebrush State* (Reno: University of Nevada Press, 2006), 40–41; Census Bureau 2005 quoted in ibid, 41.

47. For more on the minority experience and civil rights in Las Vegas, see Moehring, *Resort City*, 171–201; Moehring and Green, *Las Vegas*, 196–204; Bowers, *Sagebrush State*, esp. "Civil Rights and Liberties in Nevada"; Kraft, *Vegas at Odds*, 117–38; Elizabeth Nelson Patrick, "The Black Experience in Southern Nevada," *Nevada Historical Society Quarterly* 22 (Summer 1979): 128–40; "The Black Experience in Southern Nevada, Part II," *Nevada Historical Society Quarterly* 22 (Fall 1979): 209–20; Perry Kaufman, "The Best City of Them All: A City Biography of Las Vegas, 1930–1960" (PhD diss., University of California, Santa Barbara, 1974). A number of oral histories at UNLV SC also discuss the topic.

48. Kirk V. Cammack Jr., "Shall They Not Protest" Las Vegas Toastmasters, 1964.

49. Moehring and Green, *Las Vegas*, 200 (incl. all quotes).

50. Filed on June 4, 1971 in the U.S. District Court in the District of Nevada, the complaint is entitled "Civil LV No. 1645, Complaint" and "Civil Action LV No. 1645 Consent Decree," Court Clerk's Office, Foley Federal Building, Las Vegas.

51. Moehring and Green, *Las Vegas*, 200–1; Casinos Silent on Discrimination, *Review-Journal*, Nov. 17, 1969; Michael Lyle, "Black Community Pushed to End Racial Discrimination in Las Vegas," *Review-Journal*, Feb. 15, 2015; Bowers, *Sagebrush State*, 35. See also John N. McCarthy to Howard B. Gundersen, Nov. 10, 1969, HWC, 91st Cong., Box 30, Folder 378, UNLV SC.

52. See Murphy, *Sick Building Syndrome*, 57–59; *OSHA Technical Manual*, Sec. III: Chap. 2, "Indoor Air Quality."

53. Bureau of Labor Statistics, "Gaming Service Operations" (2010–11 ed.), DOL; Israel Posner, Lewis A. Leitner, and David Lester, "Stress in Casino Floor Employees," *Psychological Reports* 57, no. 246 (Aug. 1985); Jon Nordheimer, "Behind the Lights, Casino Burnout," *New York Times*, Aug. 5, 1994; William N. Thompson and Michele Comeau, *Casino Service the Win Win Game* (Las Vegas: Performance Unlimited, 1992), 204–5.

54. Barbara Ann Barnett interview, by Charles Moore Chesnutt, Mar. 8, 1981, UNLV SC (incl. all quotes).

55. Ravenholt quoted in Blachley, *Pestilence*, 139; Howard J. Shaffer, Joni Vander Bilt, and Matthew N. Hall, "Gambling, Drinking, and Other Health Risk Activities Among Casino Employees," *American Journal of Industrial Medicine* 36 (1999): 365–78; Lawrence S. Freidman, Nicholas F. Fleming, David H. Roberts, Steven E. Hyman, eds., *Source Book of Substance Abuse and Addiction* (Baltimore: Williams and Wilkins, 1996), 348.

56. See the Charter Hospital Collection in the UNLV SC for sources on compulsive gambling and addiction in Las Vegas, esp. in the Charter Hospital Collection, UNLV SC: Charter Hospital of Las Vegas Compulsive Gambling Treatment Program, Box 1, Folder 1; Darrell W. Bolen, "Gambling: Historical Highlights, Trends, and Their Implications of Contemporary Society" (1974), Box 1, Folder 14; Robert L. Custer, "Russian Roulette with Lives," Box 1, Folder 19; The Nevada Council on Compulsive Gambling Inc., "More About Soft Signs," Box 1, Folder 18; Robert L. Custer, "A Profile of Pathological Gamblers," Box 1, Folder 22. See also Henry R. Lesieur, Sheila B. Blume, Richard M. Zoppa, "Alcoholism, Drug Abuse, and Gambling," *Alcoholism Clinical and Experimental Research* 10 (1986): 33–38; J. Ryan, C. Zwerling, E. J. Orav, "Occupational Risks Associated with Cigarette Smoking: A Prospective Study," *American Journal of Public Health* 82 (1992): 29–32.

57. Susan Buchanan, Pamela Vossenas, Niklas Krause, Joan Moriarty, Eric Frumin, Jo Anna M. Shimek, Franklin Mirer, Peter Orris, and Laura Punnett, "Occupational Injury Disparities in the US Hotel Industry," *American Journal of Industrial Medicine* 53 (2010): 116–25.

58. Teresa Scherzer and Niklas Krause, "Work Related Pain and Injury and Barriers to Workers' Compensation Among Las Vegas Hotel Room Cleaners," *American Journal of Public Health* 95, no. 3 (Mar. 2005); Barbara J. Burgel et al., "Psychosocial Work Factors and Shoulder Pain in Hotel Room Cleaners," *American Journal of Industrial Medicine* 53, no. 7 (July 2010): 743–56; Niklas Krause, Teresa Scherzer, and Reiner Rugulies, "Physical Workload, Work Intensification, and Prevalence of Pain in Low Wage Workers: Results from a Participatory Research Project with Hotel Room Cleaners in Las Vegas," *American Journal of Industrial Medicine* 48, no. 5 (Nov. 2005): 326–37. See also "Chapter VIII—Shifting Employees to Fit Jobs," *Housekeepers' Guide to Selecting and Training Employees*, El Rancho Collection, NSMA (incl. "forbade").

59. Hopkins and Evans, "Otto Ravenholt," in *First 100*, 270–71.

60. Harold Boyer interview, by Claytee White, Nov. 15, 2000, UNLV SC (incl. all quotes); Lucius Blanchard interview, by Claytee White, Oct. 2, 2003, UNLV SC. See also Pieter-Jan Coenraads and Henriette Smit, "Dermatitis," *Epidemiology of Work-Related Diseases* (London: BMJ Books, 2000), 175–78; Pieter-Jan Coenraads, "Hand Eczema," *New England Journal of Medicine* 367 (Nov. 8, 2012): 1829–1937.

61. Kreisler interview, 16; Boyer interview, 16; U.S. Department of Health and Human Services, *The Health Consequences of Involuntary Exposure to Tobacco Smoke: A Report of the Surgeon General* (Washington DC: GPO, 2006).

62. Douglas Trout, John Decker. Charles Mueller, John T. Bernert, and James Pirkle, "Exposure of Casino Employees to Environmental Tobacco Smoke," *Journal of Environmental Medicine* 40, no. 3 (Mar. 1998): 270–76. K. Anderson, J. Kliris, L. Murphy, S. Carmella, S. Han, C. Link, R. Bliss, S. Puumala, and S. Hecht, "Metabolites of Tobacco-Specific Lung Carcinogen in Nonsmoking Casino Patrons," *Cancer Epidemiology, Biomarkers & Prevention* 23 (Dec. 2003): 1544–46; James Repace, "Respirable Particles and Carcinogens in the Air of Delaware Hospitality Venues Before and After a Smoking Ban," *Journal of Environmental Medicine* (Sept. 10, 2004). See also Earle C. Clements to Howard W. Cannon, Nov. 25, 1969; Cigarette Cancer Committee to Howard W. Cannon, Nov. 13, 1969; all in HWC, 91st Cong., Box 19, Folder 241, UNLV SC.

63. "Smoke Exposure at Work Killed Casino Dealer, Suit Says," *Westlaw News and Insight*, National Litigation (Mar. 15, 2011); Steven Green, "Casino Dealer's Suit Over Smoking Dangers at Wynn Moves Forward," *Las Vegas Sun*, Oct. 13, 2010; "Study Shows Secondhand Smoke Increases Risk of Stroke," *Reno Gazette-Journal*, Aug. 18, 1999; Trout et al., "Exposure of Casino Employees"; U.S. Department of Health and Human Services, CDC, *Environmental and Biological Assessment of Environmental Tobacco Smoke Exposure Among Casino Dealers*, Health Hazard Evaluation Report, HETA 2005-0076, 2005-0201–3080, Bally's, Paris, and Caesars Palace Casinos, Las Vegas (May 2009); Nancy L. York and Kiyoung Lee, "A Baseline Evaluation of Casino Air Quality After Enactment of Nevada's Clean Indoor Air Act," *Public Health Nursing* 27, no. 2 (2010): 158–63.

64. "Generator Exhaust Found as Hotel Disaster Cause," *Las Vegas Sun*, July 16, 1977; "Strip Hotel Becomes Towering Death Trap," *Las Vegas Sun*, July 16, 1977; "Heavy Carbon Monoxide in Hotel Guests," *Las Vegas Sun*, July 16, 1977; "Hotel Poisoning Probe Scheduled," *Las Vegas Sun*, July 19, 1977; "Gas in Las Vegas Hotel Kills One, Hospitalizes 100," *LA Times*, July 16, 1977; "900 Flee Vegas Hotel Gas," *Chicago Tribune*, July 16, 1977; "Probe Is Continuing into Toxic Death at Landmark," *Review-Journal*, July 16, 1977.

65. "Generator Exhaust Found"; "Strip Hotel Becomes"; "Heavy Carbon Monoxide"; "Hotel Poisoning Probe"; "Gas in Las Vegas."

66. Eliot Tiegel, "Call Wayne Newton Mr. Las Vegas," *Billboard*, Dec. 8, 1973; Barbara Wilkins, "'Call Doctor Ghanem' Elvis and Other Stars Gasp When They Get Las Vegas Throat," *People* 5, no. 10 (Mar. 15, 1976); "Vegas Throat Like the Plague for Some Singers," *Jet* 54, no. 17 (July 13, 1978), 61; Gina Kolata, "Body and Mind: The Lost Voice," *New York Times*, Jan. 15, 1989; "Vegas Beat—Timothy McDarrah: Dion's Caesar Show a Must-See," *Las Vegas Sun*, Oct. 23, 2002.

67. See Jeanne Mager Stellman, ed., "Entertainment and the Arts," in *Encyclopedia of Occupational Health and Safety*, 4th ed., Vol. 3 (Geneva: International Labour Office, 1998), 96.2–96.7; "OSHA Investigating Death of 'Ka' Artist: MGM Grand show closes at least through July 9," *Las Vegas Sun*, June 30, 2013; Michael Joseph Gross, "Life and Death at Cirque du Soleil," *Vanity Fair* (May 29, 2015).

68. For the Ruppert Bears, see "All in a Nights Work," *Las Vegas Sun*, Sept. 21, 1973; "Casino Attraction," *Vegas Visitor*, Aug. 30, 1974; "Casino Hit," *Las Vegas Sun*, June 27, 1975; "Bear Hug," *Review-Journal*, Oct. 5, 1974; "Dog Talk: Some Bear Facts," *Plain Dealer*, Oct. 3, 1971; photographs in the Dunes Collection, Box 9, Folder 12, UNLV SC.

69. "Siegfried and Roy Bring Illusions Into Your Home," *Review-Journal*, Nov. 6, 1994; "Tiger Attack Not Unprecedented," *Las Vegas Sun*, Oct. 6, 2003; Miguel Marquez, "Roy of Siegfried and Roy Critical After Mauling," *CNN Report*, Oct. 4, 2003; "Horn Still Critical After Attack," *Las Vegas Sun*, Oct. 6, 2003; "Roy Still Critical, Show Is

Cancelled Indefinitely," *Las Vegas Sun*, Oct. 7, 2003; "Siegfried: Tiger Confused, Tried to Protect Roy," *Las Vegas Sun*, Oct. 9, 2003; "Roy Horn: Tiger 'Saved My Life,'" *People* (Sept. 16, 2004) (incl. "I started").

70. Mark Beattie and Jacinta Gau, "Workplace Violence in Hotels," in *Hotel Management and Operations*, ed. Michael J. O'Fallon and Denney G. Rutherford (Hoboken, NJ: John Wiley & Sons, 2011), 227–28; "General Procedures—All Employees," Harrah's Entertainment Collection, UNLV SC, esp. "Conduct, Prohibited" (incl. "fighting or").

71. "Rash of Casino Robberies Tied to Trend Toward Violence," *Las Vegas Sun*, Dec. 2, 2000; Lisa Snedeker, "Lone Gunman Robs Treasure Island, Injures Cashier," *Las Vegas Sun*, Oct. 30, 2000; Jace Radke and Keith Paul, "Suspect in Casino Guard Shooting," *Las Vegas Sun*, Dec. 13, 2000.

72. "Elvis Presley in Stage Fight with Four Men," *Las Vegas Sun*, Feb. 21, 1973; "4 Try Rough Play Elvis Proves Karate Expert," *Review-Journal*, Feb. 22, 1973. Las Vegas attorneys McNamee and McNamee represented the woman who sustained an injury in the fight. See Rose Marie Leach and Lynn Leach v. Hilton Corporation and Elvis Presley et al., Eighth Judicial District Court of the State of Nevada, Filed Feb. 16, 1975, Case No. A137307 (incl. "negligently"); "Everyone Wants Millions, So Many Go Courting," (incl. "so upset" and "All I can"); both located in McNamee Collection, Box 136, Folder 45, NSMA.

73. Julie Bosman, Amy Harmon, Christine Hauser, Jess Bidgood, and Maggie Astor, "Las Vegas Shooting Victims: The Full List," *New York Times*, Oct. 2, 2017; "Rapper in Fight for Life," *Review-Journal*, Sept. 9, 1996; "Shakur Dies of Wounds," *Review-Journal*, Sept. 14, 1996; "The Death of Tupac Shakur One Year Later," *Las Vegas Sun*, Sept. 6, 1997. "Strip Killer Ammar Harris Sentenced to Death," *Review-Journal*, Nov. 4, 2015; "Why? Motive Sought after Pedestrians Mowed Down along Las Vegas Strip," *Las Vegas Sun*, Dec. 21, 2015.

74. AGVA Standard Form of Artists Employment Contract, drafted for Mary Menzies to become a Dunes dancer, Apr. 12, 1955, Dunes Collection, Box 1, Folder 14, UNLV SC; Slack, Jessie—Claim No. 61–801, McNamee Collection, Box 97, Folder 17, Nevada State Museum, Las Vegas; *Housekeepers' Guide to Selecting and Training Employees*.

75. See memorandum to All Employees, Oct. 29, 1983, Landmark Hotel and Casino, Las Vegas, Landmark Collection, Box 1, Folder 7, NSMA (incl. "good business"); and Orientation Handbook, Miscellaneous Series, Box 155, Stardust Collection; John Miner to Department Heads, memorandum, Aug. 5, 1992; Cathey Shanklin to Susan Rhodes, Dec. 6, 1991; Cathey Shanklin to Distribution, memorandum, July 24, July 30, Aug. 20, and Aug. 25, 1992; Department Series, Stardust Collection, Box 21; Fire Prevention Class, Dunes Collection, Box 2, Folder 5; all in UNLV SC.

76. The county hospital went through several name changes throughout the twentieth century. During the 1930s it was the Clark County Indigent Hospital. During World War II it became the Clark County General Hospital, and in 1956 it was renamed Southern Nevada Memorial Hospital. In 1986 hospital officials changed the name to University Medical Center (UMC) of Southern Nevada to reflect its affiliation with the University of Nevada, Reno, School of Medicine.

77. See J. C. Cherry interview, by Cheryl Mawinney, Mar. 20, 1978, UNLV SC; Southern Nevada Memorial Granted Federal Monies, Press Release, HWC, 87th Cong., Box 8, Folder 118; Hill-Burton Update, 1947–68, HWC, 91st Cong., Box 20, Folder 254, UNLV SC; "History of Southern Nevada Memorial Hospital," *News and Views* (Dec. 1968); Dee Oakey, "Southern Nevada Memorial Hospital—Its First 50 Years," *Las Vegas Sun*, May

1981; Klimek, "A History of Hospitals," 7–11; "Hospitals of Clark County," *Greasewood Tablettes* 7, no. 4 (Winter 1996–97); "Ed Koch, "Lions Burn Unit: Healing Wounds for 35 Years," *Las Vegas Sun*, Mar. 22, 2003.

78. Adele Baratz interview, by Claytee White, Mar. 19, 2007, UNLV SC; Barnett interview; Blanchard interview; Boyer interview; Joseph Rojas interview, by Suzanne Lubritz, Feb. 25, 1980, UNLV SC; John P. Watkins interview, by Brian Watkins, Mar. 4, 1979, UNLV SC. See also Klimek, "A History of Hospitals," 15–16.

79. Casino skimming entailed illegally siphoning off gambling profits to avoid paying federal taxes. Crime syndicates in Las Vegas infamously routed pretax profits across the nation throughout the 1950s and 1960s. The largest skim recorded by the Federal Bureau of Investigation occurred at the Stardust during the 1970s. By some estimates, the mob took $7 million each year from the slots alone. See Rothman, *Nevada*, 137; Michael Green, "The Jews," in *The Peoples of Las Vegas*, ed. Jerry L. Simich and Thomas C. Wright (Reno: University of Nevada Press, 2005), 167.

80. Kirk V. Cammack, "Frontier Desert Justice," *Greasewood Tablettes* (Winter 1998–99) (incl. all quotes).

81. Kreisler quoted in Blachley, *Good Medicine*, 150.

82. Barbara Wilkins, "'Call Doctor Ghanem,' Elvis and Other Stars Gasp When They Get Las Vegas Throat," *People* (Mar. 15, 1976).

83. See Baratz interview, Mar. 4, 1979; Baratz interview, Mar. 19, 2007; Barnett interview; Blanchard interview; Boyer interview; Rojas interview; Watkins interview; Klimek, "A History of Hospitals," 17–18; Michael E. Porter, *Cases in Competitive Strategy* (New York: Free Press, 1983), 257; Blachley, *Pestilence* (incl. "[It was] like getting," 113).

84. Jeff Burbank, *Las Vegas Babylon: The True Tales of Glitter, Glamour, and Greed* (Lanham, MD: M. Evans & Company, 2008), 163; "Obituary of Joseph L. Fink, M.D.," *Review-Journal*, Dec. 1, 2011.

85. Wilkins, "Call Doctor Ghanem" (incl. "A lot of").

86. Jane Ann Morrison, "Ghanem Succumbs After Long Battle with Cancer," *Review-Journal*, Aug. 28, 2001; "Nevada Boxing Official, Physician Ghanem Dies," *Las Vegas Sun*, Aug. 27, 2001 (incl. "I have to wear"); Wilkins, "Call Doctor Ghanem"; "Hundreds Bid Farewell at Services for Ghanem," *Las Vegas Sun*, Aug. 31, 2001; "Nation's Longest Strike Comes to An End," *Las Vegas Sun*, Feb. 1, 1998. For more on the boxing in Las Vegas, see Richard O. Davies, *The Main Event: Boxing in Nevada from Mining Camps to the Las Vegas Strip* (Reno: University of Nevada Press, 2014).

87. Legislature Counsel Bureau, "Workmen's Compensation Through Private Insurers," Bulletin No. 83–5 (Carson City, NV: SPO, Nov. 1982); OSHA, *Review of the Nevada Occupational Safety and Health Program* (San Francisco: DOL Occupational Safety and Health Administration Region IX, Oct. 20, 2009); NIC, "Rules of Procedure of Occupational Safety and Health Review Board," Adopted Pursuant to the Nevada Administrative Procedure Act and Chapter 591 of the Statutes of Nevada (Carson City, NV: SPO, 1973); Department of Occupational Safety and Health, *Accident Prevention Handbook* (Carson City, NV: SPO, 1978); Department of Occupational Safety and Health, *Occupational Safety and Health Standards for General Industry* (Carson City, NV: SPO, 1977).

88. For Nevada industries struggling with the new OSHA policies, see Claude Evans to Howard W. Cannon, letter, Sept. 27, 1979; Howard W. Cannon to Claude Evans, letter, Oct. 10, 1979; J. R. Henderson to Howard W. Cannon, letter, Dec. 4, 1978;

Robert B. Lagther to Howard W. Cannon, letter (n.d.); H. J. Wurzer to Howard W. Cannon, letter, Sept. 28, 1978; Kenneth E. Tobin to the president of the United States, letter, Nov. 22, 1978; Lloyd McBride to Howard W. Cannon, letter, July 6, 1979; William W. Winpinsinger to Howard W. Cannon, letter, June 6, 1979; G. R. Stewart to Howard W. Cannon, letter, Oct. 30, 1978; Howard W. Cannon to G. R. Stewart, letter, Nov. 14, 1978; Eula Bingham to Howard W. Cannon, letter, Jan. 4, 1979; J. W. Walters to Howard W. Cannon, letter, Aug. 6, 1979; Rosemary C. Smith to Howard W. Cannon, letter, Mar. 6, 1980; James H. Skaggs to Howard W. Cannon, letter, July 22, 1980; "OSHA Completes First Phase of Verticalization Process," *ACG National Newsletter* 31, no. 7 (Feb. 14, 1979); OSHA Announces Revision in Electrical Standards, Press Release, Sept. 24, 1979; all in HWC, 96th Cong., Box 57, Folder 847, UNLV SC. See also "Labor Launches Holy War on Legislators to Block Proposed Rewrite of OSHA Act," *Wall Street Journal,* Mar. 21, 1980.

89. "Architect Appointed for Las Vegas Hotel," *LA Times,* July 9, 1967; Agreement Between Carrar Marble Company of America, Inc. and Taylor Construction Company for MGM Grand Hotel, Inc., Contract No. 25, Dec. 19, 1971, MGM Grand Fire Litigation Collection, UNLV SC.

90. "Fire Destroys Plush Casino in Las Vegas," *Chicago Daily Tribune,* June 18, 1960; "Million Dollar Fire Belts Hotel Sahara," *Las Vegas Sun,* Aug. 26, 1964 (incl. "life went on"); Mary Manning, "Deadly Casino Fires Helped Rewrite Safety Standards," *Las Vegas Sun,* Jan. 25, 2008.

91. See Leland E. Backus to Alan Case, Sept. 2, 1982; Uniform Building Code (1970 ed.); Universal Mechanical Code (1970 ed.); MGM Fire Litigation Materials, esp. Vol. 1 Deli Furnishings and Restaurant Core; Vol. 2 Casino Furnishings; all in MGM Grand Fire Litigation Collection, UNLV SC. See also Ed Koch and Mary Manning, "MGM Fire Altered Safety Standards," *Las Vegas Sun,* Nov. 18, 2000; Jeffery S. Tubbs and Brian J. Meacham, *Egress Design Solutions* (Hoboken, NJ: John Wiley and Sons, 2007), 74; Chris Woodward, "MGM Nixed Improved Sprinkler System in '73," *Las Vegas Sun,* Nov. 23, 1980.

92. For employee, guest, and firefighter accounts of the disaster, see Vol. 1 in the MGM Grand Fire Litigation Collection, esp. the testimonies of Victoria Bernliner-Harris, Linda Allen, Patricia Jo Allsbrook, Alton Anderson, Emmett Barnes, Wayne Bonine, Gordon Carey, James Corbett, Peter Dobbs, Helmut Herbrectsmeir, Louis Miranti, Rex Schnleehagen, and Joseph Charles Westably, UNLV SC. See also Richard Best and David Demers, *Investigation Report on the MGM Grand Hotel Fire* (Quincey, MA: National Fire Protection Association, rev. Jan. 15, 1982).

93. Otto Ravenholt, "Eyewitness to Disaster: The Worst Fire in the City's History," in Blachley, *Pestilence* (incl. "chaotic sight," 105–6).

94. Ibid. (incl. all quotes, 106–7); "Otto Ravenholt," *The First 100,* 269–270 (incl. "bell captain," 269); Best, "Investigation Report."

95. Myocarditis is an inflammation of the heart muscle. It is the principal cause of heart disease and sudden cardiac death and is often caused by infection from a coxsackie virus. Most people recover from viral myocarditis with no ill effects, but a small number develop autoimmune myocarditis. The body's own immune system attacks the heart muscle, which eventually leads to heart failure. Panic most likely triggered this form of death during the MGM Grand fire.

96. Peggy Leen to Taylor, "Testimony Summary of Dr. Sheldon Green," Oct. 12, 1982; Alan Case to MGM Grand Litigation Team, "Deposition of Dr. Thorne Butler,"

MGM Grand Fire Litigation Collection, UNLV SC; Ravenholt, "Eyewitness to Disaster" (incl. "Only the bodies," 107); Best, "Investigation Report." See also MGM Grand Fire File, in HWC, 97th Cong., Box 30, Folder 430, UNLV SC.

97.  "Around the Nation: Las Vegas Busboy Gets Life in Fatal Fire," *New York Times*, Feb. 18, 1982; Margot Hornblower, "Eight Die in Blaze: Busboy Arrested in Las Vegas Hotel Arson," *Washington Post*, Feb. 12, 1981; "Around the Nation: Big Holes in Busboy Story of Las Vegas Fire Reported," *New York Times*, Feb. 15, 1981.

98.  "Ex-Busboy Convicted of Murder and Arson in Las Vegas Hotel Fire," *New York Times*, Jan. 16, 1982; Kraft, *Vegas at Odds*, 180–85; Jeff Simpson, "Strike Zone," *Review-Journal*, May 12, 2002 (incl. "It was an interesting").

99.  See Highlights of the Biennium, Office of the Governor, State Fire Marshal Division, in Governor's Office of Planning Coordination, *Biennial Report of Nevada State Agencies*, 60th Sess. (1980 ed.). See also Bernard J. Rothkopf to MGM Grand Employee, Mar. 24, 1981 (incl. "long trying time," "most luxurious," and "one of the"); Howard W. Cannon to the Senate Floor; "Tax Incentives for Hotel Retrofit," Washington Report from Senator Cannon (Apr. 1981); Cannon Hails MGM Grand Reopening, July 10, 1981, Press Release; The Congressional Record on MGM Grand Hotel, July 21, 1981; Alvin Benedict to Howard W. Cannon, June 29, 1981; Multimillion Dollar Life-Safety System Being Installed at Grand-Las Vegas, MGM Grand Report (Apr. 1981); all in HWC, 97th Cong., Box 30, Folder 430, UNLV SC.

100.  Arthur E. Cote, *Organizing for Fire and Rescue Services* (Quincy, MA: National Fire Protection Agency), 26.

101.  In re MGM Grand Hotel Fire Litigation, 570 F. Supp. 913 (1983); Koch and Manning, "MGM Grand Fire"; Jane Ann Morrison, "In Depth: MGM Grand Hotel Fire: 25 years Later," *Review-Journal*, Nov. 25, 2005; "Getting Insured the Morning After," *Business Week* (Aug. 17, 1981); Matt W. Holley, "The Fortuity Doctrine: Misapplying the Known Loss Rule to Liability Insurance Policies," *Texas Tech Law Review*, 41 Tex. Tech L. Rev. 529 (Winter 2009).

102.  For documents on the fire litigation, see MGM Grand Fire Litigation Collection, UNLV SC, which outlines testimonies and other materials pertinent to the case, especially American Protection Insurance Company v. MGM Grand Hotel Inc., Nos. CIV-LV-82-26, HEC CIV-LV-82-96, HEC (1983); American Excess Insurance Company v. MGM Grand Hotels Inc., 102 Nev. 601; 729 P.2d 1352 (1986). See also William M. Shernoff, "The Cases We Remember: MGM Grand 'Retroactive' Insurance Case" (Mar. 1, 2000), shernoff.com/articles (incl. "the settlement"); "MGM Grand to Battle Its Insurers: Case Expected to Last 8 to 10 Months, Cost $342,000 a Day to Try," *LA Times*, Mar. 18, 1985; David Kelley, "Settlement in MGM Grand Hotel Fire," *UPI*, Apr. 1, 1985; "Settlement Reached in Complex MGM Hotel Fire Insurance Case," *AP*, Mar. 31, 1985.

103.  In re MGM Grand Hotel Fire Litigation; Koch and Manning, "MGM Grand Fire Altered" (incl. "the things we learned"); Jane Ann Morrison, "In Depth: MGM Grand Hotel Fire: 25 years Later," *Review-Journal*, Oct. 13, 2012; Holley "Fortuity Doctrine."

104.  One-alarm, two-alarm, and three-alarm fires were categories that articulated the level of response by local authorities. The higher the alarm, the more fire stations needed. See Mary Manning, "Deadly Casino Fires Helped Rewrite Safety Standards," *Las Vegas Sun*, Jan. 25, 2008; Mark Whittington, "Unclear When Fire Damaged Monte Carlo Can Be Reopened," *Las Vegas Sun*, Jan. 25, 2008 (incl. "We have the best"); Tom Gorman, "From the Inside: How They Coped," *Las Vegas Sun*, Jan. 26, 2008.

105. For problems that employees faced when dealing with the NIC, see Margaret Howard to Mike O'Callaghan, Jan. 20, 1978; Howard W. Cannon to Margaret Howard, Jan. 31, 1978; Kenneth R. Johnston to Howard W. Cannon, Feb. 8, 1978; all in HWC, 95th Cong., Box 25, Folder 655, UNLV SC. See also Douglas D. Dailey to Howard W. Cannon, Mar. 8, 1979, HWC, 96th Congress, Box 49, Folder 683, UNLV SC; NIC v. Tropicana Garden Estates, McNamee Collection, Box 84, Folder 24, NSMA.

106. Legislature Counsel Bureau, Nevada Industrial Commission Study, Bulletin No. 104 (Carson City, NV: Dec. 1972); Legislature Counsel Bureau, Administrative Procedures Followed by the Nevada Industrial Commission and Alternative Methods of Providing Workmen's Compensation Coverage, Bulletin No. 79-1 (Carson City, NV: Oct. 1978); Legislature Counsel Bureau, Workmen's Compensation Through Private Insurers, Bulletin No. 83-5 (Carson City, NV: Nov. 1982); Legislature Commission of the Legislature Counsel Bureau, Study of Industrial Insurance, Bulletin No. 93.8 (Carson City, NV: Jan. 1993); Legislature Counsel Bureau, Legislative Committee on Workers' Compensation, Bulletin No. 01-19 (Carson City, NV: Jan. 2001); Legislature Counsel Bureau, Study of Nevada's Industrial Insurance Program, Bulletin No. 05-7 (Carson City, NV: Jan. 2005).

107. Nancy J. Niles, *Basics of the U.S. Health Care System* (Burlington, MA: Jones and Bartlett, 2011), 83–184; Philip D. Pierce, "Understanding Managed Care Health Plans: The Managed Care Spectrum," in *The Handbook of Employee Benefits: Design, Funding, and Administration*, 6th ed., ed. Jerry S. Rosenbloom, 107–15 (New York: McGraw-Hill, 2005).

108. Culinary Workers Union Local 226, Strike Bulletin #1, Picket Guidelines, Picket Pay, Apr. 20, 1984, Las Vegas Labor Unions Culinary Union Vertical File, Strikes, NSMA; Iver Peterson, "Strike Dims the Glitter of Las Vegas," *New York Times*, Apr. 22, 1984; Jess Simpson, "Strike Zone," *Review-Journal*, May 12, 2002; Culinary Workers Union Local 226, Culinary Health Fund, Brochure, Las Vegas Labor Unions Culinary Union Vertical File, Benefits, NSMA.

109. Morrison, "Ghanem Succumbs"; "Nevada Boxing Official"; "Hundreds Bid Farewell"; Niles, *Basics*, 83–184; Pierce, "Understanding Managed Care," 115; "Insurance Premiums Increase Under New Law," *Review-Journal*, June 28, 2014; Margot-Sanger-Katz, "Is the Affordable Care Act Working?," *New York Times*, Oct. 26, 2014; Robert Pear, "Health Insurance Companies Seek Big Rate Increases for 2016," *New York Times*, July 3, 2015.

110. Gregory O. Ginn and L. Jean Henry, "Wellness Programs in the Context of Strategic Human Resource Management," *Hospital Topics* (Spring/Summer 2003): 23–28; MGM "culture of health" documents at mgmresorts.com: MGM Resorts International, "Benefits: Creating a Culture of Health," Brochure (2015); MGM Resorts International, "Wellness Programs," Brochure (2015); MGM Resorts International, "Voluntary Benefits," Brochure (2015). See also Steven Moore, "Global Life Expectancy Rises, but People Live Sicker Longer," *Review-Journal*, Oct. 25, 2015.

111. Arnold M. Knightly, "A Healthy Harrah's," *Las Vegas Business Press*, Sept. 7, 2007; Press Release, "Harrah's Opens Employee Health and Wellness Center," *Harrah's News Release* (Jan. 3, 2007); Moore, "Global Life Expectancy Rises."

112. Alexandra Berzon, "A Perfect Storm," *Las Vegas Sun*, Apr. 6, 2008 (incl. "just the sheer").

113. Alexandra Berzon, "Ironworkers Want Stronger Union Action," *Las Vegas Sun*, Apr. 3, 2008; "OSHA Goes Easy," *Las Vegas Sun*, Mar. 31, 2008; AFL-CIO, "Death on the

Job: The Toll of Neglect: A National and State-By-State Profile of Worker Safety and Health in the United States," 22nd ed., AFL-CIO, Washington, DC, Apr. 2013.

114.  For more on modernizing the OSHA civil and criminal penalty system forty years after the OSH Act, see "Protecting America's Workers Act: Modernizing OSHA Penalties," U.S. House of Representatives, Subcommittee on Workforce Protections, Committee on Education and Labor, Washington, DC (Mar. 16, 2010).

115.  Alexandra Berzon, "Interpreting Protections Away," *Las Vegas Sun*, May 18, 2008; Berzon, "Pace Is the New Peril"; Allen, "Sun Wins the Pulitzer."

116.  The AFL-CIO argued that these figures, esp. the rate of accidents per year, were grossly underestimated due to underreporting. See AFL-CIO, "Death on the Job."

117.  Research Division, Nevada Legislature Counsel Bureau, "Policy and Program Report: Labor and Employment" (Apr. 2016). See also Testimony of David Michaels, Assistant Secretary for Occupational Safety and Health, DOL, before the Subcommittee on Workforce Protections, The Committee on Education and Labor, U.S. House of Representatives, Mar. 16, 2010, for views on updating the OSH Act and changes in the American workplace from 1970 to 2010.

# CONCLUSION

Roy Westerfield started his workday like any other. May 4, 1988, was a typical summer day in Henderson, Nevada—sunny and warm. At sixty-one years of age, Westerfield had late effects of polio and walked with a limp, but it did not affect his job as a comptroller for Pacific Engineering Company of Nevada (PEPCON). The company produced ammonium perchlorate, the primary oxidizer used in National Aeronautics and Space Administration (NASA) space shuttle solid rocket boosters (SRBS). Although its production was hazardous, safety experts considered ammonium perchlorate to be considerably less dangerous than mixed fuel. PEPCON conducted manufacturing operations in an industrial center west of the BMI Complex alongside a marshmallow factory, Kidd and Company, and the only other American producer of ammonium perchlorate, Kerr-McGee. The company entered the ammonium perchlorate business in 1959 at the request of the DOD, opening its factory in an isolated part of Henderson. By the 1980s developers built a new housing subdivision, Green Valley, dangerously close, increasing the nearby population to fifty thousand residents, and the risks associated with ammonium perchlorate made national headlines. On January 28, 1986, the NASA space shuttle Challenger was torn apart seventy-three seconds into flight. An O-ring seal had failed on an SRB manufactured by Morton Thiokol, igniting an external fuel tank.[1] The space shuttle disintegrated, killing all seven astronauts on board, and prompting NASA to freeze its program for thirty-two months. The freeze suspended PEPCON's shipping, but did not end the company's contract with Thiokol. Production continued as usual. Over the following fifteen months, PEPCON filled its aluminum storage bins to capacity, storing overflow in stacked, polyethylene drums around the plant site. Taken alone, ammonium perchlorate and polyethylene did not present much of a hazard. But together, according to explosion expert Dr. Michael Fox, they formed a "classic fuel and oxidizer scenario [burning] "like a roman candle."[2]

On May 4, 1988, PEPCON had accumulated more than four thousand tons of ammonium perchlorate. It also had stockpiled other hazardous chemicals, including hydrochloric acid and nitric acid. At 11:30 A.M. sparks from a welding torch accidently lit a nearby steel and fiberglass drying structure. Fires were a common occurrence at the plant, regularly caused by machinery friction, electrical and welding torches, and motor overheating. In each case, management instructed workers to extinguish the flames with a water hose. The method apparently worked well; PEPCON never felt the need to install a fire alarm or sprinkler system in the processing structures. But on May 4, 1988, the method failed. When workers attempted to douse the flames with a hose, the insufficient water pressure could not subdue it. Thanks to chemical residue contaminating the plant site and unusually high winds, the fire spread quickly to the adjacent drums. Without sprinklers to douse the flames, the situation was beyond control fifteen minutes later. Moreover, management had never established evacuation procedures in case of an emergency. As they prepared for their lunch breaks, workers saw the flames and fled for their lives, frantically running or driving into the desert. But Roy Westerfield along with wheelchair-bound Bruce Halker knew they could not escape. Instead, Westerfield called 911, telling the dispatcher, "We just had a big explosion and everything's on fire." The dispatcher said they would send somebody over and he responded, "Get 'em all out here." Those were perhaps his last words.[3]

The fire rapidly traveled along the bins toward the main storage unit. At 11:53 A.M., the first of two major blasts occurred, an explosion one hundred feet in diameter. The shockwaves shattered the windows of incoming fire response units and stopped their approach. When it subsided, a fleeing worker warned Henderson fire chief Roy Parrish about the possibility of a larger explosion. Realizing the situation was beyond his department's suppression capabilities, he ordered his firefighters to retreat. When the fire reached the main storage area, it consumed fifteen hundred tons of ammonium perchlorate. The blast was reminiscent of a nuclear explosion, the equivalent of 250 tons of dynamite and nearly four times the amount in one SRB. Spewing a mushroom cloud hundreds of feet into the air, it ripped a high-pressure gas line out of the ground, igniting a shockwave that registered 3.5 on the Richter scale in Southern California. Employees of PEPCON and Kidd and Company desperately tried to outrun it, dodging smoldering scrap metal and shards of glass. The blast and shockwaves flattened PEPCON and Kidd and Company, and spread to Green Valley, violently shattering windows, flipping cars, buckling garage doors, and buffeting a Boeing 737 as it approached McCarran Airport. It was the largest domestic, nonnuclear explosion in recorded history.[4]

After consuming nearly all the ammonium perchlorate, the explosion stopped. The incident had reduced PEPCON and Kidd and Company to warped steel and a deep crater. Response units evacuated a five-mile radius and started cleaning up, but leaking anhydrous ammonia and acid residue initially hampered their efforts. At 8:00 P.M., they found the body of a man twenty-five feet from the main entrance of the plant. It was Bruce Halker. "The clothes were blown off the body," recalled Parrish, "it was not a pretty sight." An autopsy revealed that he had died of hypoxia, the deprivation of oxygen common in bombing fatalities. They never found Roy Westerfield's body. At their funerals, the men were remembered as martyrs, facing a certain death to alert authorities. The death toll was remarkably low; it would have been worse if the fire had reached Kerr-McGee. A total of 372 people reported injuries, including lacerations, concussions, burns, and eye, skin, and respiratory irritations. A newborn suffered cuts to her eyelids after the windows shattered at St. Rose de Lima Hospital. Extensive property damage occurred as far as ten miles away, costing more than $100 million. A PEPCON attorney tried to blame the accident on Southwest Gas Company, telling reporters that nothing could ignite ammonium perchlorate because it was not flammable. The statement received considerable backlash. Critics charged that the attorney did not understand basic chemistry, and Southwest Gas Company called the theory "creative high-tech fiction." Like the MGM Grand, PEPCON did not have enough insurance, totaling only $1 million. A huge legal battle followed; more than fifty law firms represented dozens of insurance companies and corporations, ending in a $71 million settlement. Several months later, it took a jury only thirty minutes to decide that a gas leak did not cause the explosions.[5]

An investigation by the U.S. Fire Administration, the Federal Emergency Management Agency (FEMA), and the National Fire Data Center determined that PEPCON failed to observe basic safety codes. Despite sustaining repeated fires, it had not installed ventilation, sprinkler, or deluge systems, or fire sensing technology, and had never formulated evacuation procedures in case of an emergency. But one of the most glaring problems involved industrial hygiene. Management allowed a surplus of oxidizer, chemical residue, and dust to contaminate the plant site, and practiced good housekeeping only during scheduled inspections. After the incident, PEPCON retreated to Utah, adopted a new name, Western Electrochemical Company (WECCO), and built a factory in an isolated area outside Cedar City. Despite the new start, history repeated itself a decade later. On July 30, 1997, a seventy-foot explosion killed forty-eight-year-old Daniel Baldeck, a longtime maintenance supervisor for the company who survived PEPCON, and injured three others. An investigation revealed that the company did not learn much from the first event, attributing the accident to poor housekeeping, overcrowded storage, welding sparks, and high winds.[6]

The PEPCON explosion exposed to the state of Nevada the risk of urban sprawl and heavy industry situated in once unpopulated areas. Governor Richard H. Bryan toured the devastation and reacted that it was "a miracle there weren't more deaths." He assembled a commission chaired by District Attorney Bob Miller to examine heavy industry in the state. The so-called Henderson Commission held nine hearings, and received testimony on health and safety, fire prevention, zoning, insurance, and the transportation of hazardous materials. The final report detailed unsettling results. Nevada could not identify the location, use, and transportation of hazardous materials within state borders. Moreover, heavy industry rarely received inspections, and a great deal of hazardous materials were transported on state highways and streets each day, and Nevada could not completely protect its residents. The committee proposed forty-three health and safety measures, such as industrywide mandates to provide details about operations and occupational health programs, steeper penalties for violations, and a ban on hazardous industries in residential areas.[7]

Companies that refused to comply were ordered to relocate. To implement the recommendations, Governor Bryan established a task force headed by the State Fire Marshal and later, the Division of Emergency Management and, by 1991, legislative action, the regulatory agencies, and Nevada OSHA mandates had enacted most. But a follow-up investigation the same year ordered by Governor Bob Miller revealed continued problems. The biggest impediment for Nevada was policing federal lands. In the name of national security, the federal government remained evasive about its hazardous materials installations within state borders. Companies under federal contract also resisted regulation, claiming they were exempt from state laws. Another major concern was funding. Although municipal fire departments received the task of inspecting heavy industry, most had enough resources to conduct only one inspection annually. The Henderson Commission had recommended at least four.[8]

In the end, the PEPCON explosion inspired temporary interest in health and safety in Nevada. On January 7, 1998, a succession of explosions at the Sierra Chemical Company plant east of Reno killed four workers and injured six. Governor Miller responded to the incident by creating the Commission on Workplace Safety and Community Protection, outlining twenty-nine additional recommendations. It did little good. On September 17, 2001, an explosion at the Depressurized Technologies International plant in Minden resulted in another death and four injuries. An investigation revealed that the company had completely ignored most recommendations. Several weeks later, Las Vegas encountered its first major industrial incident since PEPCON. On October 15, 2001, AeroTech Inc., a manufacturer of high-powered model rockets, erupted in two explosions in a sixty-thousand-square-foot building in southeastern Las Vegas. Located in a residential neighborhood, the plant housed 2,500 pounds of ammonium perchlorate and eight hundred pounds of magnesium. When firefighters attempted to extinguish the fire with high-pressure hoses, the water seeped into a drum of magnesium, a water-reactive element. The contaminated drum flashed, resulting in a third powerful explosion. It burned all night, destroying the building and five surrounding businesses. In the aftermath, one worker died, four received burn wounds, and three firefighters were treated for smoke inhalation. The incident shocked Nevadans. Why was ammonium perchlorate, the chemical implicated in the PEPCON explosion, manufactured in a residential neighborhood? One resident summed up the sentiment: "They put our lives and our homes at risk—whoever issued those permits should have their brains examined." State Senator Randolph Townsend of Reno also commented, "They [Clark County] don't seem to have rules there. They almost grow cancerous." In truth, AeroTech Inc. did not have permits to manufacture the materials. A regulation loophole allowed the company to bypass authorization because it did not generate hazardous waste. After an investigation, Nevada OSHA determined that AeroTech Inc. did not completely disclose the complete nature of its business to county licensing and regulatory agencies. It also determined the company's health and safety program did not meet state code.[9]

Taken together, the incidents at PEPCON and AeroTech Inc. reveal the first of three major themes in the history of occupational health. First, improvements in health and safety can be temporary. The PEPCON explosion brought considerable attention to dangerous trades, prompting the establishment of strict standards that recommended regular inspections of hazardous instillations. Initially, the Clark County Fire Department complied with the recommendations, but after 1995 the inspections at AeroTech Inc. stopped. It did not receive one inspection in five years. According to Chief Earl Greene, megaresort construction on the Strip contributed to the problem. The fires at MGM Grand and Las Vegas Hilton were horrific tragedies and publicity nightmares, and inspectors needed to focus their attention on fire safety in the new megaresorts. The fire department did not have enough time or resources to evaluate Clark County's eighteen hundred high-risk facilities. According to Greene, it was virtually impossible to keep up with the growth. After the AeroTech Inc. incident, Clark County acknowledged that the system needed improvements, and increased the inspections by 50 percent, focusing greater attention on high-risk installations.[10]

This scenario occurred repeatedly in this historical study, reflecting a broader theme in the realm of occupational health. Workplace hazards always have the potential to reemerge. Historians Gerald Markowitz and David Rosner considered silicosis, a lung disease caused by the inhalation of crystalline silica dust, "a disease of the past" that the medical community stopped talking about after the 1940s when they cowrote *Deadly Dust*. But silicosis reemerged in the 1990s in the Louisiana shipbuilding industry and Latino oil field workers in Odessa and Midland, Texas. Markowitz and Rosner's book became a principal reference in numerous lawsuits and federal action to curtail the occupational disease.[11] Likewise, the risk of coal mining appeared to have been eliminated with strict federal legislation, and federal and state regulation. This assumption was proved wrong when the Massey Energy Upper Big Branch mine in West Virginia exploded in 2010, killing twenty-nine workers and seriously injuring one. The mine operator completely disregarded health and safety, ignoring important principal standards in ventilation and the application of rock dust. Moreover, management did not provide working water sprays to extinguish the initial fire. These cases, as well as continuing problems with asbestos throughout the United States and abroad, reveal that all workplace hazards have the potential to resurface.[12]

A second theme is that large-scale workplace disasters do not automatically improve health and safety. Although catastrophic events during the twentieth century motivated state and federal governments to locate and fix problems, the important lessons did not reach all work sites. This is the current relationship between the United States and the developing world, where many countries still contend with industrial dangers eliminated in the United States.[13]

In Nevada most large-scale workplace disasters inspired short-term enthusiasm, only to be abandoned months, years, or decades later. Marked failures in occupational health–carbon monoxide poisoning during the construction of Hoover Dam, atmospheric nuclear testing and the Baneberry accident, the MGM Grand and Las Vegas Hilton fires, the PEPCON explosion, and the Strip construction deaths—forced a revaluation of health and safety. Federal, state, and municipal agencies directed the investigation, reviewing existing standards and mandating new ones. However, interest quickly faded. In Nevada, a historically pro-business state, transitioning to a regulatory government was highly unpopular, and new requirements difficult to enforce. The state and municipal agencies also confronted budgetary issues, and required increased funding for inspections and enforcement. The federal government impeded improvement in Nevada as well, undermining state authority on federal lands. Still, each boom in health and safety met some success, at least encouraging the rhetoric of safety. Despite limited funding and authority, the State Inspector of Mines, NIC, and Nevada OSHA improved conditions as well. The underlying problem is that Americans are trapped in a cyclical process of remembering and forgetting about the importance of occupational health. The twelve construction worker deaths on the Strip seemed unprecedented to Nevadans in 2008, but were certainly consistent with the nation's relationship with health and safety.

A final theme is the misconception that the private sector is solely to blame for fostering hazardous workplaces, a point articulated by historians Christopher Sellers, Joseph Melling, and others. A trend in occupational health scholarship in the United States and abroad is that developing states and developed national, state, and municipal governments alike actively encouraged or assisted dangerous industries in order to promote industrial development.[14] This book presents unsettling examples of this. At Hoover Dam and the NTS, large-scale disasters occurred when the federal government condoned the contractors' methods or carried out the actions itself. During the Boulder Canyon project, Six Companies operated gasoline-powered trucks underground, an outlawed method harmful to human health. Secretary of Interior Ray Lyman Wilbur, a physician, understood the health risks and still authorized it. Moreover, he assigned federal attorneys to appear amicus curiae for the contractor during the State Inspector of Mines' failed legal attempt to police health and safety on federal land. At the NTS, the AEC, DOD, laboratories, and contractors conducted atmospheric and underground nuclear testing, exposing the American people to harmful levels of radiation. Even though most scientists recognized that prolonged, small doses increased the risk of cancers or nonmalignant diseases, the federal government willingly ignored the danger in the name of science and national security.

Throughout the twentieth century, these themes occurred repeatedly in Nevada. When I set out to write this book, I wanted to learn why the loss of human lives was an accepted risk in the state. Historians Seth Koven and Sonya Michel have argued that science in association with health reform ideology will thrive only if local and state governments allow for policy advancement and its residents to organize. The residents also must agree to the changes.[15]

This theory is helpful to understand occupational health in Nevada. Unlike most parts of the United States, the Las Vegas area never fully integrated the accumulation and business matrix with regard to health and safety, and risks of the workplace. Although residents protested after large-scale disasters, and local and state officials attempted to shift policies, not everyone consented to the adjustment. The main obstacle hindering the advancement of health and safety was that the community never developed a mission-driven culture of health to reinforce the occupational health regimes. In 2011 UMC chief executive Kathy Silver noted that there had "been a lot of dedication [in Las Vegas] to building [medical] infrastructure that generated money."[16] Its health-care system was, and always had been, a business founded by and connected to local industry. Beginning in 1905, the LA&SL built the first hospital in town for its employees, Dr. Roy Martin opened a private facility, and Clark County developed care for the poor and indigent. The system worked until a population spike inspired by Hoover Dam construction, forcing Six Companies build a hospital. The medical crisis temporarily subsided, but mobilization for World War II caused another influx in residents. BMI helped the situation somewhat, opening an overcrowded hospital that eventually became St. Rose de Lima. But people continued to migrate to southern Nevada during the postwar period to work at the NTS, on the Las Vegas Strip, or at other jobs. Once again, local medicine could not support the population, and the Teamsters provided a solution, funding the construction of Sunrise Hospital.

In the 1970s southern Nevada industry could no longer sustain the health of the community, and the region embraced nationwide trends toward corporate health care. Beginning with Sunrise Hospital, out-of-state, for-profit chains invested in local hospitals. In the 2000s Las Vegas had the most for-profit hospitals of any metropolitan area of its size in the nation. Out of its thirteen acute-care hospitals, twelve were privately owned and nine were for-profit. The national average of privately owned hospital admissions was 13 percent; in Nevada, it was 52 percent. For-profit corporations also operated 70 percent of Las Vegas's acute-care beds. Under corporate direction, the hospitals collected huge returns. During the 1980s, Sunrise reported a profit of 25 percent. In response, the Nevada legislature passed a measure that required out-of-state, for-profit chains with profits exceeding 17 percent to decrease billing charges, but the legislation had expired by the 1990s. In the process, the quality of care in Nevada diminished. Larry Matheis, executive director of the Nevada State Medical Association, blamed investor-owned hospitals for being "shaped by market forces—entrepreneurship, cutthroat competition, and the bottom line."[17]

Profit margins also led to the largest public health notification in American history. In 2008 unhygienic practices at the Endoscopy Center of Southern Nevada exposed forty thousand patients to infectious diseases, including Hepatitis C and HIV. Management had instructed its medical personnel to reuse syringes, allowing the viruses to transfer between patients. According to reports, the Endoscopy Center had authorized the practice to cut costs.[18]

At the same time, the rising cost of medical care upset the entire nation, and Nevada was particularly hard hit. In 2004 the AMA listed the state as one of nineteen in the United States experiencing a crisis in medical liability coverage. Thanks to excessive malpractice litigation, some insurance rates increased 300 percent in the year 2002. Local doctors had to raise prices, retire, or move. Most chose the latter. The crisis reached a tipping point in 2002 when nearly all of the UMC trauma center's fifty-eight surgeons resigned, forcing management to close its doors. The doctors cited as their reason the exorbitant premium costs that made it impossible to perform high-risk surgeries. The trauma center reopened ten days later, but the medical cost crisis continued. By 2010 the city's health-care problems had become notorious, leading Las Vegans to seek treatment in other states. More than $2 billion of Nevada's health-care business went to neighboring states annually. In comparison to the top one hundred metropolitan areas in the United States, Las Vegas had the smallest share of its economy tied to health services. Nevada as a whole lagged behind the nation. It had one of the lowest physician-to-population ratios, ranking forty-sixth in active primary care physicians, and its residencies covered fewer than half of all specialties. Nevada also required important liver and pancreas transplant programs, and ranked fiftieth in the number of psychiatrists per hundred thousand population. In comparison to healthier communities, Las Vegas residents were less likely to receive cancer screenings, blood sugar readings, and other forms of preventive care. They were also twice as likely to die of preventable illnesses such as childhood measles, diabetes, and colon cancer. From 2008 to 2009, 969 preventable injuries, life-threatening infections, and other damages occurred at local hospitals, as well as higher-than-expected incidents of surgical injuries, ranging 34 to 174 percent over national averages. One physician blamed the health crisis in Las Vegas on a "culture of mediocrity," comparing his coworkers to world-class sprinters satisfied with running slow. The standards were "so low" they did not "recognize a problem [that was] staring them in the face."[19]

Unlike most metropolitan areas of its size, the Las Vegas community never developed a culture that valued health during the twentieth century. The railroad founded the city's medical infrastructure, a pattern similar to many western towns. In fact, the LA&SL patterned its hospital care after one established in Sacramento, California. What separated Sacramento from Las Vegas a century later? Sacramento underwent medical crises, but its quality of care remained intact because it had several academic medical centers at its disposal, including the University of California, Davis; the University of California, San Francisco; Stanford University; and others. An academic medical center offers three important interrelated parts to a community: a medical school, a clinical trial and research division, and a sector delivering health-care services. The benefits were endless. Academic medical centers fostered state-of-the-art medicine, raising standards in innovation, excellence, and research. While training future doctors, it also studied the community's needs and developed treatments, and provided the patients with quality care. Most metropolitan areas also housed both public and private centers, promoting healthy competition. Las Vegas was the only metropolitan area of its size that did not have an academic medical center. The main campus of Nevada's only medical school, UMC, was in Reno, and acted as its own teaching hospital. But while medical students spent their third and fourth years in Las Vegas, little research occurred there. Without an academic medical center, Las Vegas did not have enough residency and fellowship programs to convince locally trained doctors to stay. The nation's best doctors also overlooked the area because its hospitals did not practice cutting-edge medicine.[20]

After a Brookings–SRI report revealed that lacking an academic medical center was one of the biggest threats to Las Vegas's economic future in 2011, its residents finally departed from historical trends to institute a research-driven health ideology in the area. In 2013 the Nevada System of Higher Education (NSHE) announced plans to open a four-year, allopathic medical school at UNLV. The NSHE Board of Regents established the UNLV School of Medicine a year later, submitting a two-year budget, and Governor Brian Sandoval signed SB514, authorizing $27 million for the project. The university raised $13.5 million in sixty days to fund scholarships, including the entire inaugural class, and began instruction in 2017. While augmenting the health of the community, the medical school was a major boost to local occupational health. It played an important role in creating a health-minded culture vital to support Nevada's workplaces. By sheer proximity, employees also gained access to higher quality of care. The eventual adoption of occupational medicine into the program could address health and safety problems as well, helping better integrate the accumulation and business risk matrix into local workplace ethic.[21]

Certainly, the development of occupational health in twentieth-century America has been marked by significant advances. No longer are employers and the government not obligated to safeguard workers, protected by outdated doctrines like assumed risk and the right to free contract. Accidents and death are not considered a part of work, and employees are now informed about dangers and given the opportunity to improve their conditions. Health and safety, and employee wellness programs, are integrated into most workplaces, and state agencies, federal agencies, and labor unions devote time to research, regulate, and advocate for American labor. Despite these improvements, the history of occupational health is not a linear story of progress. An important takeaway from this history is that working in America is still dangerous. The Bureau of Labor Statistics calculated that 4,821 workers died in 2014, an average of thirteen deaths a day. American workplaces report more deaths each year than during the nine-year Iraq War. Occupational diseases still occur, causing approximately fifty thousand deaths per year, or an average of 137 a day. More than 3.8 million employees experience work-related injuries and illnesses as well. Latino workers born outside the United States and undocumented here are the demographic most at risk; they are less likely to voice concerns about hazardous working conditions because of deportation fears.[22]

In 2018 the CityCenter operated its glamorous city within a city as a crown destination of Nevada. The twelve construction fatalities that occurred on the Las Vegas Strip a decade earlier had been forgotten in public memory.

It is important to remember that each death had a face. The workers were sons, brothers, and fathers, a fact that I am reminded of daily when I think of my two children entering the workforce. Americans need to undergo a permanent shift in social conscience, consistently placing greater value in kindness and concern for the health and safety of our workers. Only then can we end the gamble with human lives in our workplaces.

## NOTES

1. Each Space Shuttle Solid Rocket Booster (SRB) contained 550 tons of propellant; nearly 70 percent was ammonium perchlorate composite, and the remaining was aluminum fuel, iron oxide catalyst, polymer binder, secondary fuel, and an epoxy curing agent. See NASA, "From Rockets to Ruins: The PEPCON Ammonium Perchlorate Plant Explosion," *NASA Safety Center: System Failure Case Study* 6, no. 9 (Nov. 2012), 1.

2. NASA, "From Rockets to Ruins," 1–2; Karen Workman, "The Challenger Space Shuttle Disaster, 20 Years Later," *New York Times*, Jan. 28, 2016; Florence Lee Jones, "PEPCON," PEPCON Brochure, and Pacific Engineering & Production Company (Annual Report 1978) in Cahlan Collection, Box 6, Folder 41, NSMA; Warren Bates, "The Day Southern Nevada Shook"; and "Shattered Windows, Lives," *Review-Journal*, May 3, 1998; U.S. Fire Administration, "Fire and Explosion at Rocket Fuel Plant, Henderson, Nevada, May 4, 1988," *Technical Report Series*, investigated by J. Gordon Routley, National Fire Data Center (1988), 1–4; "Legislative Commission's Subcommittee on Industrial Explosions," Legislative Counsel Bureau Bulletin No. 03-9 (Jan. 2003), 5–6; Peter H. King and Henry Weinstein, "Safety at Rocket Fuel Plant Topic in Dispute,"

*LA Times*, May 6, 1988; Fox, "Rocket Fuel Plant Explosion," Chemical Accident Reconstruction Services Inc. (2008) (incl. "classic fuel").

3. Jeff German and Mary Manning, "We've Got a Miracle On Our Hands," *Las Vegas Sun*, May 5, 1988; Bates, "The Day Southern Nevada Shook"; Bates, "Shattered Windows, Lives"; Donald L. Shalmy to Richard H. Bryan, letter, July 14, 1988, in *The Governor's Blue Ribbon Commission to Examine the Adequacy of Existing Regulation Pertaining to the Manufacture and Storage of Highly Combustible Materials* (The Henderson Commission), Final Report, Presented to Governor Richard H. Bryan (Aug. 10, 1988), 93–95; "Audio from 911 call delivers news of Pepcon destruction," *News 3 Las Vegas*, May 2, 2013 (incl. "We just had").

4. NASA, "From Rockets to Ruins," 2–3; German and Manning, "We've Got a Miracle"; Bates, "Southern Nevada Shook"; Bates, "Shattered Windows"; Shalmy to Bryan, letter; Meryl Azriel, "US Examines Perchlorate Safety," *Rocket Design* (Aug. 9, 2012).

5. German and Manning, "We've Got A Miracle" (incl. "The clothes were"); Bates, "Southern Nevada Shook"; Bates, "Shattered Windows"; "In 1988, Disaster Struck as Explosions Rocked PEPCON," *Las Vegas Sun*, July 31, 1997; Warren Bates, "July Rules Against PEPCON in Blast" (Dec. 15, 1992) (incl. "creative high-tech fiction"); Azriel, "US Examines Perchlorate Safety"; King and Weinstein, "Safety at Rocket Fuel Plant Topic of Dispute"; "Jury: Southwest Pipeline Not Cause of PEPCON Blasts," *Henderson Home News* (Dec. 17, 1992).

6. Azriel, "US Examines Perchlorate Safety"; King and Weinstein, "Safety at Rocket Fuel Plant Topic of Dispute"; "One Killed, Three Injured in Southern Utah Plant Explosion," *Las Vegas Sun*, July 30, 1997; Cathy Scott, "Cedar City Explosion Kills One, Brings Back Memories of PEPCON Blast," *Las Vegas Sun*, July 31, 1997.

7. State of Nevada, Office of the Governor, Executive Order, May 12, 1988; Bob Miller, "Statement of the Chairman"; *Governor's Blue Ribbon Commission*, 1–12, 14.

8. Bob Miller to Peter G. Morros, Jan. 21, 1991, iii; Peter G. Morros to Bob Miller, Apr. 24, 1991, iv; "Report by the 1991 Governor's Task Force," 1-25; all in *Report by the 1991 Governor's Task Force on Implementation of the Recommendations of the Henderson Commission*, Presented to Governor Bob Miller (Apr. 1991), 1–24.

9. Legislative Commission's Subcommittee on Industrial Explosion, Legislative Counsel Bureau Bulletin No. 03-8 (Jan. 2003), 2–5; Keith Paul, "AeroTech Officials Criticize Handling of Blaze," *Las Vegas Sun*, Feb. 8, 2002; Adrienne Packer, "Reilly Calls County's Fire Investigation 'Horrible,'" *Las Vegas Sun*, Aug. 13, 2002; Mary Manning and Launce Rake, "Aero Facing No Criminal Charges," *Las Vegas Sun*, Feb. 10, 2003; Adrienne Packer, "Frequency of Plant Inspections Questioned," *Las Vegas Sun*, Aug. 12, 2002; Jace Radke, Keith Paul, and Mary Manning, "Fire Raises Safety Questions," *Las Vegas Sun*, Oct. 16, 2001 (incl. "They put our"); "County Criticized over AeroTech," *Las Vegas Sun*, Mar. 7, 2002 (incl. "They [Clark County] don't").

10. Packer, "Frequency of Plant Inspections Questioned."

11. Markowitz and Rosner, *Deceit and Denial*, xii–xiii (incl. "a disease of," xiii).

12. Report to the Governor, "Upper Big Branch: The Apr. 5, 2010 Explosion: A Failure of Basic Coal Mine Safety Practices," Charleston, WV (2010). See also Sellers and Melling, *Dangerous Trade*, 201, for the problem of resurfacing industrial hazards outside the United States.

13. This theme is repeatedly outlined by the various authors in *Dangerous Trade* and articulated by Sellers and Melling in their conclusion. See Sellers and Melling, *Dangerous Trade*, 200-1.

14. See Sellers and Melling, *Dangerous Trade*, 198–99, and Amarjit Kur's "Rubber

Plantation Workers, Work Hazards, and Health and Colonial Malaya," and Daniel E. Renfrew's "New Hazards and Old Disease: Lead Contamination and the Uruguayan Battery Industry."

15. See Koven and Michel, "Womanly Duties: Maternalist Politics and the Origins of Welfare States in France, Germany, Great Britain, and the United States, 1880–1920," *American Historical Review* 95, no. 4 (Oct. 1990): 1076–1108.

16. See Allen, "Why We Suffer," *Las Vegas Sun*, Nov. 14, 2010, for a discussion on the culture for seeking profits in southern Nevada medicine (incl. "been a lot").

17. Ibid. (incl. "shaped by market").

18. Allen and Richards, "Health Care Can Hurt You"; Allen and Richards, "Patients at Risk Under the Knife"; Ashley Powers, "Hepatitis C Outbreak Tied to Alleged Cost-Cutting: 40,000 Patients of a Clinic that Reused Vials and Syringes Are Told to Get Tested for HIV Too," *LA Times*, Mar. 16, 2008; "Hepatitis C Outbreak Springs for Endoscopy Center of Nevada: 40,000 at Risk," *Las Vegas Sun*, Feb. 27, 2008; Marshall Allen, "Officials: Clinic Procedures Put Thousands at Risk," *Las Vegas Sun*, Feb. 28, 2008.

19. Joelle Babula, "Medical Malpractice Crisis: Insurance Costs Driving Doctors Away with Skyrocketing Premiums as High as $200,000 per Year," *Review-Journal*, Jan. 23, 2002; Babula, "Liability Concerns: Trauma Center Closes; ER Gear Up," *Review-Journal*, July 4, 2002; "Trauma Center Reopens Doors," *Review-Journal*, July 14, 2002. See also *Las Vegas Sun*, "Do No Harm: Hospital Care in Las Vegas," series by Marshall Allen and Alex Richards, esp. the following (all in *Las Vegas Sun*): "A Breakthrough in Medical Transparency," June 27, 2010; "Health Care Can Hurt You," June 27, 2010; "A Hidden Epidemic," Aug. 8, 2010; "Patients at Risk Under the Knife," Sept. 19, 2010 (incl. all quotes); "Why We Suffer," Nov. 14, 2010. See also Noam N. Levey, "Unequal Treatment: Las Vegas Tries New Tactic to Improve City's Notorious Healthcare," *LA Times*, June 7, 2014; Tripp Umbach, "Economic Impact of Medical Education in Nevada: Economic Impact Assessment and Recommended Approach," Oct. 24, 2013; UNLV School of Medicine, "Legislative Brochure" (Spring 2015).

20. The Brookings-SRI report findings are summarized by Robert Lang, director of Brookings Mountain West at UNLV, in "The Next Chapter: Las Vegas Becomes a Global City," *Las Vegas Sun*, Sept. 8, 2013. See also Brookings Institution, "The Path Forward for Academic Medical Centers: Innovation, Economics, and Better Health," Brookings Institution, Washington, DC, Apr. 27, 2009; Henry J. Aaron, ed., *The Future of Academic Medical Centers* (Washington, DC: The Brookings Institution, 2001), 1–2; Allen, "Why We Suffer"; Allen, "Teaching hospital is slightly different from the one that teaches medical students, residents," *Las Vegas Sun*, Jan. 14, 2010.

21. Levey, "Unequal Treatment"; Umbach, "Economic Impact"; Lang, "The Next Chapter"; Paul Takahashi, "Answering Questions About a Proposed Medical School," *Las Vegas Sun*, Nov. 12, 2013; Kim Piercall and Michelle Rindels, "Sandoval Signs Bill Sending $27 million to UNLV Medical School," *Las Vegas Sun*, June 11, 2015; Jackie Valley, "Big Tasks Remain for Founding Dean of UNLV Medical School," *Las Vegas Sun*, Nov. 11, 2015. See also UNLV School of Medicine, "Summary of the Institutional Self-Study of The UNLV School of Medicine," Las Vegas, Nevada, Dec. 1, 2015, Prepared by the UNLV SOM Self-Study Summary Task Force for the Liaison Committee on Medical Education.

22. The AFL-CIO argues that these figures, esp. the rate of accidents per year, were grossly underestimated due to underreporting. See AFL-CIO, "Death on the Job: The Toll of Neglect: A National and State-by-State Profile of Worker Safety and Health in the United States," Washington, DC, 2016.

# BIBLIOGRAPHY

## Abbreviations for Notes

*Appendix: Appendix to the Journals of the Nevada State Senate and Assembly*
ATM: Atomic Testing Museum, Las Vegas
Bancroft: Bancroft Library, University of California, Berkeley
BCMHA: Boulder City Museum and Historical Association
"Chronology": "Chronology of Basic Magnesium Inc. Supporting Data," Aug. 27,
    1940–June 11, 1941, BMI Collection, UNLV SC
*Foreman Manual:* Basic Magnesium Inc., *Foreman Manual,* BMI Collection, UNLV SC
Geisel: Geisel Library, University of California, San Diego
GPO: Government Printing Office
HWC: Howard W. Cannon Papers
*LA Times: Los Angeles Times*
NARA: National Archives and Records Administration
NSMA: Nevada State Museum and Archives, Las Vegas
NTS: Nevada Test Site
NTS-OHP: Nevada Test Site Oral History Project
OHP: Oral History Project
*Review-Journal: Las Vegas Review-Journal*
SC: Special Collections
SPO: State Printing Office
UNLV: University of Nevada, Las Vegas

## Manuscript Collections

Basic Magnesium Inc. Collection, Special Collections, University of Nevada,
    Las Vegas.
Baneberry Collection, Special Collections, University of Nevada, Las Vegas.
Leonard Blood Papers, Special Collections, University of Nevada, Las Vegas.
Boulder Club Collection, Nevada State Museum and Archives, Las Vegas.
Cahlan Collection, Nevada State Museum and Archives, Las Vegas.
Howard Cannon Papers, Special Collections, University of Nevada, Las Vegas.
Charter Hospital Collection, Special Collections, University of Nevada, Las Vegas.
Jeannie Digilio Collection, Nevada State Museum and Archives, Las Vegas.
David B. Dill Papers, Mandeville Special Collections, University of California,
    San Diego.
Dunes Collection, Special Collections, University of Nevada, Las Vegas.
El Rancho Collection, Nevada State Museum and Archives, Las Vegas.
Ragnald Fyhen Collection, Special Collections, University of Nevada, Las Vegas.
Harrah's Entertainment Collection, Special Collections, University of Nevada,
    Las Vegas.

Virginia James Collection, Special Collections, University of Nevada, Las Vegas.
Frank C. "Doc" Jensen Papers, Boulder City Historical Society Museum Special
    Collections, Boulder City, Nevada.
George Knox Collection, Special Collections, University of Nevada, Las Vegas.
George Malone Papers, Special Collections, University of Nevada, Las Vegas.
McNamee Collection, Nevada State Museum and Archives, Las Vegas.
MGM Grand Fire Litigation Collection, Special Collections, University of Nevada,
    Las Vegas.
Nevada Nurses Association, Special Collections, University of Nevada, Las Vegas.
Nevada Test Site Oral History Project, Special Collections, University of Nevada,
    Las Vegas.
Sands Collection, Special Collections, University of Nevada, Las Vegas.
Six Companies Corporate Records, Bancroft Library, University of California,
    Berkeley.
Stardust Collection, Special Collections, University of Nevada, Las Vegas.
Union Pacific Collection, Special Collections, University of Nevada, Las Vegas.

## Newspapers and Periodicals

*Boston Herald*
*Chicago* (Daily) *Tribune*
*Las Vegas Age*
*Las Vegas Review-Journal*
*Las Vegas Sun*
*Life* Magazine
*Los Angeles Times*
*New York Times*
*New York Tribune*
*McClure's Magazine*
*Oakland Tribune*
*Reno Evening Gazette-Journal*
*Nevada State Journal*
*Sacramento Bee*
*San Francisco Chronicle*
*Time* Magazine
*U.S. News and World Report*
*Wall Street Journal*

## Public Documents

### Congressional Hearings

U.S. Congress. House. Committee on Interstate and Foreign Commerce. *Low-Level Ef-
    fects of Radiation on Health.* 96th Cong., 1st sess., April 23, May 24, and August 1, 1979.
————. Subcommittee on Health and the Environment of the Committee on Energy
    and Commerce. *Health and the Environment Miscellaneous—Part 2.* 97th Cong.,
    1st sess., March 9 and 24, April 1, 1981.
U.S. Congress. Senate. Special Committee Investigating the National Defense Pro-
    gram. 77th Cong., 2nd sess., Part 13, March 9, 10, 13, 14, 15, 23, and 24, 1942.

———. Special Committee Investigating the National Defense Program. *The National Defense Program*. 78th Cong., 2nd sess., Part 20, April 25; May 21 and 21; June 8, 9, 10; August 19 and 20, 1943.

———. Special Committee to Investigate the Centralization of Heavy Industry in the United States. *Centralization of Heavy Industry in the United States*. 78th Cong., 2nd sess., Part 1, March 27, 1944.

———. Special Committee to Investigate the Centralization of Heavy Industry in the United States. *Centralization of Heavy Industry in the United States*. 78th Cong., 2nd sess., Part 5, November 27 and 28, 1944.

———. Subcommittee of the Committee on Expenditures in the Executive Departments and the Subcommittee of the Special Committee to Investigate the National Defense Program, *Basic Magnesium Plant, Henderson, Nev.*, 80th Cong., 1st sess., May 29; June 24 and 25; August 21 and 22, 1947.

———. Permanent Subcommittee on Investigations of the Committee on Governmental Affairs. *Hotel Employees & Restaurant Employees International Union*. 89th Cong., 1st sess., September 20, 28, and 29; November 18, 1983.

U.S. Department of Commerce. *Health and the Environment Miscellaneous—Part 2*. 97th Cong., 1st sess., March 9 and 24, April 1, 1981.

———. Committee on Education and Labor. *Is OSHA Failing to Adequately Enforce Construction Safety Rules?* 110th Cong., 2nd sess., June 24, 2008.

### Court Cases

Allbritton v. Six Companies Inc. No. 7398 (1937).

American Protection Insurance Company v. MGM Grand Hotel, CV LV 82-26, RDF (1983).

Bulloch v. United States (D.C. Utah 1955), 133 F. Supp. 885.

Farwell v. Boston & Worcester Railroad Corp., 45 Mass. 49 (Mass. 1842).

Feres v. United States of America, 340 U.S. 135 (1950).

In Re MGM Grand Hotel Fire Litigation, 570 F. Supp. 913 (1983).

Jaffee v. United States, 663 F. 2d 1226 (1981).

Kraus v. Six Companies, Inc., Frank Bryant, and John Tacke. No. 4499 (1933).

Norman v. Six Companies, Inc., Woody Williams, and Tom Regan. No. 5256 (1934).

Lochner v. New York, 198 U.S. 45 (1905).

Roberts et al. v. United States of America (1979).

Roberts et al. v. United States of America, 887 F. 2d 899 (1986).

Roberts et al. v. United States of America, 724 F. Supp. 778 (1989).

Prescott v. United States of America, 523 F. Supp. 918 (1981).

Prescott et al. v. United States of America, 724 F. Supp. 792, 798-99 (D. Nev. 1989).

Pike v. Honsinger, 49 N.E. 760 (1898).

Six Companies Inc. v. Stinson, State Inspector of Mines, et al., No. C-191 (1931).

Six Companies Inc. v. Stinson, State Inspector of Mines, et al., 2F. Supp., 689-92 (1933).

### Federal and State Legislation

Coal Mine Safety Act (1952).

Coal Mine Health and Safety Act (1969).

Esh Act (1912).

Energy Employees Occupational Illness Compensation Program Act (2000).
The Hospital Survey and Construction (Hill-Burton) Act (1946).
Nevada Industrial Insurance Act (1913).
Nevada Inspector of Mines Act (1909).
Nevada Labor Commissioner Act (1915).
Nevada Occupational Safety and Health Act (1973).
Nevada State Board of Health Act (1883).
Fair Labor Standards Act (1938).
Federal Safety Appliance Act (1893).
Federal Employers' Liability Act (1908).
Federal Occupational Safety and Health Act (1970).
Federal Torts Claims Act (1948).
Labor Management Relations Act (1947).
Labor Relations (Wagner) Act (1935).
Metal and Nonmetallic Mine Safety Act (1966).
National Foundation of the Arts and Humanities Act (1965).
Radiation-Exposed Veterans Compensation Act (1988).
Walsh-Healey Public Controls Act (1936).
Veterans' Dioxin and Radiation Exposure Compensation Standards Act (1984).
Veterans' Health Care, Training, and Small Business Loan Act (1981).

### Federal and State Government Reports

Atomic Energy Commission. *A Summary of Industrial Accidents in USAEC Facilities.*
    Washington, DC: Government Printing Office, 1955–66.
———. *Operational Accidents and Radiation Exposure Experience Within 1943–1964.*
    Washington, DC: Government Printing Office, 1965.
———. *Operational Accidents and Radiation Exposure Experience Within 1943–1967.*
    Washington, DC: Government Printing Office, 1968.
———. *Operational Accidents and Radiation Exposure Experience Within 1943–1970.*
    Washington, DC: Government Printing Office, 1971.
———. *Operational Accidents and Radiation Exposure Experience Within 1943–1975.*
    Washington, DC: Government Printing Office, 1975.
Department of Energy. *Announced United States Nuclear Tests, July 1945 through
    December 1992.* Washington, DC: Government Printing Office, December 2000.
Hayes, Daniel F. *A Summary of Accidents and Incidents Involving Radiation in Atomic
    Energy Activities, June 1945 through December 1955.* Washington, DC: Government
    Printing Office, 1956.
———. *A Summary of Accidents and Incidents Involving Radiation in Atomic Energy
    Activities, January–December 1956.* Washington, DC: Government Printing Office,
    1957.
JAYCOR. *Summary of Radiological Safety Standards, Dosimetric Devices, & Decontami-
    nation Criteria for Atmospheric Nuclear Weapons Tests, 1945–1962.* JAYCOR Report
    2121-4-1 under DNA-79-0037, 1982.
Legislature Counsel Bureau. "Administrative Procedures Followed by the Nevada
    Industrial Commission and Alternative Methods of Providing Workmen's Com-
    pensation Coverage." Bulletin No. 79-1. Carson City, NV: State Printing Office,
    October 1978.

——. "Legislative Committee on Workers' Compensation." Bulletin No. 01-19. Carson City, NV: State Printing Office, January 2001.

——. "Nevada Industrial Commission Study." Bulletin No. 104. Carson City, NV: State Printing Office, December 1972.

——. "Workmen's Compensation Through Private Insurers." Bulletin No. 83-5. Carson City, NV: State Printing Office, November 1982.

——. "Study of Industrial Insurance, Bulletin No. 93-8. Carson City, NV: State Printing Office, January 1993.

——. "Study of Nevada's Industrial Insurance Program." Bulletin No. 05-7. Carson City, NV: State Printing Office, January 2005.

——. "Legislative Commission's Subcommittee on Industrial Explosion." Bulletin No. 03-8. Carson City, NV: State Printing Office, January 2003.

National Institute of Occupational Safety and Health. *Advisory Board on Radiation and Worker Health: Review of the NIOSH Site Profile for the Nevada Test Site*. Contract No. 200-2004-03805, Task Order I, December 13, 2005.

National Fire Protection Association. *Investigation Report on the MGM Grand Hotel Fire, Las Vegas, Nevada, November 21, 1980*. Report Revised January 15, 1982.

Report by the 1991 Governor's Task Force on Implementation of the Recommendations of the Henderson Commission. Presented to Governor Bob Miller. April 1991.

Report for Inspector of Mines. *Appendix to the Journals of the Nevada State Senate and Assembly*. Carson City, NV: State Printing Office, 1909–1977.

Report of Nevada Industrial Commission. *Appendix to the Journals of the Nevada State Senate and Assembly*. Carson City, NV: State Printing Office, 1913–1977.

Report of State Board of Health. *Appendix to the Journals of the Nevada State Senate and Assembly*. Carson City, NV: State Printing Office, 1893–1977.

Report of Commissioner of Labor. *Appendix to the Journals of the Nevada State Senate and Assembly*. Carson City, NV: State Printing Office, 1915–1977.

Science Applications, Inc. *Analysis of Radiation Exposure for Task Force Warrior Shot Smoky, Exercise Desert Rock VII–VIII, Operation Plumbbob*. Washington, DC, Government Printing Office, May 31, 1979.

State Fire Marshal Division. *Biennial Report of Nevada State Agencies*. Carson City, NV: State Printing Office, 1980.

"The Governor's Blue Ribbon Commission to Examine the Adequacy of Existing Regulation Pertaining to the Manufacture and Storage of Highly Combustible Materials (The Henderson Commission) Presented to Governor Richard H. Bryan." August 10, 1988.

U.S. Congress, Office of Technology Assessment. *The Containment of Underground Nuclear Explosions*. Washington, DC: Government Printing Office, 1988.

U.S. Department of Energy. *Operational Accidents and Radiation Exposures at ERDA Facilities, 1975–1977*. Washington, DC: Government Printing Office, May 1980.

U.S. Department of Health and Human Services. *The Health Consequences of Involuntary Exposure to Tobacco Smoke: A Report of the Surgeon General*. Washington, DC: Government Printing Office, 2006.

U.S. Department of Health and Human Services. *Environmental and Biological Assessment of Environmental Tobacco Smoke Exposure Among Casino Dealers. Health Hazard Evaluation Report*. HETA 2005-0076; 2005-0201-3080 at Bally's, Paris, and Caesars Palace Casinos, Las Vegas, Nevada (May 2009).

Western Environmental Research Laboratory (Environmental Protection Agency). *Final Report of Off-Site Surveillance for the Baneberry Event, December 18, 1970.* February 1972.

## Books

Aldrich, Mark. *Death Rode the Rails: American Railroad Accidents and Safety, 1828–1965.* Baltimore: Johns Hopkins University Press, 2006.

———. *Safety First: Technology, Labor, and Business in the Building of American Work Safety, 1870–1939.* Baltimore: Johns Hopkins University Press, 1997.

Armstrong-Ingram, R. Jackson. *Henderson.* Charleston, SC: Arcadia, 2002.

Balboni, Alan. *Beyond the Mafia: Italian Americans and the Development of Las Vegas.* Reno: University of Nevada Press, 2005.

Barth, Richard C., Patricia D. George, and Ronald H. Hill. *Environmental Health and Safety for Hazardous Waste Sites.* Fairfax, VA: American Industrial Hygiene Association, 2002.

Bayer, Ronald, ed. *The Health and Safety of Workers: Case Studies in the Politics of Professional Responsibility.* New York: Oxford University Press, 1988.

Bell, David. *The Coming of the Post-Industrial Society: A Venture in Social Forecasting.* New York: Basic Books, 1973.

Best, Katharine, and Katharine Hillyer. *Las Vegas: Playtown U.S.A.* New York: David McKay, 1955.

Billington, David P., and Donald C. Jackson. *Big Dams of the New Deal Era: A Confluence of Engineering and Politics.* Norman: University of Oklahoma Press, 2006.

Blachley, Annie. *Good Medicine: 4 Doctors and the Golden Age of Medicine.* Reno: Greasewood Press, 2000.

———. *Pestilence, Politics, and Pizzazz: The Story of Public Health in Las Vegas.* Reno: Greasewood Press, 2002.

Bluestone, Barry, and Bennett Harrison. *The Deindustrialization of America: Plant Closings, Community Abandonment, and the Dismantling of Basic Industry.* New York: Basic Books, 1982.

Botsh, Robert E. *Organizing the Breathless: Cotton Dust, Southern Politics, and the Brown Lung Association.* Louisville: University Press of Kentucky, 1993.

Bowers, Michael. *The Nevada State Constitution: A Reference Guide.* Westport, CT: Greenwood, 1993.

Boyer, Paul S. *By the Bomb's Early Light: American Thought and Culture at the Dawn of the Atomic Age.* Chapel Hill: University of North Carolina Press, 1985.

———. *Fallout: A Historian Reflects on America's Half Century Encounter with Nuclear Weapons.* Columbus: Ohio State University Press, 1998.

Brents, Barbara G., Crystal A. Jackson, and Kathryn Hausbeck. *The State of Sex: Tourism, Sex, and Sin in the New American Heartland.* New York: Routledge, 2010.

Carr Childers, Leisl. *The Size of the Risk: Histories of Multiple Use in the Great Basin.* Norman: University of Oklahoma Press, 2015.

Carson, Rachel L. *Silent Spring.* New York: Houghton Mifflin, 2002 [1962].

Cherniack, Martin. *The Hawk's Nest Incident: America's Worst Industrial Disaster.* New Haven, CT: Yale University Press, 1986.

Clark, Claudia. *Radium Girls: Women and Industrial Health Reform, 1910–1935.* Chapel Hill: University of North Carolina Press, 1997.

Commoner, Barry. *The Closing Circle: Man, Nature and Technology*. New York: Alfred Knopf, 1971.

Corn, Jacqueline Karnell. *Protecting the Health of Workers: The American Conference of Governmental Industrial Hygienists*. Cincinnati, OH: American Conference of Governmental Industrial Hygienists, 1989.

———. *Response to Occupational Health Hazards*. New York: Van Nostrand Reinhold, 1992.

Davies, Richard O. *Main Event: Boxing in Nevada from Mining Camps to the Las Vegas Strip*. Reno: University of Nevada Press, 2014.

De Ville, Kenneth Allen. *Medical Malpractice in Nineteenth-Century America: Origins and Legacy*. New York and London: New York University Press, 1990.

Duffy, John. *The Healers: A History of American Medicine*. Urbana: University of Illinois Press, 1979.

Dunbar, Andrew J., and Dennis McBride. *Building Hoover Dam: An Oral History of the Great Depression*. Reno: University of Nevada Press, 1993.

Ehrlich, Paul R. *The Population Bomb*. Cutchogue, NY: Buccaneer Books, 1968.

Engel, Jonathan. *Doctors and Reformers: Discussion and Debate Over Health Policy, 1925–1950*. Columbia: University of South Carolina, 2002.

Fernlund, Kevin J., ed. *The Cold War American West, 1945–1989*. Albuquerque: University of New Mexico Press, 1998.

Findlay, John M. *People of Chance: Gambling in American Society from Jamestown to Las Vegas*. New York: Oxford University Press, 1986.

Forbath, William E. *Law and the Shaping of the American Labor Movement*. Cambridge, MA: Harvard University Press, 1991.

Fox, Steve. *Toxic Work: Women Workers at GTE Lenkurt*. Philadelphia: Temple University Press, 1991.

Fradkin, Philip. *Fallout: An American Nuclear Tragedy*. Boulder, CO: Johnson Books, 1989.

Gallagher, Carole. *American Ground Zero: The Secret Nuclear War*. Cambridge, MA: The MIT Press, 1993.

Goodwin, Joanne L. *Changing the Game: Women at Work in Las Vegas, 1940–1990*. Reno: University of Nevada Press, 2014.

Gottlieb, Robert. *Forcing the Spring*. Washington, DC: Island Press, 1993.

Green, Michael S. *Nevada: A History of the Silver State*. Reno: University of Nevada Press, 2015.

Greenwald, Richard A. *The Triangle Fire, Protocols of Peace, and Industrial Democracy in Progressive Era New York*. Philadelphia: Temple University Press, 2005.

Hacker, Barton C. *The Dragon's Tail: Radiation Safety in the Manhattan Project, 1942–1946*. Berkeley: University of California Press, 1987.

———. *Elements of Controversy: The Atomic Energy Commission and Radiation Safety in Nuclear Weapons Testing, 1947–1974*. Berkeley: University of California Press, 1994.

Hamilton, Alice. *Exploring the Dangerous Trades: The Autobiography of Alice Hamilton*. Boston: Northeastern University Press, 1985 [1943].

Hannigan, John. *Fantasy City: Pleasure and Profit in the Postmodern Metropolis*. New York: Routledge, 1998.

Hays, Samuel. *The Response to Industrialism, 1885–1914*. Chicago: University of Chicago Press, 1957.

Helper, Allison L. *Women in Labor: Mothers, Medicine, and Occupational Health in the United States, 1890–1980.* Columbus: Ohio State University Press, 2000.

Herzberg, Frederick, Bernard Mausner, and Barbara Bloch Snyderman. *The Motivation to Work.* New York: John Wiley and Sons, 1959.

Hiltzik, Michael. *Colossus: The Turbulent, Thrilling Saga of the Building of Hoover Dam.* New York: Free Press, 2010.

Hofstadter, Richard. *The Age of Reform: From Bryan to FDR.* New York: Knopf, 1955.

Hogan, Neal C. *Unhealed Wounds: Medical Malpractice in the Twentieth Century.* New York: LFB Scholarly, 2003.

Hopkins, A. D., and K. J. Evans. *The First 100: Portraits of the Men and Women Who Shaped Las Vegas.* Las Vegas: Huntington Press, 1999.

Hounshell, David. *From the American System to Mass Production, 1800–1932: The Development of Manufacturing Technology in the United States.* Baltimore: Johns Hopkins University Press, 1984.

Hounshell, David, and John Kenley Smith. *Science and Corporate Strategy: Du Pont R&D, 1902–1980.* Cambridge, UK: Cambridge University Press. 1988.

Hulse, James W. *Nevada's Environmental Plunder.* Reno: University of Nevada Press, 2009.

———. *The Silver State: Nevada's Heritage Reinterpreted.* Reno: University of Nevada Press, 2004.

Hurst, James Willard. *Law and the Conditions of Freedom in the Nineteenth-Century United States.* Madison: University of Wisconsin Press. 1956.

Igler, David. *Industrial Cowboys: Miller & Lux and the Transformation of the Far West 1850–1920.* Berkeley: University of California Press, 2001.

Johns, Larry C., and Alan R. Johns. *The Baneberry Disaster: A Generation of Atomic Fallout.* Reno: University of Nevada Press, 2017.

Jones, R. Jay. *The Old Central Pacific Hospital.* San Francisco, CA: Western Association of Railroad Surgeons, 1961.

Judkins, Bennett. *We Offer Ourselves as Evidence: Toward Workers' Control of Occupational Health.* New York: Greenwood, 1986.

Kersten, Andrew E. *Labor's Home Front: The American Federation of Labor During World War II.* New York and London: New York University Press, 2006.

King, R. D. *Hoover Dam and Boulder City, 1931–1936: A Discussion Among Some Who Were There.* Reno: Oral History Project, University of Nevada, 1987.

Klein, Maury. *Union Pacific: Birth of a Railroad, 1862–1893.* New York: Doubleday, 1987.

———. *Union Pacific: The Rebirth, 1894–1969.* New York: Doubleday, 1989.

Kolin, Andrew. *Political Economy of Labor Repression in the United States.* Lanham, MD: Lexington Books, 2017.

Kolko, Gabriel. *The Triumph of Conservatism.* New York: Free Press of Glencoe, 1963.

Koven, Seth, and Sonya Michel, eds. *Mothers of a New World: Maternalist Politics and the Origins of Welfare States.* New York: Routledge, 1993.

Kraft, James P. *Vegas at Odds: Labor Conflict in a Leisure Economy, 1960–1985.* Baltimore: Johns Hopkins University Press, 2010.

Leavitt, Judith Walzer, and Ronald Numbers, eds. *Sickness and Health in America.* Madison: University of Wisconsin Press, 1997.

Lindee, M. Susan. *Suffering Made Real: American Science and the Survivors of Hiroshima.* Chicago: University of Chicago Press, 1994.

Lowitt, Richard. *The New Deal and the West*. Norman: University of Oklahoma Press, 1993.

Luz, Tom. *Do Nothing: A History of Loafers, Loungers, Slackers, and Bums in America*. New York: Farrar, Straus, and Giroux, 2006.

Maclean, Nancy. *Freedom Is Not Enough: The Opening of the American Workplace*. Cambridge, MA: Harvard University Press, 2006.

Markowitz, Gerald, and David Rosner. *Deadly Dust: Silicosis and the Politics of Occupational Disease in Twentieth-Century America*. Princeton, NJ: Princeton University Press, 2003.

———. *Deceit and Denial: The Deadly Politics of Industrial Pollution*. Berkeley: University of California Press, 2006.

———, eds. *Dying for Work: Workers Safety and Health in Twentieth-Century America*. Bloomington: Indiana University Press, 1987.

———. *Lead Wars: The Politics of Science and the Fate of America's Children*. Berkeley: University of California Press, 2014.

———, eds. *"Slaves of the Depression": Workers' Letters about Life on the Job*. Ithaca, NY, and London: Cornell University Press, 1987.

McBride, Dennis. *In the Beginning: A History of Boulder City, Nevada*. Boulder City, NV: Boulder City Museum and Historical Association, 1992.

McGregor, Douglas. *The Human Side of Enterprise*. New York: McGraw Hill, 1960.

Miller, Richard. *Under the Cloud: The Decades of Nuclear Testing*. New York: The Free Press, 1986.

Moehring, Eugene P. *Resort City in the Sunbelt: Las Vegas 1930–2000*. Reno: University of Nevada Press, 2000.

Moehring, Eugene P., and Michael S. Green. *Las Vegas: A Centennial History*. Reno: University of Nevada Press, 2005.

———. *Urbanism and Empire in the Far West, 1840–1890*. Reno: University of Nevada Press, 1996.

Mohr, James C. *Doctors and the Law: Medical Jurisprudence in Nineteenth-Century America*. Baltimore and London: John Hopkins University Press, 1993.

Moreno, Jonathan D. *Undue Risk: Secret State Experiments on Humans*. New York: Routledge, 2001.

Murphy, Michelle. *Sick Building Syndrome and the Problem of Uncertainty*. Durham, NC, and London: Duke University Press, 2006.

Murray, John E. *Origins of American Health Insurance: A History of Industrial Sickness Funds*. New Haven, CT: Yale University Press, 2007.

Nash, Gerald D. *The American West Transformed: The Impact of the Second World War*. Lincoln: University of Nebraska Press, 1985.

———. *The Crucial Era: The Great Depression and World War II, 1929–1945*. New York: St. Martin's Press, 1992.

———. *The Federal Landscape: An Economic History of the Twentieth-Century West*. Tucson: University of Arizona Press, 1999.

———. *The New Deal and the West*. Norman: University of Oklahoma Press, 1993.

———. *World War II and the West: Reshaping the Economy*. Lincoln: University of Nebraska Press, 1990.

Nash, Linda. *Inescapable Ecologies: A History of Environment, Disease, and Knowledge*. Berkeley: University of California Press, 2006.

Nelkin, Dorothy, and Michael Brown. *Workers at Risk: Voices for the Workplace.* Chicago: University of Chicago Press, 1984.

Newman, Katherine S. *Falling from Grace: Downward Mobility in the Age of Affluence.* Berkeley: University of California Press, 1999.

Novak, William. *The Peoples' Welfare: Law and Regulation in Nineteenth-Century America.* Chapel Hill: University of North Carolina Press, 1996.

Oughterson, Ashley W., and Shields Warren. *Medical Effects of the Atomic Bomb in Japan.* New York: McGraw-Hill, 1956.

Paher, Stanley. *Las Vegas, As It Began—As It Grew.* Las Vegas: Nevada Publications, 1971.

Palevsky, Mary. *Atomic Fragments: A Daughter's Questions.* Berkeley: University of California Press, 2000.

Pomeroy, Earl. *Search of the Golden West: The Tourist in Western America.* New York: Knopf, 1957.

Pugh, Richard G. *Serving Medicine: The Nevada State Medical Association and the Politics of Medicine.* Reno: Greasewood Press, 2002.

Reich, Robert K. *The Work of Nations: Preparing Ourselves for Twenty-First Century Capitalism.* New York: Alfred A. Knopf, 1991.

Reid, Ed, and Ovid Demaris. *Las Vegas: City Without Clocks.* Edgewood Cliffs, NJ: Prentice Hall, 1961.

———. *The Green Felt Jungle.* New York: Pocket Books, 1964.

Rifkin, Jeremy. *The End of Work: The Decline of the Global Labor Force and the Dawn of the Post-Market Era.* New York: G. P. Putnam's Sons, 1995.

Rosenberg, Howard. *Atomic Soldiers: American Victims of Nuclear Experiments.* Boston: Beacon Press, 1980.

Rosenberg, Nathan. *Technology and American Economic Growth.* New York: Harper and Row, 1972.

Roske, Ralph. *Las Vegas: A Desert Paradise.* Tulsa, OK: Continental Heritage, 1986.

Rothman, David. *Strangers at the Bedside: A History of How Law and Bioethics Transformed Medical Decision Making.* New York: Basic Books, 1991.

Rothman, Hal K. *Devil's Bargains: Tourism in the Twentieth-Century American West.* Lawrence: University of Kansas Press, 1998.

———. *Neon Metropolis: How Las Vegas Started the Twenty-First Century.* New York: Routledge, 2003.

———. *Nevada: The Making of Modern Nevada.* Reno: University of Nevada Press, 2010.

Rothstein, William. *American Physicians in the Nineteenth Century: From Sects to Science.* Baltimore: John Hopkins University Press, 1992.

Selleck, Henry B. *Occupational Health in America.* Detroit, MI: Wayne State University Press, 1962.

Sellers, Christopher C. *Hazards of the Job: From Industrial Disease to Environmental Health Science.* Chapel Hill and London: University of North Carolina Press, 1997.

Sellers, Christopher, and Joseph Melling, eds. *Dangerous Trades: Histories of Industrial Hazard Across a Globalizing World.* Philadelphia: Temple University Press, 2012.

Shaw, Robert. *Down Brakes: A History of Railroad Accidents, Safety Precautions, and Operating Practices in the United States of America.* London: Macmillan, 1961.

Sheehan, Helen E., and Richard P. Wedeen. *Toxic Circles: Environmental Hazards from the Workplace to the Community.* New Brunswick, NJ: Rutgers University Press, 1993.

Sheehan, Jack. *Quiet Kingmaker: E Perry Thomas*. Las Vegas: Stephens Press, 2009.

Short, Henry J. *Railroad Doctors, Hospitals, and Associations: Pioneers in Comprehensive Low Cost Medical Care*. Upper Lake, CA: H. J. Short, 1986.

Signor, John R. *The Los Angeles and Salt Lake Railroad*. San Marino, CA: Golden West Books, 1988.

Sklar, Martin J. *The Corporate Reconstruction of American Capitalism, 1890–1916: The Market, Law, and Politics*. Cambridge, UK: Cambridge University Press, 1988.

Smith, Barbara Ellen. *Digging Our Own Graves: Coal Miners and the Struggle over Black Lung Disease*. Philadelphia: Temple University Press, 2004.

Starr, Paul. *The Social Transformation of American Medicine*. New York: Basic Books, 1982.

Stevens, Joseph. *Hoover Dam: An American Adventure*. Norman and London: University of Oklahoma Press, 1988.

Stone, Richard D. *The Interstate Commerce Commission and the Railroad Industry*. New York: Praeger, 1991.

Tanenhaus, David S. *Juvenile Justice in the Making*. New York: Oxford University Press, 2004.

Thomson, David. *In Nevada: The Land, the People, God, and Chance*. New York: Alfred A. Knopf, 1999.

Titus, A. Constandina. *Bombs in the Backyard: Atomic Testing and American Politics*. Reno: University of Nevada Press, 1986.

Tomlins, Christopher. *Law, Labor, and Ideology in the Early American Republic*. New York and Cambridge: Cambridge University Press, 1993.

Udall, Stewart L. *The Myths of August: A Personal Exploration of Our Tragic Cold War Affair with the Atom*. New York: Pantheon Books, 1994.

———. *The Quiet Crisis*. New York: Avon Books, 1963.

Uhl, Michael, and Tod Ensign. *GI Guinea Pigs: How the Pentagon Exposed Our Troops to Dangers More Deadly Than War*. Chicago: Playboy Press, 1980.

Vernetti, Michael. *Senator Howard Cannon of Nevada*. Reno: University of Nevada Press, 2008.

Walker, Samuel J. *The Road to Yucca Mountain: The Development of Radioactive Waste Policy in the United States*. Berkeley: University of California Press, 2010.

———. *Permissible Dose: A History of Radiation Protection*. Berkeley: University of California Press, 2000.

Warren, Shields. *The Pathology of Ionizing Radiation*. Springfield, IL: Charles C. Thomas, 1961.

Wasserman, Thomas H., and Norman Solomon, with Robert Alvarez and Eleanor Walters. *Killing Our Own: The Disaster of America's Experience with Atomic Radiation*. New York: Delta Books, 1982.

Weibe, Robert. *The Search for Order*. New York: Hill & Wang, 1967.

Weindling, Paul, ed. *The Social History of Occupational Health*. London: Croom Helm, 1985.

Welke, Barbara Young. *Recasting American Liberty: Gender, Race, Law, and the Railroad Revolution, 1865–1920*. New York: Cambridge University Press, 2001.

Welsome, Eileen. *The Plutonium Files: America's Secret Experiments in the Cold War*. New York: Dial Press, 1999.

White, John. *The American Railroad Freight Car*. Baltimore: Johns Hopkins University Press, 1993.

Williams, William Appleman. *The Tragedy of American Diplomacy*. New York: W. W. Norton, 1972.

Witt, John Fabian. *The Accidental Republic: Crippled Workmen, Destitute Widows, and the Remaking of American Law*. Cambridge, MA: Harvard University Press, 2004.

## Authored Articles and Essays

Aldrich, Mark. "The Peril of the Broken Rail: The Carriers, the Steel Companies, and Rail Technology, 1900–1945." *Technology and Culture* 40, no. 2 (1999): 263–91.

———. "Train Wrecks and Typhoid Fever: The Development of Railroad Medicine Organizations, 1850 to World War I." *Bulletin of the History of Medicine* 75, no. 2 (Summer 2001): 254–89.

Berman, Daniel. "Why Work Kills: A Brief History of Occupational Safety and Health in the United States." *International Journal of Health Services* 7 (1977): 63–87.

Buchanan, Susan, Pamela Vossenas, Niklas Krause, Joan Moriarty, Eric Frumin, Jo Anna Sgimek, Franklin Miller, Peter Orris, and Laura Punnet. "Occupational Injury Disparities in the US Hotel Industry." *American Journal of Industrial Medicine* 53 (2010): 116–25.

Caldwell, Glyn G., Delle K. Kelley, and Clark W. Heath Jr. "Leukemia Among Participants in Military Maneuvers at a Nuclear Bomb Test: A Preliminary Report." *Journal of the American Medical Association* 244 (October 3, 1980): 1575–78.

Davis, Audrey. "Life Insurance and the Physical Examination: A Chapter in the Rise of American Medical Technology." *Bulletin of the History of Medicine* 55 (1981): 392–406.

Dobbs, William T. "Southern Nevada and the Legacy of Basic Magnesium, Incorporated." *Nevada Historical Society Quarterly* 34 (Spring 1991): 1–20.

Hacker, Barton C. "Radiation Safety, the AEC, and Nuclear Testing." *Public Historian* 14, no. 1 (Winter 1992): 31–53.

Johnson, Emory. "Railway Relief Departments." *U.S. Department of Labor Bulletin* 8 (1987): 39–57

Koven, Seth, and Sonya Michel. "Womanly Duties: Maternalist Politics and the Origins of Welfare States in France, Germany, Great Britain, and the United States, 1880–1920." *American Historical Review* 94 no. 4 (1990): 1076–1108.

Mancuso, Thomas A., Alice M. Stewart, and George W. Kneale. "Radiation Exposures of Hanford Workers Dying from Cancer and Other Causes." *Health Physics* 33 (1977): 369–85.

Markowitz, Gerald, and David Rosner. "More Than Economics: The Politics of Workers' Health and Safety, 1932–1947." *Milbank Quarterly* 64 (Fall 1986): 331–51.

———. "Research or Advocacy: Federal Occupational Safety and Health Policies during the New Deal." *Journal of Social History* 18, no. 3 (Spring 1985): 265–380.

———. "The Limits of Thresholds: Silica and the Politics of Science, 1935–1990." *American Journal of Public Health* 85, no. 2 (1995): 253–62.

Melling, Joseph. "The Risks of Working and the Risks of Not Working: Trade Unions, Employers, and Responses to the Risk of Occupational Illness in British Industry, 1890–1940s." Discussion Paper 12, Centre of Analysis of Risk and Regulation (CARR), London School of Economics and Political Science, London (2003).

Mittman, Gregg, Michelle Murphy, and Christopher Sellers, eds. "Landscapes of Exposure: Knowledge and Illness in Modern Environments." Special Issue, *Osiris* (2004), 1–17.

Nugent, Angela. "Fit for Work: The Introduction of Physical Examinations in Industry." *Bulletin of the History of Medicine* 57 (1983): 578–95.

Rocha, Guy. "The I.W.W. and the Boulder Canyon Project: The Death Throes of American Syndicalism." In *At the Point of Production: The Local History of the I.W.W.*, edited by Joseph R. Conlin. Westport, CT: Greenwood Press (1981): 213–34.

Rodgers, Daniel. "The Search of Progressivism." *Reviews in American History* 10, no. 4 (Dec. 1982): 113–32.

Scherzer, T., and N. Kraus. "Work Related Pain and Injury and Barriers to Workers' Compensation Among Las Vegas Hotel Room Cleaners." *American Journal of Public Health* 95, no. 3 (March 2005).

Schofield, Richard O. "Industrial Medicine in Nevada as Practiced in the Construction of Boulder Dam." In *A Life's Review and Notes on the Development of Medicine in Nevada*, edited by M. R. Walker, 86–92. Reno: n.p., 1944.

Sellers, Christopher. "Factory as Environment: Industrial Hygiene, Professional Collaboration and the Modern Sciences of Pollution." *Environmental History Review* 18, no. 1 (1994): 55–83.

Shaffer, H. J., J. V. Bilt, and M. N. Hall. "Gambling, Drinking, and Other Health Risk Activities Among Casino Employees." *American Journal of Industrial Medicine* 36 (1999): 365–78.

Tomlins, Christopher L. "A Mysterious Power: Industrial Accidents and the Legal Construction of Employment Relations in Massachusetts, 1800–1850." *Law and History Review* 6, no. 2 (Fall 1988).

Turk, Michelle Follette. "Dead Roses and Blooming Deserts: The Medical History of a New Deal Icon." *Nevada Historical Society Quarterly* 50 (Fall 2007): 239–64

Usselman, Steven. "Air Brakes for Freight Trains: Technological Innovation in the American Railroad Industry, 1869–1900." *Business History Review* 58 (1984): 30–50.

Walker, J. Samuel. "The Atomic Energy Commission and the Politics of Radiation Protection, 1967–1971." *History of Science Society Isis* 85, no. 1 (March 1994).

———. "The Controversy over Radiation Safety: A Historical Overview." *Journal of the American Medical Association* 262 (August 4, 1989): 664–68.

Warren, Shields. "Hiroshima and Nagasaki Thirty Years After." *Proceedings of the American Philosophical Society* 121, no. 2 (Apr. 29, 1977).

## Theses, Dissertations, and Unpublished Papers

Dobbs, William. "Working at BMI: Reflections on Life and Labor at America's Largest World War II Magnesium Plant." Unpublished paper, 1984, Special Collections, University of Nevada, Las Vegas.

Edwards, Susan. "Atomic Age Training Camp: The Historical Archeology of Camp Desert Rock." Master's thesis, University of Nevada, Las Vegas, 1997.

Foster, Jonathan Lavon. "Stigma Cities: Dystopian Urban Identities in the United States West and South in the Twentieth Century." Doctoral dissertation, University of Nevada, Las Vegas, 2009.

Klimek, Sandra. "A History of Hospitals: Clark County, Nevada." Unpublished paper, 1985, Special Collections, University of Nevada, Las Vegas.

Murphy, Don R. "The Role of Changing External Relations in the Growth of Las Vegas, Nevada." Doctoral dissertation, University of Nebraska, Lincoln, 1969.

Sadovich, Maryellen. "Basic Magnesium, Incorporated and the Industrialization of Southern Nevada." Master's thesis: University of Nevada, Las Vegas, 1971.

Wammack, Mary D. "Atomic Governance: Militarism, Secrecy, and Science in Postwar
   America, 1945–1958." Doctoral dissertation, University of Nevada, Las Vegas, 2010.

## Interviews

Baratz, Adele. Interview by Steve McClenachan. March 4, 1979. SC, UNLV.
———. Interview by Claytee White. March 19, 2007. SC, UNLV.
Barnett, Barbara Ann. Interview by Charles Moore Chesnutt. March 8, 1981. SC, UNLV.
Beam, William. Interview by Mary Palevsky. January 20, 2005. NTS-OHP.
Blanchard, Lucius. Interview by Claytee White. October 3, 2003. SC, UNLV.
Boyer, Harold. Interview by Claytee White. November 15, 2000. SC, UNLV.
Campbell, John F. Interview by Robert Nickel. July 23, 2004. NTS-OHP.
———. Interview by Mary Palevsky. January 14, 2005. NTS-OHP.
———. Interview by Charlie Deitrich. January 31, 2006. NTS-OHP.
Campbell, Robert "Doc" Jr. Interview by Suzanne Becker. March 12, 2005. NTS-OHP.
Chadburn, Louis A., and Debbie Endsley. Interview by Dennis McBride. May 18, 1999.
   Boulder City Museum and Historical Association, Boulder City, NV.
Cherry, J. C. Interview by Cheryl Mawhinney. March 20, 1978. SC, UNLV.
Curran, Robert Joseph. Interview by Suzanne Becker. July 18, 2005. NTS-OHP.
Dill, David Bruce. Interview by Lusie A. Soholt. March 13, 1975. SC, UNLV.
———. Interview by R. C. Turner. May 4, 1976. SC, UNLV.
Flangas, William. Interview by Mary Palevsky. November 12, 2004. NTS-OHP.
Friedrichs, Robert. Interview by Mary Palevsky. February 25, 2005. NTS-OHP.
Johnson, Viola. Interview by Claytee White. March 12, 1996. SC, UNLV.
Jones, Mazie Martin. Interview by Jane P. Kowalewski. November 3, 1978. SC, UNLV.
Kreisler, Leonard. Interview by Suzanne Becker. April 20, 2005. NTS-OHP.
McDaniel, John R. Interview by Daniel Malloy. October 24, 1974. SC, UNLV.
Merlino, James. Interview by Suzanne Becker. Nov. 7, 2004. NTS-OHP.
Rojas, Joseph. Interview by Suzanne Lubritz. February 25, 1980. SC, UNLV.
Rymer, Mary Kennedy. Interview by Mary Fitzgerald. May 4, 1977. SC, UNLV.
Sowder, Elmer. Interview by Mary Palevsky. April 29, 2004. NTS-OHP.
———. Interview by Mary Palevsky. June 23, 2004. NTS-OHP.
Watkins, John P. Interview by Brian Watkins. March 4, 1979. SC, UNLV.
Witt, Rosemary. Interview by University of Nevada, Las Vegas. November 17, 2006. SC,
   UNLV.
Woodbury, Clare. Interview by Ralph Roske. September 12, 1974. SC, UNLV.

## Web Pages

Census Bureau Quick Facts, census.gov/quickfacts
Centers for Disease Control and Prevention, The National Institute for Occupational
   Safety and Health, cdc.gov/niosh
Las Vegas Convention and Visitors Authority, lvcva.com
Lawrence Livermore National Laboratory, llnl.gov
Los Alamos National Laboratory, lanl.gov
Nevada Test Site Oral History Project, digital.library.unlv.edu/ntsohp
Nevada State Library, Archives and Public Records, nsla.nv.gov
Nevada State Museum, Las Vegas, nvculture.org/nevadastatemuseumlasvegas

Office of Disease Prevention and Health Promotion, health.gov

Online Nevada Encyclopedia, onlinenevada.org

Sandia National Laboratories, sandia.gov

State of Nevada Department of Business & Industry, Occupational Safety & Health Administration, dir.nv.gov/OSHA/Home

State of Nevada Department of Business & Industry, Office of the Labor Commissioner, labor.nv.gov

University of Nevada, Las Vegas Digital Collections, digital.library.unlv.edu

University of Nevada, Las Vegas Special Collections and Archives, library.unlv.edu /speccol

U.S. Bureau of Reclamation, usbr.gov

U.S. Department of Energy National Laboratories, energy.gov/maps/doe-national -laboratories

U.S. Department of Energy OpenNet, osti.gov/opennet

U.S. Department of Health and Human Services, hhs.gov

U.S. Department of Labor, dol.gov

U.S. Department of Labor, Bureau of Labor Statistics, bls.gov

U.S. Department of Labor, Occupational Safety and Health Administration, osha.gov

# ABOUT THE AUTHOR

MICHELLE FOLLETTE TURK is a historian of occupational health and the state of Nevada. She has authored scholarly articles on health, safety, and labor at the Hoover Dam, and is a lecturer on Las Vegas medical history and Hoover Dam labor history. Professor Turk earned her doctorate in the history of the twentieth century American West with specialties in public history from the University of Nevada, Las Vegas. She served as a founding deputy director of Preserve Nevada, a statewide nonprofit organization dedicated to the preservation of Nevada's cultural, historical, and archeological heritage, and currently teaches history at the University of Nevada, Las Vegas. Professor Turk is the granddaughter of Kirk V. Cammack Jr., MD, the second board-certified surgeon in Nevada and cofounder of the Lion's Burn Care Center at University Medical Center (UMC) in Las Vegas. She lives in Las Vegas with her husband and two children.

# INDEX

absenteeism, 144
academic medical centers, 313–314
Accident Reports Act, 26
acute radiation syndrome, 194–95
Adams, Harry, 207
addictive behaviors, 256
Adrian Dominican Sisters, 158
AEC. *See* Atomic Energy Commission
AeroTech explosion, 307–8
AFL. *See* American Federation of Labor
African Americans: Oscar Allbritton's
    medical malpractice case, 104–8; BMI
    employee housing and, 135; in the BMI
    workforce, 130, 131–32; Boulder Dam
    construction and, 69, 111n13; employ-
    ment discrimination and desegregation
    during World War II, 130–32; employ-
    ment discrimination on the Las Vegas
    Strip, 252, 253–54; railroad laborers, 27;
    residents in Nevada and Las Vegas, 131
Aikman, Duncan, 68
Alabama Dry Dock and Shipbuilding
    Company, 130–31, 162n33
Aladdin casino, 245
Alcoa Aluminum, 124
alcohol, 41, 42, 83, 144, 211
Aldrich, Mark, 22–23, 44, 100
Allbritton, Oscar, 104–8
*Allbritton v. Union Pacific*, 103–8
Allen, Marion, 78
Allis-Chalmers Manufacturing, 67
ambulances, 73
Amchitka island, 204
American Association for Cancer
    Research, 184
American Engineering and Industrial
    Standards, 97
American Federation of Labor (AFL), 65,
    74, 146–47
American Guild of Variety Artists, 267
*American Journal of Tropical Medicine*, 87, 88
American Legion, 54–56
American Magnesium Corporation, 124

American Medical Association, 217
American Medicorp, 270
American Railway Association, 26
ammonium perchlorate, 303–5, 307–8
Anaconda Copper Company, 138, 150
Anderson, Frank Desmond, 74
Anderson Brothers Supply Company, 82,
    83–84, 139, 143, 164n63
animal acts and attacks, 262–64
Anthony, Robert, 260
Apcar, Frederic, 252, 262
Arcade saloon, 41
*Archives of Environmental Health*, 217
Arizona Club, 41
Arizona Industrial Commission, 90
Armed Forces Special Weapons Project, 187
Army Air Corps, 123, 125
Army Air Force, 127
*Arrows into the Sun* (Lauritzen), 127
arson, 278, 282
Arsphenamine, 81, 113n46
assumed risk doctrine, 8–9
Atkinson, H. H., 94
atmospheric nuclear testing: American
    postwar pursuit of, 187–88; ban on, 186,
    204; Exercise Desert Rock, 185, 192, 193,
    202–4, 218–20; first tests at the Nevada
    Test Site, 188–89 (*see also* Nevada Test
    Site); occupational health regime at the
    Nevada Test Site, 193–99, 200–204
Atomic Bomb Causality Commission, 184,
    185
atomic bombs: dropped on Japan, 158–59;
    studies of the effects of radiation expo-
    sure in Japan, 183–85. *See also* Nevada
    Test Site; nuclear testing
atomic demolition munitions, 204–5
Atomic Energy Act (1946), 187
Atomic Energy Commission (AEC): atmo-
    spheric nuclear testing and, 186, 187,
    188, 189; Baneberry test/disaster and,
    214, 215–16; creation of, 187; Division
    of Biology and Medicine, 185, 186, 198,